SPOILED

ARTS AND TRADITIONS OF THE TABLE

ARTS AND TRADITIONS OF THE TABLE
PERSPECTIVES ON CULINARY HISTORY

Albert Sonnenfeld, Series Editor

The Fulton Fish Market: A History, Jonathan H. Rees

The Botany of Beer: An Illustrated Guide to More Than 500 Plants Used in Brewing,
Giuseppe Caruso

Gastronativism: Food, Identity, Politics, Fabio Parasecoli

Epistenology: Wine as Experience, Nicola Perullo

The Terroir of Whiskey: A Distiller's Journey Into the Flavor of Place, Rob Arnold

The Chile Pepper in China: A Cultural Biography, Brian R. Dott

Meals Matter: A Radical Economics Through Gastronomy, Michael Symons

Cook, Taste, Learn: How the Evolution of Science Transformed the Art of Cooking,
Guy Crosby

Garden Variety: The American Tomato from Corporate to Heirloom, John Hoenig

Mouthfeel: How Texture Makes Taste, Ole G. Mouritsen and Klavs Styrbæk,
translated by Mariela Johansen

Chow Chop Suey: Food and the Chinese American Journey, Anne Mendelson

Kosher USA: How Coke Became Kosher and Other Tales of Modern Food,
Roger Horowitz

Taste as Experience: The Philosophy and Aesthetics of Food, Nicola Perullo

Another Person's Poison: A History of Food Allergy, Matthew Smith

Medieval Flavors: Food, Cooking, and the Table, Massimo Montanari,
translated by Beth Archer Brombert

For a complete list of books in the series, please see the
Columbia University Press website.

SPOILED

The MYTH of MILK
as SUPERFOOD

ANNE MENDELSON

Columbia University Press
New York

Columbia University Press
Publishers Since 1893
New York   Chichester, West Sussex
cup.columbia.edu

Library of Congress Cataloging-in-Publication Data
Names: Mendelson, Anne, author.
Title: Spoiled : the myth of milk as superfood / Anne Mendelson.
Description: New York : Columbia University Press, 2023. | Series: Arts and
traditions of the table | Includes bibliographical references and index.
Identifiers: LCCN 2022037361 | ISBN 9780231188180 (hardback) |
ISBN 9780231547703 (ebook)
Subjects: LCSH: Milk as food—History. | Milk consumption—History. |
Milk—Pasteurization—History. | Advertising—Milk—History. |
Milk—Health aspects. | Milk trade—Environmental aspects.
Classification: LCC TX379 .M46 2023 | DDC 641.3/71—dc23/eng/20220922
LC record available at https://lccn.loc.gov/2022037361

Columbia University Press books are printed on permanent
and durable acid-free paper.
Printed in the United States of America

Cover design: Julia Kushnirsky
Cover image: P Maxwell Photography/Shutterstock.com

To the memory of my friend Nach Waxman:
bibliophile, champion of good food and
honest research, irreplaceable mensch.
He took a lively interest in this project
but did not live to see it completed.

CONTENTS

Preface   ix

INTRODUCTION
1

1 MILK: SOME SCIENTIFIC INS AND OUTS
14

2 FROM THE CRADLE OF DAIRYING
TO THE ENGLISH MANOR
31

3 THE RISE OF DRINKING-MILK
53

4 SETTING THE STAGE FOR PASTEURIZATION
70

5 PASTEURIZATION: THE GAME-CHANGING YEARS
AND NATHAN STRAUS
104

6 SOUR MILK, BRIEFLY RETHOUGHT
140

7 MILK FOR THE MASSES: THE PRICE TO BE PAID
177

8 TECHNOLOGY IN OVERDRIVE I: THE ANIMALS
208

9 TECHNOLOGY IN OVERDRIVE II: THE MILK
241

10 REVIVING THE RAW MILK CAUSE
274

11 THE FUTURE
311

Acknowledgments 341
Notes 343
Select Bibliography 375
Index 385

PREFACE

T his book never would have existed without the efforts of three distinguished editors. Elisabeth Sifton welcomed my proposal for a report on the state of the milk industry some forty years ago and we worked on it together for several years before I realized that I simply didn't know enough to complete the massive survey I'd promised. Much later, Judith Jones skillfully saw me through a completely different project: a cookbook exploring the uses of fresh milk and dairy products, with a brief sketch of its route from the prehistoric Near East to today's supermarket shelves. Most recently, Jennifer Crewe listened to some of the obstinate ideas that had grown on me since the cookbook was published and not only didn't laugh them out of court but encouraged me to turn them into a book.

Curiously, writing about milk from a cook's perspective steered me to a historical puzzle that I could not have noticed otherwise. Eating and shopping in new immigrant communities of the Greater New York City area—Balkan, Turkish, Indian, Central Asian—I grasped, first, that their cuisines were linked by an intense devotion to yogurt under many names and in many culinary roles and, second, that their home countries contained some of the most ancient centers of dairying. To quote myself:

Slowly it dawned on me that in simple fermented yogurt I was tasting something that might have been eaten or drunk by Old Testament patriarchs, Sumerian lawgivers, Homeric heroes, Hindu gods, or the flower of Persian chivalry. The uses I saw it being put to in modest little eateries made me realize how little I'd known about cooking with milk and dairy products.[1]

It also dawned on me that the peoples of these regions had no tradition of drinking fresh milk—in fact, little or no genetic history of being able to digest lactose. Fermented milk from dairy animals really predated fresh—that is, full-lactose—milk as a crucial food resource for humans. Why doesn't it share the exalted rank of fresh milk in modern Western nutritional belief systems?

I began to glimpse some answers when another gifted editor, Darra Goldstein, asked me to review two important books, Andrea S. Wiley's *Re-imagining Milk* and Deborah Valenze's *Milk: A Local and Global History*, for the magazine *Gastronomica*. As far as I know, nobody has argued more forcefully than Wiley against the timeworn misconception that nonfermented fluid milk is an absolute necessity in human diets; Valenze seems to have been the first researcher to note that modern medical theories about the nutritional value of fresh milk were critically influenced by an eighteenth-century English milk-drinking cult.

The book I'd written for Ms. Jones had also set me rethinking the tangled history of controversies over raw versus pasteurized milk. In fact, that was another subject on which Ms. Goldstein had invited me to write for *Gastronomica*. And it was the subject that I meant to tackle when Ms. Crewe and I began discussing the present book.

In short order, however, I became absorbed in the prehistory of dairy animals' milk, from their steppeland and Fertile Crescent origins through their northwestward travels to the far edge of the Eurasian continent. The puzzle of fresh milk's supremacy in Western nutritional hierarchies also continued to disturb me. I came to see today's colossal fluid milk industry, with its effects on animal health and environmental resources, as more blight than blessing.

Eventually the raw milk wars became a subsidiary issue. The book now covers far more historical ground and scientific questions than I had originally meant to deal with. It is also much more polemical. It argues that influential nutritional theories about fresh and fermented milk took a disastrously wrong turn in the eighteenth century. The reason is that the founders of modern Western medicine had no way of understanding the genetic fluke that allowed them, unlike most of the world's peoples, to digest lactose from babyhood to old age. In other words, today's mega-industry stemmed from a lack of scientific perspective.

That lack turned the one form of milk that is most fragile, perishable, difficult to produce on a commercial scale, and economically pitfall-strewn into a supposed daily necessity for children and, to a lesser extent, adults. The highly processed end product now retains little of the original chemical makeup and physical structure of milk from a cow (or any other dairy animal). It reaches retail purchasers at unrealistically low prices that keep dairy farmers struggling to survive.

The present book doesn't pretend to be an encyclopedic global history of milk, though it does begin with an introductory sketch of issues with strong global ramifications. After a short summary of the chemical and biological background that will be necessary to understand the various stages of human relationships with milk, it presents a rapid summary of crucial events from the Neolithic Near East to eighteenth-century England, the scene of some watershed developments. By roughly 1800 state-of-the-art nutritional theory held unfermented cows' milk to be the purest and most nourishing possible food for young children. Soured (i.e., lactose-reduced) milk rapidly came under suspicion as being harmful to their delicate systems.

The stage was set in the technologically advanced West for a tremendous expansion of fresh unfermented milk as an article of commerce, unfortunately long before the means of safely producing and transporting it on a large scale had been developed. The book's subsequent focus is on the United States, where shifts in attitudes toward the role of government in an increasingly urbanized nation helped to bring about greater professionalization and specialization in farming, as well as calls for heightened regulation of food safety, in the course of the nineteenth century. Drinking-milk as a business gradually emerged from the ghastly era of "swill milk" in cities. By the 1890s milk was being contentiously discussed as a possible target for the application of the pathogen-inhibiting technique that Louis Pasteur had shown to be effective with wine and beer.

Early debates over milk pasteurization chiefly centered on tuberculosis as the most intractable of all the milk-borne illnesses then known. They came to be dominated by Nathan Straus, the idealistic but self-glorifying apostle of a movement into which he infused lasting rancor and partisanship. The cause of raw milk certified as clean through painstaking inspection gradually fell into medical disrepute. But in a development possibly spurred by sudden publicity about koumiss (or imitation koumiss) after it had been administered to the fatally wounded President James Garfield, fermented milk began to enjoy a certain rehabilitation in scientific opinion. Following the turn of the twentieth century, microbiologists made the surprising discovery that when milk went sour through fermentation by lactic acid bacteria, the drop in pH (or increase in acidity) had a strong inhibiting effect on most of the major milk-borne pathogens.

Shortly thereafter, popular interest in the microbiology of the intestinal tract—especially the colon—was roused by Élie Metchnikoff's claims about yogurt as the secret of Bulgarian peasants' longevity and John Harvey Kellogg's experiments with milk therapy at the Battle Creek Sanitarium. Nonetheless, unfermented drinking-milk never lost its supremacy in mainstream nutritional opinion.

Farmers who expected the towering prestige of drinking-milk as a superfood to translate into surefire profits were in for many successive shocks. Nobody had foreseen that the explosive industrial-scale growth of the entire business during and after World War I would beget labyrinthine mysteries in the wholesale prices paid to producing farmers by processors and distributors. Though nutritionists were surer than ever of drinking-milk's miraculous powers, policy-setters took this as a reason for keeping retail prices as *low* as possible. Where dairy farmers were concerned, drinking-milk was invariably a buyer's and not a seller's market. Their predicament deepened with the increasing regulation of milk production and the imposition of costly on-farm sanitation and safety requirements. The industry had devolved into near-chaos when it was temporarily bailed out by World War II.

The most striking feature of the postwar scene has been a race toward gigantism, aided by progressively more and more complex industrial technologies that have had devastating effects on both dairy cattle and the milk they produce. An unrelenting focus on wringing the greatest possible yield from every animal at the lowest possible cost per pound of milk has created the bizarre spectacle of nearly perpetual milk surpluses from a continually shrinking number of animals, nearly all Holsteins. Intensive breeding and feeding practices keep their lives short and illness-ridden. As for the milk, intensive processing deprives it of much resemblance to the original substance. My chief examples are the technologies of homogenization and refrigeration. The first is a gratuitous interference with the basic structure of milk. The second, though it is vitally necessary for preventing the growth of pathogens, is now proving to be less foolproof against them than was previously thought, as shown by recent outbreaks of *Listeria monocytogenes*.

While the drinking-milk business expanded, certified raw milk generally faded from the scene. The raw milk cause, however, began a defiant comeback in the 1990s and became the subject of noisy political debates. Current arguments against pasteurization are strongly rooted in the naturopathic movement that began asserting the health benefits of raw foods in general about a century earlier. The contemporary activist who has done most to promote arguments for the medical rehabilitation of raw whole milk is Sally Fallon Morell, leader of a backlash against advocates of low-fat, low-cholesterol diets. The organization that she founded, the Weston A. Price Foundation, presents a peculiar synthesis of claims for the traditional dietary wisdom of preindustrial peoples and attacks on modern medical and public health authorities. "Food Freedom" is the best-known objective championed by the foundation—especially the freedom to buy and consume raw milk.

In 2000, raw milk supporters witnessed the arrival of an implacable opponent, John Sheehan, at a Food and Drug Administration food safety division. A series of unenlightening battles between angry ideologues has ensued, unfortunately coinciding with the emergence of still more "new" (meaning previously unidentified) food-borne pathogens, particularly *E. coli* O157:H7. I strongly contend that civil discussions across usual party lines are essential for mapping out the best route to milk safety.

Meanwhile, raw milk dairy farmers are bypassing the frustrations of the mainstream drinking-milk market system in favor of direct sales to consumers—an example that can be profitably followed by other small-scale producers of milk and various dairy products. In addition, a new demographic wrinkle has to be taken into account as immigration from many parts of the world starts to alter the genetic makeup of the U.S. population: In future, dietary advisers must reckon with an increasing proportion of Americans who cannot easily digest lactose. This development suggests that some of these people's favorite fermented milk products also deserve green cards. It also shows the timeliness of a novel research project meant to call attention to milk-fermenting organisms as an extraordinary—and now endangered—microbiological legacy that connects us with the ancient origins of dairying.

SPOILED

INTRODUCTION

This book deals with the food I'll call drinking-milk, meaning dairy animals' milk that is consumed in fluid form rather than as some kind of fermented sour milk or cheese. No other food product is as staggeringly difficult and expensive to get from source (in this case, a cow) to destination (milk glass on table) in something loosely approximating its first condition. If one existed, it would be treated as an astounding luxury.

As preamble to my historical survey, let me briefly sketch two profoundly important scientific discoveries about people and milk. The first occurred in the mid-1960s, when fresh milk was considered a peerless nutritional mainstay in the United States and all industrialized nations of northern Europe. Dietary authorities in these regions had long asserted that it would be a great improvement to average diets in many non-Western countries where it was little used.

The dietary-improvement idea rested on an apparently rock-solid assumption: Any healthy human being could easily digest the major constituents of drinking-milk from cows. What would eventually shatter this consensus was the role of lactose, or milk sugar.

Lactose occurs in milk as a double sugar, formed from one molecule of glucose linked with one molecule of another sugar, galactose. For many years, usual medical teaching held that it is easily absorbed into the bloodstream after being broken down into its two component sugars by lactase, an enzyme that normal people were thought to secrete in the small intestine throughout their lives. No researcher had suggested otherwise until a young resident at the Johns Hopkins School of Medicine became involved in a program that treated many indigent people in Baltimore, and thus many Black people in Baltimore, at around 1963–1964.

Pedro Cuatrecasas made it his business to understand as much as he could of his patients' personal backgrounds. Interviewing them about their dietary habits and histories, he soon was struck by how often Black people mentioned disliking milk. He was seeking an explanation when he came across an article about congenital lactase deficiency, a rare but life-threatening condition in which an inability to secrete lactase makes newborns unable to digest their mothers' milk. The coincidence sparked a hunch. In 1964 Cuatrecasas persuaded two colleagues, Dean H. Lockwood and Jacques R. Caldwell, to collaborate on an experiment to determine whether a lesser degree of lactase deficiency might occur in adults, particularly Black adults.[1]

The subjects were sixty people identified in the study, by then-standard racial terminology, as "18 women (13 negro, 5 white) and 42 men (28 negro, 14 white)." Once the investigators had measured each person's response to specific doses of lactose and correlated it with a carefully recorded medical history, they realized that they had stumbled on an issue of revolutionary importance—revolutionary enough for the three novice researchers to boldly submit their findings to the august British medical journal *The Lancet* and be rewarded with prompt publication in the first issue of January 1965.[2]

The title of the article pointed to its paradigm-shattering implications: "Lactase Deficiency in the Adult: A Common Occurrence." Not only was congenital lactase deficiency extremely *un*common in infants, but the ability to secrete lactase had previously been considered as universal for healthy adults—regardless of race—as it was for healthy babies. Nobody, including the three authors, could account for the fact that thirty of the forty-one Black subjects demonstrated difficulty in absorbing lactose, as contrasted with three of nineteen white subjects. In addition, Cuatrecasas's original intuition had led him to question participants about their milk-drinking habits. Confirming his guess, nearly all of the Black "non-absorbers" reported that they didn't drink milk because it gave them some form of digestive distress like diarrhea or colicky pain. The medical histories provided to the investigators repeatedly indicated that *at some point between infancy and puberty, these subjects had at least partly lost the ability to digest lactose.*

All observers saw that the explanation had to be genetic. The tools of analysis available in the mid-1960s were inadequate for anything beyond the authors' suggestion that "a genetic polymorphism" might be involved. ("Polymorphism," at the time, hadn't acquired a meaning in genetic studies much more precise than some inheritable variant form of a gene.) But the Cuatrecasas-Lockwood-Caldwell findings soon inspired further population studies gradually establishing that Asian Americans, Native Americans, and Black Americans all usually experienced mild or serious abdominal discomfort on consuming more than small amounts of unfermented milk.

The stunningly consistent findings about the reaction of nonwhite subjects to fresh fluid milk—that is, full-lactose milk—might well have raised medical doubts then and there about the normality of unimpaired lactase secretion from infancy to old age, or the wisdom of recommending fresh fluid milk as an indispensable cradle-to-grave food for the entire human race. In fact, the basis of the enormous modern drinking-milk industry might have been called in question. Nothing of the sort happened.

About thirty-eight years after Pedro Cuatrecasas's first hunch, a team of researchers chiefly working from Helsinki pinpointed the operative genetic discrepancy through the new tools of DNA sequencing analysis. In an article published in 2002 in *Nature Genetics*, they identified a precise location on one particular chromosome where a single "letter" of the four nucleotide bases adenine, cytosine, guanine, and thymine switches places with another to create a "single-nucleotide polymorphism," a genomic variant occurring as Mendelian dominant-recessive alternatives. By either permitting or suppressing the activation of another gene, it determines the secretion or nonsecretion of lactase throughout adulthood in certain populations.[3]

By then students of population genetics were inching toward a consensus that had once looked improbable: adult lactase persistence, or the ability to go on secreting enough lactase for untroubled lactose digestion throughout life, is unquestionably a minority condition. The 2002 study provided the wherewithal for confirming this conclusion. Adult lactase persistence now is known to occur with overwhelming frequency in a certain genetic contingent: white people of northwest European ancestry. Otherwise, only a few pockets crop up in nonwhite groups. In other words, lactase nonpersistence after childhood is not a medical "problem" or genetic abnormality, but the default or ancestral condition; adult lactase persistence appears to be a fairly recent anomaly.

Again, a scientific breakthrough might have appeared to threaten the ultimate rationale of the drinking-milk industry—and again, the industry shrugged off any apparent conflict with reality. This book was spurred by my curiosity about the bizarre disconnect between the global distribution of a genetic quirk and the global reach of a vast enterprise that treats the quirk as the norm.

The advances in evolutionary genetics and paleoarchaeology that became possible in the wake of the Johns Hopkins and Finnish experiments have firmly established that the first humans to consume the milk of dairy animals could not have digested it fresh from the udder. Dairying was invented in the Late Stone Age by Western Asian and Middle Eastern peoples who today would be classified as "lactase nonpersistent" or "lactose intolerant." What allowed milk to become an important part of their diet, long before the polymorphism governing lactase production had appeared, was fermentation.

Fermentation has recently acquired the reputation of an intriguingly esoteric craft. For reasons to be explored in later chapters, it was no such thing for the first societies to practice milking. Local climatic conditions alone ensured that during the spring-summer milking season, when ambient daytime temperatures reached sweltering point, hordes of lactose-loving and warmth-loving bacteria would swarm around lactating goats, sheep, cows, and their nurslings. Invading any pot of freshly drawn milk, they would speedily produce some form of sour milk by converting their favorite sugar into lactic acid.

This book seeks to trace the journey from the prehistoric cradle of dairy husbandry, with its built-in reliance on fermentation to make milk usable by people who couldn't digest lactose, to the contemporary dairying scene, with its illogically preferential treatment of unfermented full-lactose milk. No previous history of drinking-milk as a major modern industry has examined the ramifications of what is now known about lactase persistence or nonpersistence—often popularly called lactose tolerance or intolerance—in either the remote past or the present.

The sheer vastness of today's drinking-milk industry makes it difficult for consumers to understand much about milk itself—for instance, the extraordinary perishability that for many thousands of years prevented it from being an article of commerce. Fermentation into yogurt or other versions of sour milk allows it to be kept a little longer without spoiling. Transformation into fresh cheeses prolongs its useful life further; ripening into older cheeses still further. Fresh milk was manifestly more impractical than any of these. Considering the many obvious obstacles to the idea, how did such a thing as a drinking-milk industry come into being, much less become a revered institution?

The conclusion I have come to is that fresh milk's rise to the status of nutritional mainstay—the first scientifically anointed superfood of the modern industrialized world—was one of the great flukes of food history. I trace its beginnings to the late eighteenth and early nineteenth centuries: the Age of Enlightenment and the start of the Industrial Revolution. The most remarkable center of progress, Great Britain, was then hurtling into both an epoch of colonial expansion and a dominating role in science and medicine that seemed more brilliant with every passing decade.

I argue that in the case of drinking-milk's merits or demerits, early modern medical authorities' unquestioning faith in their own advanced knowledge lured them into misguided teachings destined to form the flawed basis of a huge—and soon troubled—undertaking that is now on the thin edge of unsustainability. From the Enlightenment era on, the seeds of many future dairy industry crises lurked in an unavoidable bit of historical mistiming: Medical authorities arrived at a supposedly up-to-the-minute belief that "sweet" (unfermented, and thus full-lactose) drinking-milk was purer and more healthful than sour milk, well before scientific evidence to the contrary.

Northwest Europeans, not gifted with foreknowledge about the racial distribution of traits carried on some human chromosomes, were for better or worse the genetic group elected by destiny or accident to conquer most of the globe during the eighteenth and nineteenth centuries. One of their resulting roles was that of dietary oracles authorized to decide on priorities that, as far as they knew, were solidly based in science and must hold good for all races. Where milk was concerned, their well-meant but ignorant assumptions left an imprint that has yet to be erased.

Second thoughts might have arisen in some quarters when turn-of-the-twentieth-century scientists began observing the action of harmful and benign microorganisms in milk. They soon grasped an unexpected fact: when the major lactic acid bacteria colonize fresh milk and convert enough lactose into lactic acid to make it go sour, the increased acidity forms a fairly strong defense against many pathogens.

But by this time drinking-milk had already assumed phenomenal economic importance in most technologically advanced nations, above all the United States. The new discoveries did make some forms of soured milk marketable as niche products after about 1880—but without disturbing anyone's faith that fresh cow's milk was humanity's greatest bulwark against childhood malnutrition. That dogma had already become one of the most unshakably internalized beliefs of modern Western consumers, along with their nutrition advisers and family physicians. No discoveries about the potential benefits of fermentation had any effect on ever-faster growth in production and per capita consumption of drinking-milk, generally pasteurized in order to be safely distributed on an enormous commercial scale. And in 1900 nobody could have predicted that the barely fledged discipline of genetics might in any way touch on people's milk-consuming habits.

The most startling thing about the 1965 Cuatrecasas-Lockwood-Caldwell experiment, and the later discovery of the single nucleotide polymorphism that accounted for its results, is how little they have affected the status quo. Not even an accumulating weight of genetic evidence has shaken the conviction of industry-backed and most government-backed nutritional policy-setters that unfermented drinking-milk is the most important of all dairy products for all people. This is the firm assumption of the pasteurized milk industry and its medical allies—nor is it questioned by the small, vocal minority who place their trust in raw milk.

Among several large drawbacks, one is a Catch-22 paradox: everything that fits freshly secreted milk for its biological role as the sole life support of newborns also unfits it for functioning as a commercial article matched to ordinary laws of supply and demand. Simply put: price instability is a given in any free-market system of drinking-milk production. For this reason, trying to make a living from dairying became a road to bankruptcy in the early twentieth century for many hopeful farmers attracted by publicity about the profits to be realized by sending milk from country pastures to a continually expanding clientele of city families.

Why doesn't a supply-and-demand equilibrium work for drinking-milk? The answer is that profiting from lactation is not really comparable to profiting from the life cycles of potatoes, wheat, apples, or olives. Because of milk's great bulkiness and great perishability, a creature who produces it can't be temporarily relegated to the back burner of day-to-day bookkeeping after the harvest in the same way as a field where potatoes are planted. She requires to be milked at least once a day, *every day*, from start to finish of the current lactation cycle. Farmers in 1890 knew that if one day's output of milk from all cows couldn't be gotten off the farm in time for the milk train, they could do nothing but dump it in order to make room for the next day's output.

Another facet of the same booby trap was that dairy herds simply didn't produce uniform amounts of milk at all seasons. Like the Stone Age ancestors of all dairy animals, a pre-twentieth-century cow nearly always gave birth in the spring, worked up to peak production while the grasses were still flourishing in early summer, and gradually ceased lactating by late summer or fall. At that point the grass was drying up, the spring calves were mostly weaned, and it was time to breed again for the next round of spring births. This biological timetable meant recurrent surpluses of milk at peak season—a nightmare illustrating the unbridgeable distance between drinking-milk and any other article of commerce. Every summer, prices would collapse, leaving the farmers helplessly dependent on dealers and distributors to take each day's output off their hands for a pittance. From the turn of the twentieth century, farmers who had been lured into the drinking-milk business viewed contractors and milk processing companies as enemies eager to shave their profit margins to the bone.

The outlines of the quandary started to emerge while the new discipline of dairy science, including research on dairy stock husbandry and milk chemistry, was unfolding at the first publicly funded agricultural schools and experiment stations in the developed world. A corps of freshly minted bureaucrats in government offices charged with representing agricultural interests helped to shape these institutions. Celebratory histories of dairying routinely treat the new arrivals as friends to the farmer and contributors to every glass of health-giving milk reaching the family breakfast table. As with so much in the usual narrative, there is a measure of justice in this description. But the facts can also support an alternative scenario in which the benefits of both drinking-milk and experts' advice to farmers have been appallingly exaggerated.

In both conventional story and counternarrative, professionally schooled reformers eager to rescue dairy farming from what they saw as a jumble of backward, counterproductive efforts began planning models of more rational, efficient, orderly, and profitable operations. Simultaneously, colleagues in the laboratory learned to understand the chemical basis of commercially desirable milk qualities while rethinking milk-handling safety in the light of ongoing discoveries in bacteriology. One result among many was the stirring of interest—first in Denmark and Germany, then in the United States—about pasteurization as a weapon against pathogens.

These initiatives have been credited with saving many millions of lives. The claim can't be refuted if one takes millions of quarts of drinking-milk safely consumed by millions of families as an absolute imperative. But to what degree did these same efforts actually square the circle—that is, magically abolish an inherent property of milk, the cascade of microbiological and chemical changes it starts to undergo the instant it leaves a lactating mother's system? The answer is that various newly devised measures could get partway there, but only at a great cost in technical infrastructure whose fiscal (and to an extent, societal) burdens would fall more and more heavily on the farmer.

One advance followed another from the 1880s on, allowing the new trade to expand into a sector of the agricultural economy as enormous as "soft" commodities like wheat and corn. Experts drilled into farmers the need for rigorous sanitation, which involved new expenses starting with soaps, disinfectants, and an endless supply of clean water to wash the cow's flanks and udder as well as the milker's hands and all utensils. Decade by decade, professors of dairy science at prestigious agriculture schools, state extension agents, and public health authorities kept piling capital-intensive new demands onto farmers' budgets: scientifically approved field crops and scientifically calculated feed rations, scientifically bred cows and bulls (later, frozen semen), scientifically designed milking machines hooked up to elaborate piping and refrigeration systems.

At every stage, small dairy farms closed down and the average scale of operations became bigger—but never big enough to painlessly keep up with the newest supertechnology or solve the unending surplus problem. No matter how frantically drinking-milk producers and processors have pushed themselves to cancel out the biological inconveniences of milk and pursue economies of scale like those favored by bulk commodity producers, they have never really managed to square the circle.

Commercially produced drinking-milk has always been bound up with impossible dreams. Hailed in the late nineteenth century as an unprecedented moneymaking opportunity for farmers, it no sooner started flowing from country to city on something like an industrial scale than it faced *unrelenting downward pressures on retail prices*. To tack on a few extra cents, the popular argument ran (and still runs), was to profiteer from the lifeblood of needy children. This obtuse, inflexible public mentality turned dairying into financial ruin for numberless farmers in the twentieth century and continues to do so today.

Again and again, industry leaders and agricultural school gurus have churned out advice about survival of the biggest and most tech-savvy. Again and again, the smallest farms have been the least able to cope with the ultimate consequences of a disastrous, but never seriously re-examined, historical mistake. That mistake was a taken-for-granted faith that drinking-milk from cows must be privileged above all other foods—as pure, nourishing, and obligatory for every child as the breast milk that it clearly had been designed to replace after weaning—while at the same time it must always remain cheaper than other highly nourishing foods. (The raw milk business escapes the fiscal insanity of the mainstream enterprise by being obliged to operate on a tiny scale, usually through direct sales to customers willing to pay premium prices. But it rests on the same unfortunate belief in fresh milk's unique virtues.)

Though people in First World countries are now in a position to see the original genetic fallacies—or racial blind spots—that gave rise to the primacy-of-drinking-milk doctrine, it has triumphantly resurfaced elsewhere. To grasp the sheer daftness of this new development, it's important to think about some historical relationships of food, empire, and race. Alt-right extremists have recently garnered headlines by trying to turn milk into a malignant symbol of white supremacy. Half-witted though that notion may be, it is rooted in just these relationships. So were the now-discredited claims of the eugenics movement that passed as cutting-edge science between about 1900 and 1940.

The eugenicists rejoiced in the thought that the people they hailed as direct ancestors were also the Northwest European segment of the white race whose towering achievements had triumphantly transformed the planet. They categorized this racial "stock"—a favorite word drawn from purebred livestock rearing—as "Nordic" and liked to point to such superior traits as tall stature, blond hair, blue eyes, and fair skin.

Nobody realized, or *could* have realized, that these genetic paragons were exactly the human stock in which lactase persistence was most prevalent. On the other hand, everybody recognized that they had founded the mightiest globe-spanning empires in the history of mankind. The eugenic reasoning was that they had done this by having not only magnificent physiques but brains more highly developed than anybody else's—brains that had enabled them to invent steam engines, lay transatlantic telegraph cables, and command the world's most self-evidently superior diet.

Surveying the rise of white-founded modern world powers from a non-eugenic perspective, we can grasp that food has always been intricately linked with empire, and empire with encounters between different races or genetic "stocks." (Salted fish, for instance, was sent to ancient Rome after being harvested and processed by local peoples of varied ethnicities in Iberian, North African, and Black Sea provinces.) After about 1500 the rulers of Spain and Portugal began launching long-distance exchanges of foods (notably sugar) on a far greater scale than would have been possible without slave labor drawn from Africa. It was nearly two centuries before Northwest Europeans—Frenchmen, Netherlanders, and above all Britons—came to dominate the scramble for colonial possessions around the globe. With the Dutch and very conspicuously the British, more rigid and imperative assumptions about skin color and who deserved to rule whom—foreshadowing eugenic theories—became part of the colonial rationale.

It is impossible to separate the dietary fallout of British imperialism from the fact that the white-skinned conquerors of North America, India, Australia, and several African and Far Eastern possessions were also the inventors of modern science, including medical science and nutritional theories. At first they wasted little time on trying to convert plantation slaves or conquered populations to supposedly improved dietary habits like milk-drinking (though they did establish "military dairies" to supply fresh milk to army bases in Africa and India). Nor, after the War for Independence, did American slaveowners. Such efforts came later, when slavery as such had been abolished, colonial economies were shrinking, and public health bureaucracies were growing in all industrialized nations.

In the twentieth century and particularly after World War II, Western experts earnestly began working to modernize the diets of non-Western peoples, who often accepted the advice at face value. But gradually it began occurring to nutritionists acquainted with advances in evolutionary genetics that they might have known less than they'd assumed they knew. It is now clear that some of their well-meant advice was deeply if unintentionally mired in outmoded assumptions about one racial group's right to impose its own norms on the rest of humanity. Large doses of white-man's-burden thinking were involved in telling people in every corner of the globe to drink milk by the pint or quart—thinking whose evil twin spawned "scientific" race theories still happily embraced by American political extremists chugging milk as a badge of white supremacy.

By horrific irony, the drinking-milk gospel is now roaring to new life in areas of widespread lactase nonpersistence (or lactose intolerance). China—where nutritional policy-setters have built monumentally polluting mega-dairy operations while also offering a timely remedy for surpluses in Western nations—and India—where a long and rich tradition of fermenting milk to yogurt now takes a back seat to campaigns for pouring drinking-milk into every child—are the biggest examples. But the gospel is being preached to all developing countries.

The purpose of this book is not to portray drinking-milk from dairy animals as a dangerous poison or the vehicle of racist plots. It is to debunk the idea that milk in unfermented fluid form is a food of unique virtues whose use goes back to remote prehistory. In the first place, if the earliest livestock-domesticators hadn't lived in regions where hot summers offer ideal conditions for spontaneous fermentation, they couldn't have invented dairying, because they couldn't have drunk copious amounts of milk unfermented. Milk's greatest usefulness to the greatest number of people begins once it is soured by lactic acid bacteria and stops being fresh milk. In the second place, the enormous drinking-milk industry built in modern times by people who do have the right genes for digesting lactose would crumble to ruins without outlandish expenditures of technology as well as dysfunctional government price support systems. In other words, it is ultimately unsustainable.

The drinking-milk mythos that fueled the growth of Big Milk robbed consumers of a valuable piece of knowledge: drinking-milk is not and never has been a superfood. It is just one potentially valuable food among many other valuable foods. It deserves to be reappraised in a spirit of common sense, neither demonized nor deified.

The industry as it stands is not a pretty spectacle. But milk is worth reclaiming from the false position into which it has been thrust through no fault of its own.

Everything that makes drinking-milk near-impossible to produce, process, and sell on a colossal scale at low retail prices without the whole edifice simply collapsing under its own weight is rooted in biological, chemical, and other scientific facts of life. There is no grasping its staggering challenges, puzzles, and frustrations—the numberless factors that complicate the match between fresh milk and the requirements of a super-gigantic, super-mechanized enterprise—without tracing parts of the root system.

For several decades, specialists at universities and research institutes around the world have been seeking to explore the tangled history of people's relationships with animals' milk, including drinking-milk, from dozens of different angles. Biochemists, reproductive physiologists, and microbiologists are just a few of those with fingers in a very large and mystery-ridden pie. Chapter 1 is a crash course in aspects of what they have learned: a sketch of some major questions connected with milking and milk use. How is milk secreted? What makes it digestible or indigestible to animals and people? What differentiates one creature's digestive system, or one creature's milk, from another's? How do fermenting organisms enter the picture? Every crucial development in the long history of dairying can be better understood after, rather than before, an introduction to the essential scientific framework.

1

MILK

Some Scientific Ins and Outs

By far the most chemically complex food any person ever consumes is milk straight from the source, meaning a human breast. The reason is that at one point in our lives it is the most urgently *necessary* food, called on to supply the entire A-to-Z range of our nutritional needs when it is the only food we can digest. Until the milestone known as weaning makes it unnecessary, it is completely responsible for the development of an infant's body and brain.

But milk quite removed from this source assumed great importance in some civilizations many thousands of years ago, when adult humans began using milk formerly consumed only by the young of other species. In recent centuries, nonhuman milk acquired still greater importance for a certain genetic segment of the human race while undergoing more and more difficult journeys between the animals that produced it and the persons who pressed it into service. The milk of these animals was just as complex as that of human mothers. But exploiting it for human purposes introduced other tangled factors.

This chapter explores some of the chemical, biological, and microbiological issues that have been a formative and enduring backdrop to the history of dairying as a human activity. The varied interactions among people, livestock, and milk over the course of millennia left traces that can now be ferreted out and interpreted by scientists belonging to a fantastic spectrum of different disciplines. Though all scientific approaches to the story of milk have been revolutionized in the last few decades by high-speed computing and gene sequencing, most of what is covered here precedes the cyber-age.

SQUARE ONE: LACTATION

Anyone who had to memorize the historic kingdom-to-species rankings of plants and animals in high school biology will remember that *class* is one of the earlier pigeonholes, between *phylum* and *order*. The Swedish taxonomist Carl Linnaeus, who hammered out the first usable version of the system between 1735 and 1758, lumped together several thousand species of four-limbed, warm-blooded creatures as a class. From aardvarks to zebras, they still bear the general label that he assigned them: "Mammalia." Linnaeus's reasoning was that the females of each kind have *mammae*—Latin for breasts or teats.

It's tantalizing to wonder what name he would have chosen had he decided that dependence on drinking mother's milk (behavior shared by both sexes) was a more important qualification than producing it (a purely female capacity). As it is, the defining characteristic of the entire class is *lactation*: any new mammal mother's secretion of the food that must keep her helpless newborn alive to a later stage of growth. Whether she is a panda, dolphin, guinea pig, or lioness, her milk is targeted to her own off-spring's particular needs for certain nutrients headed by fats, proteins, and carbohydrates. We will return to them repeatedly, especially the unique carbohydrate called *lactose*, or milk sugar. It is a *disaccharide*, meaning a double-barreled molecule composed of two simple sugars.

In many ways, lactation is the raison d'être of this book—the biological context, and the key to understanding a host of issues. The first thing to grasp is that it is a *finite process*—and needs to be. It has a beginning (parturition) and an end (weaning). No female is innately programmed to continue a single lactation indefinitely after the infant she has nursed is big enough to survive on an adult diet.

Many people have seen an impatient mother cat or dog let a brood of strapping youngsters know that they're on their own. Once they get the point and start eating like grownups, an irreversible change occurs in their digestive relationship with milk: they stop secreting lactase, the enzyme that enables nurslings to break down the difficult lactose molecule into a more easily assimilated source of energy.

For all nursing infants, lactose digestion takes place in the center section, or *jejunum*, of the small intestine. Its internal walls are lined with a dense outgrowth of microscopically thin projections known as *microvilli* that collectively form a surface called the brush border. (Supposedly the microvilli-covered surface reminded some observer of a bristle-covered brush.) In newborns of all species, the tips of the "bristles" secrete lactase as they come in contact with lactose moving past the brush border. Dissolving the bond between the halves of the lactose molecule, the enzyme cleaves it into its component sugars glucose and galactose, which are then sent on to the liver for further breakdown and absorption into the bloodstream. But at some point after the young one is weaned, the microvilli receive a genetically programmed signal telling them to shut off lactase production, putting an end to the animal's ability to digest lactose.[1]

Mammals that have been weaned do not consume the milk of their own species for the simple reason that it would make them sick. This reaction—now often labeled lactose intolerance or more correctly adult lactase nonpersistence—is just as important as the fact of lactating in the first place. It means that hungry adult members of any mammal species cannot compete with the most helpless members for a valuable food. Nor do they try helping themselves to the milk of any other species.

Milk avoidance by the young after weaning has another consequence. By allowing the mother to shut down milk production, it ensures that after one cycle of conception, pregnancy, delivery, and lactation, she ordinarily will not be lactating to feed a singleton or a litter when she gets pregnant with another, and will be spared having to meet the physical demands of gestation and milk production at the same time.

Several of the above rules have been challenged or jettisoned, since the Late Stone Age, by one two-legged mammal. Lactose-intolerant humans first started using several other animals' milk in fermented (i.e., mostly lactose-free) form between 10,000 and 8,000 BC. Some millennia later, a small genetic cohort destined for future political and economic greatness unknowingly acquired the ability to digest full-lactose milk without fermentation because the brush border in their gut never stops secreting lactase. Still later, members of this group made drinking-milk from cows into a business enterprise, eventually disconnected from any environmental or seasonal context, that can rejigger reproductive schedules so as to keep a cow producing milk from the start of one cycle almost up to the end of a successive pregnancy.

The evolution of this vast industry is bound up with a tangled skein of questions. What is milk, anyhow? How does it meet the needs of a newborn giraffe, muskrat, or chimpanzee? Why did people choose some mammal species and not others as dairy animals? How do these creatures digest foods that we can't, and how do we digest the milk that they produce?

Every one of these questions touches on some branch of science— for instance, reproductive physiology. A new human mother doesn't need to be told that it all starts here. She knows, or has had it explained to her, that for nine months a placenta has been linking her circulatory system with that of the growing presence inside her womb, pumping lifeblood into its body through the umbilical cord. At the time of delivery, this source of prenatal nourishment shuts off and she begins channeling blood elsewhere, into a system of tiny sacs and ducts in her breasts. Milk can be most simply understood as the postnatal food source that takes over from the placental blood supply. Lactation furnishes infants new to the job of breathing air through their own lungs with another blood-derived substance delivered by a unique route: the nipple-to-mouth connection, replacing the placenta-to-umbilical-cord connection. Or to state the case differently: pregnancy takes the fetus up to the limits of growth that the mother's circulatory system can directly support without letup. What's needed afterward is a transitional food with strategically different chemical properties, delivered at intervals instead of nonstop.

MILK CHEMISTRY: THE BASICS

The chemical makeup of milk is at least as intricate as that of the blood from which it's concocted in a nursing mother's mammary system. Like blood, milk is thicker than water—but also like blood, it starts with water. Both are essentially water with a multitude of other substances swimming around in it.

No one needs a degree in hematology to recognize that blood contains more water than anything else, and that water is the medium in which dissolved elements like sodium and potassium, elaborate structures like red and white blood cells, lipids like triglycerides, and many other substances are distributed. Many of the same realities apply to milk.

To visualize the grand structure of cow's milk, human milk, and all other mammals' milk, it is easiest to start by picturing a glass of clear water and imagining the other contents being added to it in stages. They exist in three basic kinds of structural arrangements called *phases*. In all cases, water is the *continuous* phase and the other substances the *dispersed* phase, or matter infused into this aqueous medium.

The main thing that makes the originally transparent water opaque is *casein*, which occurs as millions of microscopic structures vaguely suggesting Christmas-tree ornaments redesigned under the influence of some psychedelic substance. They are spheres composed of many smaller subspheres, with innumerable hairlike projections waving from their surfaces. These strange shapes are *micelles*, or assemblages of molecules, containing most of the protein and calcium in milk. They are its heaviest, densest component. But in apparent disregard of gravity, they permeate it in a suspended state, kept from clustering together by repellent electrical charges on the projecting filaments. Thus they form the dispersed phase of a *suspension*. Hovering as if weightless in our glass of water, they refract beams of light in different directions instead of allowing them to pass through it. By themselves, they would render the water a thin bluish off-white color.

As the bizarre "Christmas ornaments" with their manes of filaments hang in the water medium, they share space with much larger but less dense orbs bobbing around like innumerable balloons. These consist of extraordinarily thin but complex membranes encasing globules of milkfat or butterfat, the principal lipid in milk. Reinforcing the light-refracting effect of casein, the membrane-surrounded milkfat globules lend a cream-colored tint to the whole along with a richer, more unctuous consistency. Though fat is much lighter than either water or the casein micelles, the microscopic balloons also seem to defy gravity, remaining evenly distributed, or emulsified, throughout the milk as long as it remains inside the mother's system. That is, they are the dispersed phase of an *emulsion*.

The third of the basic milk phases does not conjure up visual metaphors as evocative as casein or milkfat. If there is a handy analogy, it would be something like water-color paints minus the color: *solutes* capable of diffusing through a *solvent* (water, in this case) in an absolutely homogeneous manner, not interrupting it like suspended Christmas trinkets or emulsified balloons. Milk is chock-full of solutes, possibly more than have ever been identified. Most are electrolytes like sodium and potassium that can travel across cell membranes or capillary walls as ions, or electrically charged particles. But the solutes include some larger molecules—for example, several water-soluble milk proteins and enzymes as well as lactose, the all-important milk sugar. All are technically *dissolved* as the dispersed phase of a water-based *solution*.

This biological and chemical picture more or less holds true across the entire mammal class, though we have to figure in some eccentricities including the systems of non-placental creatures like marsupials. But it doesn't begin to hint at the spectrum of differences that became obvious once biochemists learned to analyze the makeup of other animals' milk. They saw that milk is no more interchangeable than blood between one species and another. For this reason, no mammal would ordinarily come into contact with the milk of another species; even humans didn't stumble on that idea until about the ninth or tenth millennium BC.

The interspecies differences in milk composition are literally countless. The largest ones reflect the dissimilar environments that nursing infants will have to cope with as they grow to maturity. For the young of herd animals that evolved to range across grassy terrain ahead of predators, it is vital to reach something close to adult size and stamina between spring and the end of the grass season. Their mothers' milk logically enough contains large amounts of protein. Humans, on the other hand, are born much more helpless—a baby may not master walking for as many months as it takes *minutes* for a newborn foal to stagger to its feet—and don't approach full growth until their mid- or late teens. The ratio of protein to other constituents is lower in human milk than in that of any other mammal. Romulus and Remus never would have grown up to start a fatal quarrel over the founding of Rome if a shepherd hadn't chanced to stumble on them after a few days in the custody of the helpful she-wolf, who undoubtedly didn't know that her milk (like that of other carnivores) supplied about ten times as much protein as a human infant's kidneys can long tolerate. Dolphins, sea lions, whales, and other aquatic mammals have still other needs. Newborns couldn't survive immersion in water unless they instantly started building a protective layer of blubber generated from the huge amounts of fat in their mothers' milk.

Interestingly, fat content tends to vary less widely than protein in most land mammals' milk. But lactose content shows striking differences, with the highest amounts occurring in humans and other primates as well as horses and their close relatives. The milk of cud-chewers like cows is much less rich in lactose, as is that of most carnivores. No one has fully determined why infant humans, chimpanzees, and gorillas need such high concentrations of lactose, though some researchers hypothesize that in primates it or its component galactose may be a more finely calibrated source of caloric energy for early brain development than protein or fat.[2]

Since people took up consuming other mammals' milk, they have concentrated solely on grass-eaters. Primates, the creatures whose milk is most chemically similar to ours, were never in the running. Nor were carnivores or omnivores like pigs. It was herbivores such as cows, sheep, goats, and horses whose milk proved most chemically adaptable to adult human purposes. Furthermore, competition for the same food sources could never exist between prehistoric peoples and their chosen dairy animals. It was precisely because cows and horses thrived on grass that their ecological niches so beautifully complemented those of human custodians with completely different digestive tracts. The animals' systems had room for a form of intervention not available to humans: bacterial fermentation on a massive scale. And their milk, once sidetracked from its original purpose and sent into the outside world, was excellently suited to other versions of fermentation that would revolutionize Neolithic diets.

GRASS-EATERS AND GRASS-FERMENTERS: A MUTUAL-ADVANTAGE PARTNERSHIP

Though it may seem complicated to humans, the human gut is simplicity itself compared to the systems of the herbivores whose milk various societies have been using since Neolithic times. If you were to stretch out the entire digestive tract of a five-and-a-half-foot man or woman in a straight line, it would measure about thirty-eight feet from mouth to anus, or about seven times the person's height. The alimentary canal of a cow measuring eight feet from nose to tail would be close to twenty times her length, or a hundred sixty feet. The difference reflects the fact that digesting grass and most leaves is a more demanding task than digesting the staples of human diets. The great hurdle is cellulose.

Cellulose belongs to the tribe of complex carbohydrates, or *polysaccharides*, which are fashioned from many linked glucose molecules. In cellulose, the bonds between these simple sugar units are especially strong and stubborn. They are almost indissolubly locked together in *microfibrils* that cannot be directly unfastened by an animal's own digestive enzymes. But loosening the obstinate connections is no trouble for certain other organisms, most of them microbes whose most conspicuous role in the lives of herbivores is to permanently occupy particular sectors of the digestive tract and ferment cellulose. (Since no natural forage is pure cellulose, the diverse microbial armies ferment plenty of other things, but cellulose is the greatest single source of energy for the host animal's needs.)

There are many kinds of fermentation. But all involve a biochemical assault on a particular food source, or *substrate*, by devouring legions of microbes that digest it by secreting enzymes neatly targeted to the makeup of whatever substance they're attacking. Their action is so necessary to the lives of all dairy animals that whole areas of their alimentary canals have been enlarged into enormous fermenting vats where bacteria secrete a range of enzymes—most critically, cellulase, the enzyme that unlocks the available energy of cellulose by cleaving it into its component glucose units. Only after this chemical dissection can fodder be turned into flesh, milk, and the wherewithal of all the animal's life processes.

Students of animal anatomy broadly map any beast's digestive tract into several different sectors of highway. Everything located between a herbivore's mouth and small intestine can be considered the *foregut*. Everything on the other side of the *midgut*, or small intestine, is the *hindgut*. From reindeer to rhinos, all fall into one of two groups defined by where their bacterial guests carry out the work of cellulose fermentation. Most dairy animals—cows, sheep, goats, water buffa-loes, camels—are foregut-fermenters, meaning that the most important stages of digestion take place in a spectacular succession of stomach chambers. A few, however, postpone the crucial breakdown of cellulose to the hindgut.

Cows and their closest relatives are *ruminants*, or cud-chewers. Their mouths, unlike ours, are not designed to masticate food thoroughly as soon as it is bitten off. Grass and leaves get rapidly swallowed down with the help of floods of saliva—a cow secretes about forty-five gal-lons a day—until the animal has finished a meal. After that, the food is regurgitated into the mouth in installments, a mouthful at a time, and chewed at leisure. Ruminants have no teeth in the upper jaw, only a hard, tough, but toothless structure called the dental pad. They chew by an odd sideways motion of the lower against the upper jaw that grinds every mouthful of cud between the lower teeth and the dental pad, slowly reducing pieces of grass or leaf to smaller particles.

Beyond the mouth lies a very large, complex stomach divided into four chambers. The first two, the *rumen* and the *reticulum* (which actu-ally adjoin each other like a big room and a smaller alcove) together form the main fermenting vat. The walls of the rumen are covered with papillae like larger versions of those on a cat's tongue, while those of the reticulum are segmented into a corrugated lattice pattern.

The rumino-reticular space is huge in proportion to the rest of the animal, by far the largest organ in the body. In an adult cow, it usually has something like a fifty-gallon capacity. The stomach lying south of the human esophagus can hold about one gallon when stretched to its limits—but a mid-sized cow is only eight or ten times as large as a mid-sized woman or man, certainly not fifty. A human stomach might be comparable to a large swimming pool, while a cow's rumen and reticulum would be more like a township water tank.

Traveling from the mouth into the rumen, the re-swallowed wad or *bolus* of cud is greeted by a microbial welcoming committee: trillions of bacteria and other microorganisms that together with the chewed cud form a coarse-textured greenish-brown sludge continually fed by more saliva. This is where the real heavy lifting of cellulose digestion takes place, along with breakdown of many other dietary components.

Beyond the rumino-reticular area lies a third chamber officially titled the *omasum*. It has also historically gone by such names as manyplies, psaltery, or bible, all referring to the dozens of papillae-studded, closely packed page-like folds that it contains. Food that has been mostly broken down in the rumen now gets squeezed through the omasal folds before being propelled on to the *abomasum*, the fourth and last stomach chamber.

Only then does the animal's latest meal start to be digested in the same way as food entering a human stomach: by hydrochloric acid and an enzyme named *pepsin*, both secreted in the walls of the abomasum. In fact, this is the only true stomach in a ruminant's gastric system—that is, the only one of the four chambers in which arriving food is exposed to the action of digestive juices directly supplied by the animal. The acid and enzyme together bring about decisive chemical breakdowns without which food would not be ready to enter the small intestine.

But significantly, this description doesn't apply to the youngest ruminants. In fact, nursing calves and other members of the suborder Ruminantia don't ruminate until they start eating grass. The reason is casein. Milk from the udder is shunted straight past the rumen, reticulum, and omasum. It goes into the abomasum, whose walls secrete a special enzyme called *chymosin*, once known as *rennin*, able to disarm the repellent electric charges on the filaments projecting from casein micelles and allow the separate micelles to cluster together in a curd. The stomach contents then move on to the small intestine. The first three stomach chambers are undeveloped at birth and in cattle take six months or more to become fully functional, though a calf may explore grass almost from birth.[3] (At least, that was true when farmers didn't start day-old calves on milk-replacement formulas designed to trigger ruminal development as fast as possible, with a view to weaning them from a liquid diet in three to five weeks.) Chymosin, or rennin, was one of the earliest aids to making simple cheeses when people learned to harvest the abomasum of an unweaned calf, kid, or lamb after slaughtering; salt and dry it; and obtain rennet by soaking a small piece in water to extract the curdling enzyme.

Horses are less familiar to most of us as dairy animals than cattle, goats, and sheep. But they have been historically central to some of the most milk-dependent Old World societies. Together with their donkey and zebra cousins, horses belong to the family of *equids*. Like ruminants, they are grass-eaters who depend on microbial tenants to digest cellulose for them. Equids, however, are hindgut-fermenters with drastically dissimilar alimentary arrangements. The differences start at the front end: Equids have mouths filled with upper and lower teeth for cropping and chewing grass before sending it down into a single-chambered enzyme- and acid-secreting stomach. But with only brief exposure to gastric juices, the food rapidly moves on to the hindgut. After a fairly quick passage through the small intestine with some uptake of nutrients, it reaches the threshold of the large intestine, where a pouch called the *cecum* is located. In humans and many other mammals, this is a minor blind alley (*caecum* means "blind" in Latin). In hindgut-fermenters, however, it is enlarged into a microbial workshop more than twice the size of the stomach. Here for the first time the transit of food through the system slows down enough to allow for prolonged digestion of cellulose and many other constituents. As with ruminants, the animal itself acts only as host to innumerable microbes capable of untying the obstinate bonds that fasten together the myriad simple sugar molecules in cellulose. After about seven hours in the cecum, food is finally propelled to the colon (also greatly enlarged in equids, and also home to platoons of fermenting microbes).

The different kinds of bacterial colonies in a cow's rumen or a horse's cecum have never been fully catalogued. In fact, the word "bacterial" is misleading. Strictly speaking, "bacteria" now are considered just one group within the great empire of microorganisms, a taxonomic challenge unknown to Linnaeus. (In common usage, the name still covers microorganisms in general.) It is now known that the rumen or cecum contains not only life forms that fall within the official domain of bacteria but also others including diverse kinds of archaea, fungi, protozoa, and more. No dairy microbiologist can ever dream of tracking down and conclusively labeling each variety. They all work together somewhat like a hive mind, inadvertently regulating the host animal's metabolism through their different food preferences and ever-changing population balances.

MICROBIAL ECOLOGIES

Most people who follow ecological issues now know that any given environment is made up of many diverse living creatures in intricately shifting dynamic equilibrium. It is not an enormous mental stretch to grasp that plants and animals in Yellowstone National Park form an ecosystem, living in a state of interdependence on each other as well as local water supplies and climatic patterns. Remove or intensify one factor, and others are rapidly thrown out of balance. Try, for instance, to eliminate wolves, and in short order an expanded population of elk and deer will overgraze their particular food supplies enough to start dying from starvation (especially under environmental stresses like drought or unusual cold) and trigger a cascade of effects on other species.

Students of livestock animals' digestion now see the contents of the rumen or the cecum as a microbiological ecosystem, or *microbiome.*

Just as in larger land-based ecosystems, different subcommunities act out their parts within a diversified landscape where each group hungrily seeks its appointed substrate while also constantly interacting—like the Yellowstone elk and wolves—with other groups under particular environmental conditions. Some inkling of these complexities began to dawn after the late 1930s, when veterinary experimenters perfected a surgical procedure called *fistulation*. It involved cutting a circular opening in the ruminal wall of a (previously anesthetized) cow, plugging it with a tightly fitted plastic ring like the frame of a porthole, and closing it with a removable cap. (A horse's cecum can also be fistulated, but it's a trickier operation.) Fistulated cows, apparently untroubled by the arrangement, eventually became a sight unnerving only to newcomers on agricultural school campuses. The fistula allowed a researcher to plunge a gloved arm into the enormous cavity, retrieve gobs of partly digested fodder at any stage in a day's feeding routine, and study what was happening. No more dramatic example exists of a microbiome in action.

Fistulation showed beyond question that the rumen and reticulum housed a fantastically complex microbiology lab with many different organisms pursuing their own metabolic agendas. Think of the space as an anaerobic (oxygen-free) fermentation chamber where shipments of chewed cud arrive at intervals. An animal that crops wild grasses, or browses tender shrub and tree leaves, lets its highly diversified microbial lodgers *ing*est and *dig*est all this vegetation—but in constant competition with each other for niches in the overall microbiome, much like animals seizing varied dining opportunities within the ecosystem of Yellowstone. And to continue the parallels, some microorganisms are predators that devour others. But grass-eaters, when left to their own devices in their preferred environments without unusual stresses, generally manage to maintain an overall equilibrium of microbial kinds.[4]

Modern dairy farming profoundly altered the internal ecosystems of cows and other domestic ruminants—with serious implications for their long-term health—in order to increase milk production. (Equids like horses and donkeys were not affected to the same extent because farmers in the industrialized West were never particularly interested in them for either milk or meat purposes.) The rearrangement of animals' internal microbiota is only one instance of much-touted progress among many others that will be traced in this book.

A brief flash-forward: experts on bovine metabolism now know that grass and leaves furnish a low-energy (that is, low-calorie) diet and that boosting these rations with more concentrated formulas stimulates higher milk yields. Unfortunately, it also alters group relationships among the many different species that live in the ruminal microbiome. The most troublesome change is in pH: the relative acidity or alkalinity of any water-based solution, with 7 representing a neutral state.

The normal pH of a cow's rumen on a cellulose-rich diet of grass and hay is just slightly acid, fluctuating between a little more and a little less than 6.5. The microbes that prefer a substrate of cellulose and that play such a crucial role in a ruminant's life are incredibly sensitive to any lower dip. At a pH below 6 they lose their competitive edge over organisms that multiply in more acid conditions, and cellulose digestion almost comes to a standstill.[5] Later chapters will discuss in more detail how commercial planners of dairy cow rations eventually came to treat risky balancing acts between normal rumen conditions and borderline acidosis as indispensable management practice.

LACTIC ACID BACTERIA
AND PREHISTORIC DAIRYING

Fermentation within the hospitable warmth of a ruminant's digestive tract sustains large, diverse populations of microbes able to digest the otherwise indigestible. By remarkable good fortune, when people began investigating the milk that goats, sheep, and cows produce, microbial fermentation again provided a bridge over the limitations of human digestive capacities. But this time the substrate was the dissolved lactose mentioned above. In the open air, lactose happens to attract bacterial invaders more powerfully than any other component of milk. From the first prehistoric days of dairying in the Near East and western Asia, it exercised an irresistible fascination on swarms of lactic acid bacteria, or LAB, that became invisible allies of lactose-intolerant humans.

It may not be self-evident to consumers who encounter cow's milk only when filled into cartons or jugs after drastic industrial processing that no mammal's milk is designed to enter the outside world. Before humans invented dairying, milk existed only as part of an exclusive two-party, one-way flow shielded from external forces. The complementary gateways formed by the mother's nipple and the suckling infant's mouth allow the living fluid to travel straight from mammary system into digestive system with no detours. If it is diverted into an external environment, its intricate structure instantly comes up against foreign agents.

We all know that blood quickly begins to clot and discolor on exposure to the open air; milk is equally susceptible to change the instant it has left the closed nipple-to-mouth pathway. A recent book on cheesemaking by Bronwen and Francis Percival perceptively comments that milk, once milked, is "a moving target. It is constantly evolving, its bacterial populations and balance a reflection of its life history up to that point."[6] For human purposes, its reluctance to stand still poses endless difficulties to anyone who wants to convert it into uniform, standardized products. But this same readiness to absorb influences is a major reason that it so easily managed to become a prominent feature in prehistoric human diets.

Invading the water-based solution that is one of milk's principal phases, LAB that hung around cows' teats and nursing calves' muzzles in Neolithic settlements avidly devoured lactose, their appointed substrate. A large tribe with diverse talents, LAB secrete enzymes capable of snipping the bond between the two halves of the lactose molecule, as well as breaking down each of the now-separated sugars and commandeering most of its caloric energy. What's left is a lactic acid solution. As the lactose content diminishes and lactic acid accumulates, the original pH of the fresh milk (very slightly acidic, at 6.5 in roughly the same range as a grass-fed cow's rumen[7]) quickly declines. The Neolithic peoples who first saw milk go sour in summer heat reaped the benefit of several biochemical consequences.

For one thing, the increased acidity or lower pH of the *solution* kicks off changes in the *suspension*. It causes the casein micelles to partly shed the electric charge that allows them to repel each other and remain suspended in the milk. At about pH 5.5, the casein partly gathers together or *flocculates*, a marvelous piece of chemical terminology derived from the Latin word for tufts of wool.[8] Home yogurt-makers will recognize the soft flocculent mass as the stage where the milk is loosely set. If the acidity increases much more it will completely neutralize the original electric charge and the casein micelles will do what floating droplets of water vapor do when they come together in large enough drops to fall out of a cloud by gravity: precipitate. At that point the milk is visibly separated into curd—the precipitated casein, which has taken the emulsified fat with it—and whey—the remaining water-based lactic acid solution. (This is also what happens through the action of chymosin as described earlier, except that chymosin precipitation occurs without changes in pH, leaving all the lactose in the whey.)

In either flocculation or complete curdling through lactic acid fermentation, the milk loses all or most of the original lactose—a tremendous dietary advantage to peoples who could not easily digest lactose. From a practical standpoint, it was the yogurt-like flocculated version of fermented milk that was easiest to keep producing on a daily basis in the Neolithic Near East and western Asia.

As everyone knew, lactating sheep, goats, and cows reached peak flow during the hottest months of the year and began drying off as fall approached. The combination of fierce, dry summers and ambient legions of LAB that particularly loved temperatures between 105°F and 115°F/40.5°C and 46°C had historic consequences. It ensured that milk drawn from the udder into a bowl in the morning would be pleasantly sour and partly thickened in a matter of hours and that it could be freshly made every day as long as the weather and the milk supply lasted. After that, people waited until the next spring brought in the lactation cycle again with a spate of new births.

Since milk disagreed with adult digestive systems to a greater or lesser extent until it went sour, these early dairyists happily consumed it in that state without knowing that ten or twelve thousand years later, lactose fermentation and lactose digestion would greatly preoccupy scientists throughout the developed world. By 1900 AD, microbiologists would begin to grasp a second great benefit of lactic acid fermentation: the low pH of fermented milk discourages many common pathogens from invading it and spreading lethal contagions. This advantage is not shared by unfermented drinking-milk.

It took a long time for modern food science to perceive any concrete reasons for the primacy of fermented milk in many dairying societies. Not until the late twentieth century would researchers from many disciplines start confronting the belated discovery that the ability to comfortably digest large doses of lactose in adulthood is not shared by most of the human race and that the trait of "adult lactase persistence" chiefly belongs to white people of northern European genetic background. The wherewithal for arriving at this unexpected truth hadn't existed before James Watson and Francis Crick managed to map the structure of DNA in 1953. By then dairying had been a major human activity for many millennia. To trace its beginnings and development we must go back to the Late Stone Age, or indeed the aftermath of the last Ice Age, in several ecosystems of the Old World.

2

FROM THE CRADLE OF DAIRYING TO THE ENGLISH MANOR

GRASSLANDS, ANIMALS, PEOPLE, AND MILK

When the last ice sheet had finished riding roughshod over large tracts of the Northern Hemisphere and melted back to the Arctic Circle, animals and plants beyond number began moving into available ecological niches like so many Noah's Flood survivors climbing out of the ark and looking for anchoring spots. Many life forms found the homes that suited their needs in or close to an immense east-west stretch of open ground running from Manchuria to the Danube, or about 5,000 miles. Geographers call this vast sky-canopied expanse the Great Steppe of Eurasia.

The Eurasian steppe resembles our New World counterpart, the North American Great Plains, in being windswept and for the most part semiarid, with fiercely cold winters and hot summers. But it is far larger and has figured more dramatically in the global history of food.

In places the Great Steppe is only about 200 miles wide from north to south, in others more than 500 miles. To the north, it merges into mixed forest-steppe terrain followed by tremendous boreal forests. To the south, it borders some of the world's most forbidding deserts. Despite a few mountain barriers, it has always functioned as a natural highway, or biological—and cultural—pipeline through which the eastern and western edges of Asia have exchanged influences in more dynamic and diverse ways than might seem possible to an observer unexpectedly set down in these grass-clad wilds.

Grasses, or Poaceae to botanists, were the family of plants that most dramatically seized the ecological initiative throughout the steppe as the planet began warming up after the last glacial epoch. Along its main body, river valleys and lake borders are almost the only places with enough water to support tree growth. But grasses, with their tough and many-branched roots, can make efficient use of limited rainfall, the chief factor that always kept many other kinds of plants from colonizing the sweeping corridor.

Grasses were the making of several complicated relationships between people and their food along the Great Steppe and in some mountainous areas abutting it. They may be the most important reason that nonhuman milk ever entered human diets—starting with the fact that these regions are, or until modern times were, ideal environments for wandering herds of grass-eating animals. The herbivores in turn attracted an array of predators unequipped to digest grass themselves but able to profit from it in the flesh of nearby herbivores. The most effective of all predators would be *Homo sapiens*.

The first stages on the path to the milking revolution emerged long before milking as an actual practice. They started when Neolithic peoples found that by usefully meddling in the reproductive cycles of certain wild grasses and animals, they could create a cushion against seasonal food shortages. The setting for these discoveries was a well-watered swathe of West Asian terrain some 500 miles south of the steppe, encompassing what is often dubbed the Fertile Crescent. Researchers who study the beginnings of farming now map its earliest centers not only in the originally identified Fertile Crescent—a curving belt lying between the Zagros Mountains of modern Iran on the east and the Taurus Mountains of Turkey on the west—but also in several other sites of human activity farther west and south, on the Anatolian Plateau and close to the Levantine coast of the Mediterranean. These areas had their own scattered pieces of grassy terrain that would figure lastingly in global foodways.

At some point close to 10,000 BC, local hunter-gatherers took note of an important fact: not only would grasses that escaped being eaten by animals eventually bear seeds, but some of the seeds in question were worth searching out and collecting as food for humans.

Over an unknown number of centuries, people began encouraging likely specimens to reseed themselves in one spot and ripen on a fairly systematic schedule for easier gathering. At the same time, they learned to single out individual plants with unusual qualities like especially large seeds, or whole seed-heads that tended not to shatter when ripe and (inconveniently, from a human viewpoint) spill the contents on the ground before they could be efficiently harvested. By degrees, a focus on such traits shaded into planned cultivation, which in turn shaded into actual domestication. There are various definitions of domestication, but all agree that it replaces natural selection with artificial selection for qualities desired by human custodians, eventually creating strains of true-breeding descendants that can rarely survive in their altered form without being planted, harvested, and maintained by people. The earliest resulting plants in the greater Fertile Crescent were what are now labeled cereal grasses or grain crops, ancestors of today's wheat and barley. The last centuries before 10,000 BC appear to have seen the emergence of truly domesticated strains.

Meanwhile, the hunting sector of the Near Eastern hunter-gatherer economy had long depended on the vast populations of hoofed and horned grass-eaters that roamed the Great Steppe and the foothills of neighboring mountain regions. Swift and agile enough to usually outrun predators, they traveled in herds to avoid being picked off singly. Such itinerant groups were superbly equipped to rove across dozens or hundreds of miles throughout a year, cropping one range before moving on to another. Since wild grasses can grow back quickly and feed migrating herds more than once in the course of a year, the animals and their food supply were usually able to exist in stable ecological balance.

The West Asian ungulates (as zoologists call hoofed mammals) included Old World bison, assorted gazelles and antelopes, and four other great lineages that in time would beget the first domesticated milk-givers: goats, sheep, cattle, and horses. Horses, the outlier in the quartet, were domesticated long after the others and would not cross their paths for several thousand years—though they would then become a game-changing factor in human relationships with the other three.

Students of Neolithic civilizations believe that as with plants, the domestication of wild goats, sheep, and cattle occurred in stages over centuries or millennia rather than being the result of one bright idea. As the anthropologist David W. Anthony has observed, "Animal domestication, like marriage, is the culmination of a long prior relationship"[1]—undoubtedly one that had begun with hunting and killing these creatures for their meat, along with gazelles and the rest. Successful hunters knew how to track a herd's movements and corner it at some vulnerable point.

As people learned to coordinate group efforts and reliably steer herds into massive ambushes, they began to deplete some wild populations. Eventually somebody would have tried capturing and penning up a few young members of a herd, to be raised to maturity before slaughter. This approach had some success with individual captives, which often allowed themselves to be tamed. But real domestication required something far more difficult: getting the captives to reproduce so as to keep renewing the supply. Even today, no one fully understands why some creatures resist breeding in confinement much more stubbornly than others—one of the chief factors that hinder zoos from replenishing the numbers of many species now endangered in the wild.

For whatever reason, the first grazing animals of suitable size—that is, small enough for one or two strong men to tangle with them —that were finally persuaded to mate under permanent human custody were local wild goats and sheep. In them, late Neolithic peoples of the Fertile Crescent and its mountainous fringes had managed to find two of the very few hoofed mammals that can be chaperoned down the path to domestication. Over many generations, probably starting at or before about 10,000 BC, selected groups of goats and sheep not only accepted human control in preference to freedom but began to deviate from their ancestral morphology (structure and outward appearance). Zooarchaeologists are not always sure whether bones recovered from the early transitional period belonged to wild or domesticated goats and sheep, but the final differences are so unmistakable that the animals are now classified in their own species, *Capra hircus* and *Ovis aries*. The coat of curly, crimped hairs—"wool"—that domesticated sheep acquired while losing an ancestral outer coat of longer hairs is only one example of morphological change.

A third target of Neolithic hunters was a much more terrifying candidate for domestication: *Bos primigenius*, the huge wild ox or aurochs (plural "aurochsen," as in "oxen"). This ancestor of all domesticated cattle breeds was among the largest and fiercest creatures of the Old World grasslands. For sheer bulk, aurochsen would have presented greater challenges than wild goats or sheep. Almost no modern breeds suggest the size of full-grown aurochs bulls. The towering Italian Chianina, which is often six feet high at the shoulder and can weigh as much as 3,500 pounds, gives an idea of how unanswerably an aurochs must have stacked up against any human. The bulls were at least as aggressive as Spanish fighting bulls, though these are deliberately bred for less fearsome size and rarely reach five feet or 1,500 pounds.

Nevertheless, this powerful creature turned out to be one of the few herbivores that people finally managed to mold into a domesticated species, *Bos bovis*. The first domesticated cattle—selected for undersized dimensions—were considerably smaller than aurochsen, an obvious advantage for handlers. Nobody ever managed to completely breed the original ferocity out of bulls. But cows became habituated to conceiving and giving birth in captivity, if human helpers could introduce them to a sire without being mowed down in the process. Few domestic mammals show more striking male-female differences than today's cattle, in either physique or behavior.

It is impossible to pinpoint a place or date where some inquisitive person first tried to milk one of the animals being kept for meat. The idea must have occurred to people in more than one corner of the general region, though adopting it as standard practice may have taken many centuries. Two things are certain: the subjects of early experiments did not have the large, capacious udders of today's dairy animals, and did not share their compliant attitude toward being milked. Not only is shoving oneself between a nursing mother and her young a good way to get attacked, but simply yanking on a teat will do nothing but agitate her more.

Like human mothers, lactating goats, sheep, and cows have an instinctive need to see, touch, and smell the nurslings who depend on their milk. These sensory cues reinforce the particular combination of suction and pressure that the infant's mouth exerts in suckling, helping to stimulate production of the hormone oxytocin, which governs the "letdown reflex." The first humans who managed to trick the mother into letting down her milk had to allow the little one an initial few moments of nursing and then keep it as close to her as possible, usually by tethering it to her front leg or neck, while cleverly mimicking the suckling rhythm with their fingers wrapped around a teat in a particular grasp. (A later refinement in prompting the hormonal trigger was to have a helper blow air through a pipe inserted into the animal's vagina or anus.[2]) Another certainty is that by comparison with modern norms, these efforts would have yielded much smaller amounts of milk—though milk more naturally concentrated than anything one can buy today.

We do not know in what forms prehistoric peoples consumed milk, except that they could not have easily digested it fresh from the udder. Nonetheless, milking skills seem to have become well advanced by late Neolithic times (possibly about 6,500 BC) in the greater Fertile Crescent.

As living with the results of both plant and animal domestication became second nature to people, some intractable conflicts arose between the demands of the two enterprises. The old hunter-gatherer life allowed bands of humans to move around synchronously with both the annual migrations of animals and the seasons of wild fruits, vegetables, and anything else that can be reaped with two hands. Tending crops meant a break with this mobility and either rapidly or by slow degrees imposed a sedentary life on the tenders. Sedentism, however, was an abnormal condition for herbivores used to eating their way from range to range. For them, survival had always been contingent on grazing one patch of grass, then moving on to the next. Where grass was plentiful, they could linger a while; where it was scarce, they had to cover wider areas. Goats were somewhat flexible in their needs, since they could readily browse on shrub or tree leaves. Sheep and to some extent cattle depended more heavily on grass. And as people soon found, any restricted pasturage on which a herd is kept grazing without letup is soon depleted, often with serious damage to the ground itself.

The dilemma for two-legged keepers moving on foot was how to either provide these instinctive wanderers with everything they needed (including protection against animal predators and human thieves) in an artificially confined space or travel as far and fast as they did. Sedentism-versus-mobility choices were an early example of a quandary that has never gone away: how to use land resources to balance a community's food demands against the environmental costs that come with raising animals—or, to state the issue another way, mismatches between food consumption and sustainable food production. Complex modern economies have not so much solved these problems as displaced them beyond the everyday view of the consuming public, especially since the growth of cities began shunting the people who consumed perishable products into living spaces far distant from the site of production.

LIVING WITH DOMESTICATED ANIMALS: SEDENTISM, NOMADISM, AND HORSES

By the time stone-based technologies gave way to experiments with copper (roughly 5,500 BC) and bronze (by about 3,300 BC), the systems of plant and animal control that had first appeared in the greater Fertile Crescent had already started to be carried elsewhere throughout an ever-widening geographical span. Of course they pushed some societies in the direction of sedentism, eventually leading to highly specialized uses of space and human abilities. Over time, animals would receive dedicated pasturage and stabling, while specific food-handling tasks would be apportioned to different workers. This is the model of animal husbandry most familiar to modern humans, though, as we shall soon see, not the only possible one.

Livestock management in Neolithic and Bronze Age societies had already been enriched by an interest in what have been called "secondary products."[3] People had long used the carcasses of slaughtered meat animals to obtain leather, bones (for making tools and needles), and sinews (for sewing together animal hides). Eventually they began to recognize the benefits of keeping large numbers of goats, sheep, and cattle alive. (Nobody ever found a way of extracting extra value from another early domesticate—the pig—while it was still breathing.) The dung of all made excellent fertilizer for crops, and could serve as fuel for cooking fires. Sheep and sometimes goats were prized for shearable fleeces. The unique advantage of cattle, for the pioneers of sedentary agriculture, was muscle power. Even a cow could carry loads too heavy for most men, or pull the simple stick plows that had appeared by about 4,000 BC or possibly earlier. But still more efficient were young bullocks castrated before maturity, which lost the murderous instincts of intact bulls and grew into the most powerful aid to crop cultivation devised up to that point: oxen.

Among the reasons for valuing goats, sheep, and cattle on the hoof rather than when roasted for dinner, one differed from all others: their milk was *the only renewable food resource* that could be extracted from living animals on a daily basis. And though domestic animals' milk fresh from the udder was somewhat indigestible to adult humans, climatic conditions in early milking regions allowed lactic acid bacteria to solve the problem within hours. There is no reason to think that fresh milk figured significantly in human diets unless perhaps as a transitional weaning food for children. (To put it another way, the burden of proof should rest with anyone trying to argue that it was commonly used by adults.)

We know that the oldest sedentary civilizations both prized milk in everyday uses and associated it with mighty goddesses. Images from the Bronze Age cultures of Sumer and Egypt clearly depict cows and goats being milked, with calf or kid almost invariably tethered to the mother to encourage letdown. Tending animals and collecting their milk for a caste of priest-rulers seems to have been a regular occupation in Sumer. But since we have few reliable ways of matching operative words with translations into any modern language, guessing just *how* ancient civilizations used milk is treacherous ground. Apparently there were Sumerian words for many different kinds of cheese, though reconstructing the specifics is probably beyond the powers of any food historian. Interpretations of Egyptian texts mentioning milk and milk products are also subject to much doubt. Actual cheese remains have been recovered from a few Egyptian sites—but it must be understood that in the hot, dry climates of Egypt and Sumer, cheesemaking would have depended on simple lactic acid or rennet coagulation, not complex extended ripening.[4] Only limited variations (such as added flavorings, or preservation by salting or brining) would have been possible.

Domesticated livestock had become closely integrated into sedentary farming systems in the Fertile Crescent and some neighboring areas by 5,500–5,000 BC. But in the next few thousand years, sharply contrasting relationships with animals began to penetrate into western tracts of the Great Steppe north of the Black and Caspian seas. Long stretches of grassland in regions that ancient Greek observers would later call Scythia and Sarmatia formed an ideal environment for another hoofed creature: the horse.

For hunter-gatherers in these regions, wild horses had long been a major meat source. With growing exposure to other examples of domestication, they came to see that the animals' extraordinary combination of speed, stamina, and intelligence might be (literally) harnessed. No documentation exists of just when during the centuries-long process of engineering the domesticated species *Equus caballus* some innovator managed to scramble up onto a horse's back and stay there. But the skills of riding first mastered by the steppe peoples would convert horses, and later a few other animals, into remarkable instruments of human purpose.

The physical and mental bond between horse and rider was unlike any prior animal-human relationship. Their shared motion, opening up the new experience of tapping into the energies of a creature stronger than any human but able to intuit human wishes, was one of the great transforming thrills of mankind. The steppe riders were the first peoples to feel the adrenaline surge of superhuman speed, and to exploit its practical uses. And as this first transportation revolution worked back to Bronze Age centers of sedentary farming in the Near East, it formed a lasting marriage with the recently invented wheel—or more precisely, pairs of wheels joined by axles.

From then on, horses were destined to become invaluable adjuncts to expanded trade and warfare. They made at least as good pack and draft animals as oxen and were incomparable as steeds for messengers and fighting men. We can also easily see how the horse example eventually inspired people to recruit donkeys (equid cousins first domesticated in Africa) and still later camels (the toughest of hoofed animals in desert and near-desert environments) to some of the same uses. But it was left to assorted peoples living in the great transcontinental grass corridor to bypass sedentary animal husbandry and forge notably milk-dependent societies on entirely new models.[5]

Since the steppe horsemen had no written language, the first accounts of their ways come from Greek-speaking outsiders. Zeus in the *Iliad* briefly turns his gaze from the Trojan assault on the Greek ships to far-away peoples including the "horse-riding Thracians," "Galactophagi" (Milk-Eaters), and "illustrious Hippemolgi" (Mare-Milkers).[6] Much later writers mention horse-riding tribes living north of the Black Sea, toward the European end of the Great Steppe. The best-known were the Scythians, whose skill as mobile cavalrymen without permanent headquarters for enemies to target gave them a frustrating advantage against opponents like King Darius I of Persia. The historian Herodotus, who chronicled Darius's much-thwarted campaigns, relates that crews of blinded slaves were responsible for milking the Scythians' mares with the aid of a pipe stuck into the vagina (see above); the milk was held in casks and agitated into some kind of churned beverage.[7] (All these details ring true except for the blinding, which may represent some misunderstood Scythian word. The walls of the casks undoubtedly served as a reservoir of bacteria for quickly fermenting the milk.) The geographer Strabo (c. 64 BC–c. 24 AD) also notes the strange peoples' dependence on mare's milk in different fermented forms; as explained in chapter 6, the chemical makeup of mare's milk allows it to undergo especially rapid and complex fermentation. Strabo singles out several local tribes as "Nomades" (from a Greek word for pasturing) who had no fixed homes and spent their lives on horseback tending their animals throughout wide areas of grazing land, with women, children, and portable property carried in horse-drawn wagons that served as mobile homes.[8]

This way of life—pastoral nomadism—would support some of the world's most intensely milk-centered societies from perhaps 3500 BC to the present. Horse-powered travel enabled people, for the first time, to keep up with animal peregrinations far and wide over the Great Steppe and other grasslands. Horses themselves proved to be the ideal instrument for managing horses—and as horse-riding nomads soon realized, other dairy animals. A couple of men on horseback could do more than many men on foot to direct a large herd of mares, goats, ewes, or cows from one grazing range to another. For several millennia the nomads of Central Asia found in their horses, as one nineteenth-century European traveler described it, their alter egos.[9]

While sedentary husbandry became more solidly established in Near Eastern and other city-states, pastoral nomadism diffused into many steppe regions as well as the plentiful grasslands of Africa. In fact, many versions of nomadism gradually developed in all areas of the Old World where animals could be grazed. Among other shared features, nomadic societies prized livestock as a measure of wealth, took the animals' quests for grass and water as a template for communal planning, and used milk—though not in fresh form—as a dietary mainstay. They also ignored, or came late to, written language.

Nomadic herding was an entirely different ecological bargain from sedentary farming and livestock raising. Modern agronomists generally evaluate given areas of land by "carrying capacity," meaning the largest number of units belonging to some species (tons of soybeans, head of cattle) that an acre or other measure of land can support without starting to degrade soil and water resources through pollution or overuse. The simplest forms of nomadism, however, distributed both people and animals across areas too wide to bring carrying capacity into question—at least, over many centuries while population growth remained low. Some nomads, notably in East Africa, were able to accompany migrating animals on foot without benefit of horses. Some achieved their own flexible balances between mobility and limited cultivation of a few crops. But milking was always a defining part of the package. And it was always true that societies devoted to giving their animals and themselves extensive seasonally planned *Lebensraum* incurred less localized pollution or depletion of grass than sedentary counterparts.

Settled farmers and nomads alike understood milk not as an uninterrupted year-round resource but as something that came and went with changing seasons. The great limiting factor was the availability of grass, which began drying up in late summer. This signaled the end of the year's milking, as the animals finished weaning their young, stopped lactating, and went on to mate before or during autumn. The pregnant mares, she-goats, ewes, and cows survived for the next several months on whatever meager herbage remained until spring grass brought back the season of births.

It should be understood that in the cradle of prehistoric dairying nobody had to *invent* fermented milk. Ordinary daytime temperatures during late spring and summer far exceeded 95°F/35°C, at which level ambient lactic-acid bacteria spontaneously colonized freshly drawn milk. Converting fresh into sour milk didn't require elaborate techniques. People did, over time, learn how to direct the process and maintain particular bacterial communities with great skill. But under the circumstances, it would have been unnatural for milk *not* to ferment within hours of being drawn. In other words, lactic-acid fermentation by warmth-loving organisms (also forming a partial defense against many pathogens) is as old as milking itself.

MILK IN A COLD CLIMATE: NEW DIMENSIONS

Long before the founding of Egypt and Sumer or the emergence of steppe nomadism, some Neolithic peoples of the greater Fertile Crescent had imported themselves and their farming skills from Anatolia, or "Asia Minor," into the most southeasterly corner of Europe. Crops including wheat and barley, and livestock including goats, sheep, and cattle, had appeared in Greece by around 7,000 BC. (Whether milking was already a common practice among the new arrivals is not known.) It took another three or four millennia for descendants of these farmers to work their way north and west through the Balkans and Central Europe to the northern shores of Europe and the British Isles—a meandering, uneven progress that undoubtedly threw the newcomers into unplanned contact with native hunter-gatherers or peoples possibly taking their own first steps toward farming.

By the time these epic journeys brought Near Eastern domesticated crops and animals to the North Sea and Baltic coasts, many changes had overtaken all of Europe. Stone Age technologies had given way to copper and bronze. Some horse-centered communities of the steppes, now frequently trading with settled civilizations of the Near East and southeastern Europe, had increased in numbers enough to overtax former resources and start moving westward. Waves of nomadic peoples sporadically penetrated into the eastern reaches of Central and Northern Europe, bringing their genes and their languages into regions being traversed by the northbound farmers.

The custodians of wheat, barley, cows, sheep, pigs, and other resources inched forward in unsystematic increments, picking up new cultural, technological, and genetic baggage as they went. Every degree of latitude brought them deeper into ecosystems radically unlike the regions of torrid summers in which plants and animals had been domesticated. Reaching the edge of the continent in today's north Germany, southern Scandinavia, and neighboring lands, they were greeted with much yearly precipitation, many different soil types, distinctive patterns of vegetation including towering forests, and above all some of the world's shortest summers and longest, coldest winters.

This northerly climate effactually redrew the outlines of settled animal husbandry for many future members of the white race—and, in ages to come, all other races. It reshaped milk and milking in ways that would have been impossible anywhere else in the Old World, but that after a few thousand years would be glorified in every corner of the globe as enlightened models for people of all cultural and racial backgrounds.

From the start, cattle had a critical advantage at North Sea and Baltic latitudes. Their size alone meant that in the act of ruminating to digest their food they generated a great deal of heat. In fact, most strains of cattle have difficulty dissipating enough body heat to remain healthy in hot climates without constant access to shade and water. Being tolerant of all but the most extreme cold, the large beasts rapidly became the preeminent regional livestock animal. Oxen were indispensable for plowing and hauling, cows for milk. Raising animals specifically for the table was a great luxury, so meat often came from worn-out plough stock or milking stock. Even so, beef enjoyed immense prestige for the large amounts of meat that could be furnished by a single animal. A similar consideration made cows the dairy animal of choice. People also valued sheep as a thrifty triple-threat asset providing wool, milk, and (in old age) mutton. Ewe's milk was incomparably rich and concentrated—but also forbiddingly labor-intensive to collect, since it took only one cow to match the yield of eight or ten ewes. When North European communities thought of milk, they thought of cow's milk. Goats and their meat or milk came a poor third in usual calculations, while horseflesh and mare's milk never gained great regional importance.

Northern environments were determinative in other ways. We have no written record of local societies until Julius Caesar's legions marched into the newly named Gallia Transalpina, Germania, and Britannia after 58 BC. The accounts that filtered back to the Greco-Roman world shed only scanty and confused light on the barbarians' use of milk. But the four-century occupation left a serious imprint on livestock husbandry, including dairying.

The role of cultural interpreter had no interest for Caesar. He tersely mentions in Book IV of *The Gallic Wars* that the Suebi, one of the chief German tribes, consumed "milk and livestock" (*pecus*), and in Book VI describes the Germans in general as largely depending on "milk, cheese, and flesh," but doesn't clarify either "milk" or "cheese."[10] But Pliny the Elder, who about a century later spent several years as a military officer in the northern provinces, plainly says that though the "barbarous peoples who live on milk" used it to prepare butter—a puzzling novelty to Romans—and a pleasant tart substance that may have been sour buttermilk, they were ignorant of cheesemaking.[11] Pliny's contemporary Tacitus speaks of the Germans eating milk in a thickened or condensed state (*lac concretum*) but conspicuously fails to use the ordinary word "cheese" (*caseus*); Strabo comments that the Britons were well provided with milk but too backward to use it for cheese.[12]

As it happens, the Romans had been the first civilization to develop what we can unequivocally recognize as hard or semihard cheeses: those aged at cool enough temperatures over long enough periods of time to undergo complex, sustained chemical changes. They were able to do this because much of northern Italy offered well-watered grazing shielded from the hot, dry Mediterranean summers and favored with comparatively cool autumns and chilly winters. In northwestern Europe and Britain, the occupying armies found equally fine cheesemaking conditions. They also enlarged on the local peoples' earlier success in carving limited clearings out of the dense, enormous primeval forests, creating tillable fields and pockets of mixed grazing land as well as lush meadows.

The Romans had a lively appreciation of meadows (*prata*) and their usefulness in supplying hay to help feed livestock through the winter. Both haymaking and aging hard cheeses are efforts requiring skill, proper equipment, and attention to detail. It is not clear that the far northern subjects of the empire had ever flirted with either accomplishment before the Romans arrived. But both proved ideally suited to North European climates. By the time the last legions departed in the early fifth century AD, household economies reliant on these two defenses against winter shortages were in place in all future northwestern European nations.

But there is a gaping hole in our knowledge. What (if anything) did the Gauls, Germans, and Britons use milk for *besides* butter, the sour or coagulated products mentioned by several ancient writers, and the aged cheeses probably introduced by the Romans? Did they drink unfermented fluid milk as casually as their twenty-first-century descendants in, say, today's United States? There is a hitch in trying to even ask the question: Neither the Romans nor their conquered subjects in Northern Europe knew that a crucial genetic difference separated them.

Roman food-lovers were quite aware of not always sharing foreigners' gastronomic preferences. Butter for them was an unacquired taste, and cow's milk for cheese was less desirable than goat's and ewe's milk. But they didn't think to tell future scholars whether the northerners had or lacked an everyday postweaning habit of drinking any animal's milk in its original noncheese state, a practice never adopted by the Romans. Of course fresh milk was there for Roman and Greek writers to comment on, or even to recommend for occasional medical uses. But their digestive systems could not comfortably handle it in more than very small amounts.

The northern barbarian farmers, however, had acquired a particular genetic quirk or polymorphism—a novel dominant-recessive pair of genes governing a trait—at some point in their journey from Asia Minor to the North Sea. The result was that an ability to digest fresh milk into adulthood eventually became widely distributed through the population.

Archaeologists and geneticists believe that the polymorphism in question originated somewhere in an area of eastern Central Europe including the Hungarian Plains, Slovakia, and southeastern Austria, and went north with farming communities. It governed the production of lactase after weaning and was inherited as a dominant trait, though this is a case where we don't always find mutually exclusive dominant/recessive alternatives; many people displayed (as people do today) incomplete versions of the ability or inability to digest fresh milk. Early estimates of when it emerged were in the general neighborhood of 5,500 BC, but more recent data seem to indicate something close to 2,300 BC or still later. (Some researchers speculate that it may have been carried to Europe by one of the nomadic groups that kept sweeping in from the steppes while the farmers were making their slow way north, but no conclusive evidence has come to light.)[13]

The puzzling thing is that though we know that the northbound farmers *could* have relied very heavily on fresh drinking-milk after the critical shift appeared, it has yet to be established that they *did*. To suppose that people usually able to digest fresh milk would never have tasted it is clearly unreasonable. But we have no evidence that they at once took up regularly drinking fresh milk in large amounts.

Regardless of that unsolved mystery, the appearance of the new trait in the European gene pool was one of the most consequential monkey wrenches ever thrown into the gearbox of world history. This is not because the genetic variation in question was unique. It was not, and is not. A handful of similar polymorphisms involving lactase persistence exist elsewhere in the Old World—and curiously enough, the people affected sometimes prefer fermented milk. What sets the European deviation apart is that a few thousand years after it had first appeared, two nations in which a majority of the population possessed it became world powers on a scale dwarfing imperial Rome. Great Britain, and later the United States of America, came to enjoy not only global military and economic preeminence but the privilege of setting scientific agendas (including theories of nutrition) for the rest of the planet, long before anyone knew that most humans did not share Britons' or North Americans' common ability to digest large amounts of fresh milk.

We cannot simply project modern milk-drinking practices back into Neolithic, Bronze Age, or even early Iron Age times. Today's everyday habits require a year-round industrial-scale milk supply completely divorced from the seasons and dependent on an enormously complex technological infrastructure that didn't exist even a century and a half ago, much less seven thousand or four thousand years. For all the differences in climate, early northwestern European farmers operated under natural limitations on milking and milk use just as strong as those in the Near Eastern cradle of dairying. Under and after the Romans, milking still depended on yearly cycles of grass growth and animal reproduction. The supply still reached its peak during the months most favorable to spontaneous or culture-assisted fermentation and started to decline in late summer as the next mating season approached. Just as before, cows, ewes, and goats would ordinarily be dry (and pregnant) by autumn.

Much useful insight into English dairying can be gleaned from both Latin and vernacular records after about 800 AD. By far the most important uses of milk were for cheese and butter. Under the manorial system, both of these were produced on an estate-wide scale to supply the domestic needs of a lord (or monastery or convent), but also on an individual scale by peasant families who had the privilege of grazing one or more cows on the estate. Some seasonal use of fresh milk for drinking in both great and small households is also documented in manorial or abbey records and a scattering of other sources.

Surveying the general picture: there is no doubt that in England, as in nearly all of northwestern Europe, most dairying on both a manorial and a small-householder scale was cow dairying. Sheep were important only on large estates in wool-producing areas where ewes were also milked for cheese; Essex and the North Holland island of Texel were long famous for sheep cheeses. (Late in the Middle Ages, as multipurpose animal husbandry lost ground to less labor-intensive commercial priorities, sheep dairying was abandoned in many wool-growing regions.) Goats, the least popular of the three chief dairy animals in England and other northern strongholds of milking, hung on in a small way as "the poor man's cow" for those who couldn't upgrade to the real thing.

The cool climate and the chemical makeup of cow's milk allowed it to be transformed into an amazing number of products, most of which were regarded more as peasant mainstays than delicacies. The most important, because the least perishable, were hard cheeses and butter.

Cheese sometimes appeared on a lord's table, but it had stronger associations with the peasantry. Its great virtue was that it was generally available, whether in good or bad condition, at all times of year. A morsel of dry bread and almost equally dry cheese together with a little ale might be a complete breakfast (or other meal) for the poor tenants on a manor, in winter or summer. Butter represented one of the lucky results of cow dairying. Milkfat, the emulsified chemical phase of milk described in chapter 1, performs an especially neat trick in cow's milk, whose comparatively large milkfat globules don't remain reliably emulsified for long after milk leaves the udder. If the milk stands for a day or longer, it separates by gravity into a fatless bottom layer (skim milk) and a fat-rich upper layer (cream). During the main milking season, both would have undergone either spontaneous or controlled bacterial action by the time the cream was churned, leaving both small householders and manor cowherds or dairymaids with naturally fermented skim milk, buttermilk, and ripened butter. The butter was commonly worked together with heavy doses of salt, the preservative of choice, and packed into tubs, casks, or other convenient containers. It kept for months.

Besides the two commonest uses, milk also entered peasant households in the form of simple fresh (green) cheeses made by curdling skimmed or whole milk, either with rennet or by prolonged lactic-acid bacteria souring, and draining the whey from the curd before lightly pressing the cheese and mixing it with salt and/or herbs. People also relished soft curds and whey eaten as is, without draining. Whey itself (either "sweet" or sour, and including the whey from making aged cheeses) was prized as a refreshing drink, as was the sour buttermilk left from buttermaking.

Consuming milk in its own right instead of turning it into something else was not invariable practice, but we know that both sour and fresh milk appeared on medieval tables. The "poor widow" in the Nun's Priest's Tale of Chaucer—prosperous enough to keep three cows and a few other farm animals—was acquainted not with fripperies like red or white wine but with "Milk and broun breed [brown bread], in which she foond no lak [found no deprivation]."[14] In loftier circles a few centuries earlier, the monks of Abingdon Abbey in Berkshire were unequivocally recorded as getting *lac acidum* (sour milk) from "Hokeday" just after Easter to the feast of Michaelmas on September 29, and *lac dulce* ("sweet" milk) from then until Martinmas on November 11.[15]

That distinction tells us much about the realities of medieval milk-drinking. Milk expectably went sour in spring and summer, remained fresh somewhat longer in autumn temperatures, and then vanished from consideration until next Hokeday—or in some cases, next May. In fact, no dairy products except hard cheese and butter commonly reached the table out of season. The limiting factors were two: the availability of fodder for the animals, and their breeding cycles.

The haymaking probably introduced by the Romans helped to eke out nourishment for cows between the last summer grass and the first spring grass. But only large estates with very generous allotments of meadow in proportion to the livestock inventory could easily get through the winter without worrying about losing some cows. Haymaking allowed large manor farms, and perhaps smallholders able to purchase hay, to partly close the forbidding annual forage gap. But since manor farms also had to feed oxen and horses, decisions about which beasts to provide for first didn't necessarily favor cows.

Another seasonal constraint was the chancy interval between the end of one lactation cycle and the beginning of another. Like ewes and goats, cows are genetically programmed to come into milk after giving birth in spring and dry off in time for autumn mating and winter pregnancies. For this reason, some farm managers didn't allow any cow to be milked or suckled after Michaelmas, which in the words of one thirteenth-century authority will "make the cows lose flesh and become weak."[16] It is easy to see why medieval kitchens were usually bare of drinking-milk and milk products other than cheese and butter throughout the cold months.

COUNTRY, CITY, AND CONSUMER

Throughout the Middle Ages, nearly all dairying was based in the countryside, because that was where the grass was. Dairying is inherently a rural enterprise, linked to the needs of creatures that evolved as herd animals moving over grazing ranges on steppes and other grassy terrain in the same way as bison moving over the American Great Plains. The countryside was also where most people were; medieval England and all North European countries were overwhelmingly rural.

It is not hard to understand why most milk-derived foods were consumed by the people who had produced them, and on the estates where dairy animals lived, instead of changing hands in cash transactions elsewhere. The manorial system was based on a labor economy, not a money economy. Fresh drinking-milk, of course, was far too perishable (and heavy) to be transported over any distance. It could not have existed as a commercial product in the same way as timber or cloth. The only forms in which milk could travel over long distances, or more than a few miles at any time other than spring and summer, were as hard cheese and butter.

Nonetheless, medieval city-dwellers did want some access to fresh milk and fresh milk products. Since neither could be transported from the countryside, a limited trade in milk as well as curds and whey was permitted to sellers who had found some way to house and feed a cow, or a handful of cows, in town. The name of Milk Street in London is the last surviving vestige of centuries when milk vendors plied their trade there in a corner of the great Cheapside Market. Purchasers who didn't want to buy prewatered milk passed off as new milk were wise to bring their own container and insist on seeing the cow directly milked into it rather than letting the seller dip milk out of a bucket.

Country life, meanwhile, had undergone deep disruptions by the end of the fifteenth century. Since the Crusades, foreign trade had become steadily more important. The star of overseas commerce in the English economy was wool. Sheep farming had begun to take over wide expanses of land after the Black Death reached England at about 1350, leaving labor shortages (leading to higher cash wages) throughout the depopulated rural landscape. The manorial system never recovered. But independent farms operated for profit multiplied. The wool boom, far from fostering a sheep-cheese boom, encouraged entrepreneurial farmers to manage the flocks only for fleeces.

Lands formerly designated as commons for peasants on manor farms were progressively swallowed up by enclosures for sheep and to an extent cattle farming. From the fifteenth century on, the rural poor began to be driven off the land. Towns and cities that ran on money rather than labor or payment in kind mushroomed, creating a widening divide between places where food was produced and consumed.

What this meant for poor cottagers who might once have supplied many of their own wants with the help of a family cow was summed up many years later by the Elizabethan dramatists Robert Greene and Thomas Lodge in their play *A Looking Glass for London and England* (c. 1590), a thinly veiled jeremiad against a Mammon-worshiping English society set in the Biblical Nineveh at the time of Jonah. A poor peasant, found to have been one day late in repaying thirty shillings that he has unwisely borrowed against his cow, expostulates with the usurer who insists on sending his family into ruin by confiscating the animal: "Why, sir, alasse, my Cow is a Common-wealth to me; for first sir, she allowes me, my wife and sonne, for to banket our selues withal [for regaling ourselves on], Butter, Cheese, Whay, Curds, Creame, sod [boiled] milk, raw-milke, sower-milke, sweete-milke, and butter-milke . . ."[17]

In the new economy, aged cheeses and sometimes butter began to be marketed on a commercial scale as regional specialties, partly in response to an enormous volume of butter and cheese being produced and exported by a successful dairying-for-profit movement in the Netherlands. A more surprising effect of the new order was to create a fast-growing upscale market for perishable or semiperishable milk products that a few centuries earlier had not had either commercial importance or high culinary reputation.

3

THE RISE OF DRINKING-MILK

I t is hard to establish just when drinking-milk started to take on some aspirational cachet in its own right instead of being casually lumped in with other common uses of milk. The young Swiss physician and diarist Thomas Platter, who disembarked at Dover on a visit to England in 1599, noted that as he and his brother traveled along a much-used route through Canterbury and Sittingbourne to Rochester, "in various places we were given nothing but milk to drink in tankards instead of beer," presumably at inns and taverns where they stopped.[1] The implication is that it was offered as a bracing and enjoyable quaff, or to use a word then coming into currency, "refreshment."

Cream (which did not appear in cookbooks before the tail end of the Middle Ages) also acquired new prestige in the sixteenth and seventeenth centuries, as did "sweet" or "fresh" butter (as distinguished from long-stored, heavily salted butter). They and fresh milk were still intrinsically linked with the countryside, and getting them from country to city was either chancy or impossible. But even as London solidified into an ever-larger, denser metropolis, one solution to the problem of burgeoning urban demand materialized—that is, for the upper echelons.

The great city still contained a number of royal "parks." These were sizable expanses of partly wooded ground that earlier monarchs—chiefly

Henry VIII—had set aside specifically to allow more scope for the royal pastime of deer-hunting within convenient reach of their London palaces. The public was granted some access to Hyde Park, one of the largest of these hunting-grounds, under King James I. It seems to have been a familiar playground for diversion-seekers for some years when Charles I completely opened it to visitors in 1637.

Seizing the moment, the playwright James Shirley revived his five-year-old comedy *Hyde Park*, which choreographed several romantic entanglements against a raucous background of sporting events in the park. Act IV has a milkmaid, amid the excitement of an offstage horse race, fetching one of the female leads a treat from "the Lodge." Formerly occupied by a royal gamekeeper, this building was now a refreshment stand for the rich and fashionable. The delicacy in question is a bowl of "syllabub," which at the time usually meant a drink made by combining milk with a sweetened and flavored wine or cider mixture. The finest effect, obviously not practical in city households, was thought to come from directly milking the cow into a bowl containing the other ingredients. One character in *Hyde Park* wants to know if the milk is good and is told that it's "of a red cow,"[2] a recommendation that makes sense in the light of the agricultural writer Gervase Markham's opinion (in *Cheape and Good Husbandry*, 1614), "The red Cow giueth the best milk."[3] This scene is early proof that by about 1630 a stretch of the park adjoining the Keeper's Lodge had been turned into urban pasture for a herd of cows, and the Lodge into a fashionable showcase for their output.

After the convulsions of the English Civil War, the Keeper's Lodge was again going strong by the 1660s, when celebrity-worshipers like Samuel Pepys clearly regarded it as a place to see and be seen during the months favorable to both fresh milk and open-air recreation. Among the chief refreshments were syllabubs and "cheesecakes," the name for a family of tarts featuring fresh curds baked in pastry with various combinations of sugar, spices, eggs, and butter, now wildly popular in à-la-mode society. But milk on its own was just as much of an attraction, and one that Pepys repeatedly notes having enjoyed. In April 1669, he writes, "I carried my wife to the Lodge, the first time this year, and there in our coach eat [ate] a cheesecake and drank a tankard of milk."[4]

On other occasions he treated himself to "a cup of milk" or "a cup of new milk." He also frequented an establishment called the Whey-House that had premises in the New Exchange, a Restoration precursor of the modern indoor shopping mall located on the Strand in Westminster.[5] (If Pepys's allusions are anything to go by, a drink of whey at the Whey-House served a function for men of business and fashion not unlike a drink of coffee at one of the early London coffeehouses.) During his lifetime, fresh milk products of all kinds were in their early heyday, partly from a general image of milk as a natural, health-giving food evoking innocent country pleasures.

But curiously enough, there are a few moments where Pepys records the effects of milk or whey as highly unpleasant. One occurred on a July day in 1666 when he "drank a great deale of small beere" before making an excursion with his wife and friends "away into the fields, to take the ayre, as far as beyond *Hackny*," a country town that was later subsumed into London. On the way home an attack of heartburn ("wherewith I have of late been mightily troubled") drove him into "drinking a great deale of milke"; soon he started to "breake abundance of wind behind," and for some reason to think he was coming down with a cold. There followed an awful night: "and so to bed in some pain and in fear of more, which accordingly I met with, for I was in mighty pain all night long of [because of] the winde griping of my belly and making of me shit often and vomit too, which is a thing not usual with me, but this I impute to the milke that I drank after so much beer, but the cold, to my wash-ing my feet the night before."[6] He recorded a lesser mischance in May 1668 after going with a friend to the New Exchange: "and so down to the Whey house and drank some [whey] and eat some curds, which did by and by make my belly ake mightily."[7]

Another unfortunate incident, in May 1667, involved not Pepys but the superior to whom he reported as Secretary of the Navy: Vice Admiral Sir John Mennes, Comptroller of the Navy: "Up, and with Sir W. Batten [William Batten, Surveyor of the Navy] and J. Mennes to St. James, and stopped at Temple Barr for Sir J. Mennes to go into the Devil tavern to shit, he having drunk whey and his belly wrought [become disordered]."[8]

Perhaps Pepys, the admiral, or both had contracted gastroenteritis caused by some milk-borne pathogen. Such illnesses may not have happened every day, but neither they nor much more dangerous contagions spread through unfermented milk can have been nonexistent in seventeenth-century London.

There may be, however, another plausible explanation. Most English people, like most Northwest Europeans, could consume fresh milk or derivatives like unsoured curds and whey with no digestive aftereffects. But as noted above, the genetic trait that would later be called lactose tolerance or adult lactase persistence was not always inherited in a complete, unalloyed manner. Even in populations where a large majority of people had no trouble drinking any amount of "sweet" (unsoured) milk or whey, traces remained of the ancestral condition— shared by all mammals except humans—that had stopped the first Neolithic dairyists from consuming milk in unprocessed forms. The result would be colicky diarrhea and sometimes nausea. Already in the seventeenth century medical observers were aware that milk seemed to disagree with some digestions. Today students of the lactose question recognize that in places like Great Britain and the United States, intolerance and tolerance are often a matter of degree. Some people wouldn't be bothered by drinking a gallon a day; others may have varying limitations of tolerance.

The most noticeable effect is looseness of the bowels, or frank diarrhea, accompanied by abdominal cramps and sometimes vomiting. People with incomplete tolerance (which must have occurred more often than complete intolerance) might suffer much distress by gulping large amounts of fresh milk in haste, though there is no telling whether that was actually the cause of Pepys's misery after the visit to Hackney. The effects of unfermented whey are more intense because it contains proportionally much more lactose. In fact, during Pepys's lifetime and for more than a century afterward, doctors often recommended whey as a useful laxative less drastic than the mineral or vegetable cathartics then prescribed for a large grab bag of ailments. Both Sir John Mennes and Pepys clearly viewed the admiral's dose of whey and urgent need of a tavern privy as a simple case of cause and effect. Their peers well might have thought the same of the bellyache that Pepys himself developed after a visit to the Whey-house.

The occasional digestive contretemps notwithstanding, a vogue for milk and fresh dairy products took an even stronger turn in eighteenth-century England and France, with an upper-crust (and sometimes royal) fan club leading the way. Some high-ranking personages—Marie Antoinette being the best-known—went so far as to set up their own elegantly appointed dairies, complete with live maids a-milking and airy, sparkling-clean marble and tile interiors. In England, dozens of noble families with country estates built what were known as "ornamental dairies" or "pleasure dairies" in which the lady of the house and her children could enjoy the result of a working herd's lactation, and a working staff's labor, in all its innocent ivory goodness. Meanwhile, the Hyde Park Keeper's Lodge and another dairy in St. James's Park continued to bring fresh milk to well-off Londoners.

Scattered attempts to make milking more independent of seasonal limitations were another ongoing development. For several centuries, few farmers would be able to dream of an uninterrupted twelve-month supply of livestock fodder. But improved hay-meadow management augured improved strategies for overwintering livestock, at least on large and prosperous estates. Dairy herders had long recognized that unlike sheep and most goats, cows not infrequently had out-of-season pregnancies and lactations. This flexibility couldn't be exploited by everybody, but had started to be noted by agricultural writers. Though no prophet yet envisioned either seamless year-round dairy production independent of the seasons or unfermented drinking-milk as its primary raison d'être, it was becoming possible to glimpse advantages in staggered breeding schedules.

Drinking-milk had now acquired an association with privileged reproductions of country pleasures that soon would disappear from quasi-pastoral urban playgrounds and dwindle in actual rural landscapes. What it had not yet acquired was a medical rationale for becoming a nutritional mainstay unquestioningly revered across all strata of society.

Broad acceptance of medical rationales does not necessarily depend on hard evidence, logical argument, or employment of what is commonly called the scientific method. A much more important trigger is a charismatic, highly visible advocate. And a striking member of the breed appeared in Great Britain at a pivotal moment.

THE APOSTLE OF MILK-DRINKING

One winter day in 1707 or 1708, an English clergyman happened to fall into conversation with a thirty-something physician who looked as if he himself needed medical help in the worst possible way. Dr. George Cheyne (1671?–1743) had left his native Aberdeenshire in 1701 to establish a London practice. Big, fleshy, talkative, gregarious, and fun-loving, he had thought to pursue a useful professional networking strategy by joining a set of "Free-Livers" given to frequent binges in taverns or at each other's amply stocked supper tables. But after a few years of happy indulgence Cheyne (pronounced "Cheney") had found himself blindsided by physical and psychological torments that he could not seem to shake off.

A confused barrage of symptoms gradually climaxed in "a constant violent *Head-ach, Giddiness, Lowness, Anxiety* and *Terror,* so that I went about like a *Malefactor* condemn'd, or one who expected every Moment to be crushed by a *ponderous* Instrument of Death, hanging over his Head."[9] He had spent several years seeking spiritual and medical deliverance when the sympathetic clergyman (whose name Cheyne doesn't record) chanced to mention "a wonderful Cure, which Dr. *Taylor* of *Croydon* had wrought on himself in an *Epileptick Case,* by a total *Milk Diet.*"

At once Cheyne recalled that some leading authorities of the last century had testified to milk's fighting powers against intractable diseases. Resolving "to advise with Dr. *Taylor* personally," he set out on the wintry roads to Croydon, at that time a market town just southwest of London. "I found him at home, with his full Quart of Cow's Milk (which was all his dinner)."[10]

Taylor, the "Milk Doctor of Croydon," was helpful and forthcoming. His own epileptic seizures, he said, had been constant and—on some terrifying occasions when he toppled unconscious from his horse into the road while making the rounds of his country practice—life-threatening. But taking clues from the works of an illustrious medical predecessor, he had found a path back to health by progressively eliminating everything but fresh milk from his diet. He had been free of seizures for seventeen years and had cured many patients of "inveterate Distempers" through the same system.

Cheyne was fascinated. With the details of Taylor's recovery fresh in mind, he eagerly went back to London to quaff milk in copious amounts and rescue his foundering practice. Since he tended toward morbid obesity as well as morbid imaginings and managed always to be his own worst patient, he did not achieve a complete and lasting return to health. But he produced something a great deal more remarkable: one of modern England's first celebrity diets. In London and his later base of operations, Bath, the enormous and witty transplanted Scot cut a memorable figure among swarms of physicians aggressively competing for the patronage of the rich and famous. Milk would assist his path to fame.

The kindly Dr. Taylor's inspiration had been Thomas Sydenham (1624–1689), the most revered English medical authority of the late seventeenth century. His celebrated Latin treatise on gout had pointed to "galacto-pousia"—printed in Greek letters, and meaning a strict milk-drinking regimen—as a powerful remedy. Sydenham, however, had couched that recommendation in decidedly cautious terms. Far from decreeing that all gouty patients should commit to a permanent course of nothing but milk, he had warned his readers that the diet was not for everybody, since any deviation from the strait and narrow throughout the patient's life would bring on a ghastly relapse.[11] Cheyne, the unabashed product of a more publicity-conscious age, wrote in English rather than Latin and was less interested in addressing fellow physicians than a coterie of the London and Bath elite. He began making himself into an expert on "nervous complaints," a cluster of newly fashionable ailments seldom diagnosed among the lower orders.

The aspiring medical superstar could not insist that all his patients live on milk alone, but it was often the central element in the diets he worked out for individual cases. This emphasis was partly tied to a strain of Christian thought that abhorred killing fellow creatures for food and that had caused Cheyne to give up meat and alcohol during some of his personal mind-body crises. His medical opinions were closely bound up with strong religious convictions that became palatable to his patients because he was also voluble, funny, and charming. Frankly counting himself among the number of sufferers from overstrained nerves, he had the gift of making fellow victims feel that he spoke from firsthand experience of their distress.

The diets that Cheyne devised for nervously afflicted patients rarely went as far as Taylor's exclusive reliance on milk. Instead, they often verged on what we now might call lacto-vegetarianism. Though he knew better than to flout majority medical opinion by openly calling for a strict vegetarian regimen, he firmly steered many people to an approach that in his scheme of things spared the nerves by placing as little strain as possible on the digestion. His favorite regimen in advanced cases of nerves concentrated on large daily doses of fresh milk discreetly supplemented with "seeds" (grain-based foods like bread and porridge), certain "light" garden vegetables, and—for people free of alarming symptoms— possibly a few "light" meats.

Lightness was to be measured by both color and age. Pale, tender new vegetables, for instance, had a less unwholesome influence than overgrown, showily pigmented specimens. Big joints of beef or mutton were more taxing to the digestion than young chicken or veal. Everything should be prepared with the least possible culinary folderol, since pungent seasonings and elaborate mélanges of ingredients ("mixed" dishes) ruined pure foods and were dangerously stimulating to disordered nerves.

By all such criteria, new milk—meaning that drawn from the cow a few hours or minutes earlier—clearly surpassed any other everyday substance except water, another polestar in Cheynean diets. What food could be more calming to the nerves than milk, or freer from guileful human interference? For polite English society during Cheyne's career, nothing more convincingly proclaimed its lightness and innocence at first glance and first taste. All circumstances seemed to confirm that the more new milk you drank, the shorter would be the path to glowing health.

Cheyne summoned contemporary biochemical theories to prove the efficacy of his favorite food. The milk of animals like cows, he explained, was essentially *"Vegetables* immediately cook'd by *Animal Heat* and *Organs"*—i.e., plant substances metabolized in the creatures' digestive and mammary systems—and "the lightest and best of all Foods, being a *Medium* between *animal* Substances and *Vegetables*."[12] In one of his last works, he would ask readers to imagine milk as "white Blood already made, adjusted to all the *Meanders* of *Circulation,* and prepar'd by the Hand of Nature" as a divinely intended panacea.[13] The lacto-vegetarian regimen that he liked to urge on the nervously afflicted was also tinged with quasi-religious hints about establishing something like the happy fellowship of beasts and humans in the lost Eden or the millennial Peaceable Kingdom.

There was just one thing wrong with Dr. Cheyne's white wonder food: it made some patients sicker.

No one in Augustan England was systematically collecting and analyzing numerical data about adverse reactions to food or medicine. But contemporary discussions of milk for therapeutic purposes seldom failed to mention that here and there, patients reported unpleasant effects from the recommended doses. For some, new milk was too unpalatable to get down and keep down. It gave others such painful colic or diarrhea that they had had to give up the miracle cure.

The problem wasn't a complete surprise. Earlier physicians who prescribed a milk-only diet for gout and some other chronic conditions had at times encountered complaints about nausea, stomach cramps, flatulence, and loose stools. Reaching for logical reasons, the medical profession at large had concluded that any setbacks should be blamed on the patient, not the milk.

At the time, scientific tools for disputing this verdict could not be imagined. It seemed impossible that fresh, pure cow's milk could upset sound constitutions. To all appearances, it was *made* to be naturally, easily digested by tender infants of any species; failure to tolerate it showed the sufferer's system to be chronically disordered from unwise eating and drinking. As Cheyne would explain in *The Natural Method of Curing the Diseases of the Body, and the Disorders of the Mind,* the digestive distress that milk seemed to provoke in some people "entirely proceeds from the ill state of the *Stomach* and *Bowels*, that by a Distemper are loaded with *Wind, Choler* and *Phlegm* . . . and not from the Nature of *Milk*, which is the mildest, softest, most nourishing, and salutary of all Foods."[14] He insisted that by repeated tries with the aid of a well-stocked medicine chest, virtually anybody could overcome initial bad reactions and reap full benefits from the gentle panacea.

Cheyne died in 1743 at seventy-one or seventy-two, disdained by some medical colleagues as a peddler of dietary gimmicks but sincerely mourned by a large circle of patients. None felt his loss more deeply than the printer-turned-novelist Samuel Richardson, who had actually written *Pamela* while under his care. As a private memorial of their friendship, he had his beloved physician's letters to him copied in a fair hand along with a smattering of other documents and bound in a small volume now in the Edinburgh University Library. One entry is an anonymous poetic tribute in both Latin and English versions that imagines Cheyne arriving in the sector of the afterlife best suited to his genius:

> Open thy shining Gates, thou Milky Way!
> And to thy Stars a kindred Star convey.

The benevolent healer's steadfastness in the spare routines he prescribed to others is admiringly noted:

> This his sole Precept—*On a little live*
> And follow'd what he did so justly give.

The unnamed poet (we do not know whether it was Richardson himself) went on to praise the departed for two godly habits:

> For, while on earth, from Carnage and from Wine
> Abstaining, he on harmless Milk would dine.[15]

The historian Deborah Valenze has pointed out that Cheyne's ideas of simple, virtuous eating were destined to reverberate far beyond his own fashionable practice. They also traveled thousands of miles beyond Great Britain, thanks to the fact that at one time Cheyne's patients included at least four seminal figures in the forging of Methodism, a creed then emerging from the spiritual struggles of evangelical revivalists disillusioned with existing Anglican forms of worship.[16]

The milk diet as such never put down deep roots in Methodism. But John Wesley himself rejoiced to find the general outlines of an innocent, natural, frugal dietary creed being praised by one of the age's most sought-after authorities as both godly and therapeutic. He singled out Cheyne as a profound influence in his own health guide *Primitive Physick*, first published in 1747 and eagerly read by newly convinced revivalists in the English-speaking American colonies.[17] (Milk diets make only a few brief appearances.) The celebrity diet created by Cheyne faded from memory, but meanwhile it had helped to confer up-to-date scientific validation on some eighteenth- and nineteenth-century convictions about morally praiseworthy diets.

With or without knowing it, Cheyne had come along just in time to help infuse lasting energy into the concept of an Edenic, blameless diet— but for a purpose that he had paid little if any attention to. The next generation of medical experts was developing emphatic doctrines about cow's milk as nature's innocent, ideally designed provision for children.

A belief in the moral dimensions of "natural" diet fitted remarkably well with new ways of thinking about childhood that had sprung up in the late eighteenth century. England proved especially welcoming to ideas that Jean-Jacques Rousseau's semi-novelized treatise *Émile* (1763) had set in motion throughout Western Europe. As the British social historian J. H. Plumb astutely observed, the growing tendency of upper- and middle-class families to treat little ones as repositories of human potential asking to be developed through loving encouragement opened up important moneymaking avenues. It effectually made children into "a trade, a field of commercial enterprise for the sharp-eyed entrepreneur."[18] Food and medicine do not figure in Plumb's survey of consumer goods and services aimed at the burgeoning parental market. But they deserve to be examined as part of what he calls "the new world of children."

The early Romantic cult of the little child fresh from "the glory and the dream" of its heavenly home beautifully paralleled the medical-moral reputation of new milk fresh from the dairy. Each was the very image of purity and naturalness in a radiantly unspoiled state, and each could be profitably exploited through products and services targeted to caring parents. The services included the branch of medicine now called pediatrics. From the late eighteenth century on, specialists in treating childhood diseases increasingly stressed the importance of George Cheyne's wonder food, though in a context he may not have foreseen. It acquired and never has lost a uniquely exalted status as a life-giving proxy for mother's milk, a concept not closely related to any nutritional reality.

How much direct inspiration did the child-care specialists who began emerging in the "long" eighteenth century (roughly 1675 to 1825) draw from Cheyne's paeans to the all but heavenly purity of drinking-milk fresh from the cow? We can never have clear-cut answers to such a question. But it would have been impossible for the precursors of pediatrics to have been unaware of the milk-diet vogue popularized by Cheyne and his celebrity patients, as well as his arguments about milk's calming and restorative effects on delicate systems.

The child-care pioneers were soon busy laying down the law to parents about proper and improper foods. Inveighing against addiction to "high diets" or alcohol by breastfeeding women (nursing mothers and wet nurses alike), they also sought to banish ignorant and unprofessional female advisers. Over time, respectable people learned to assume that the only party qualified to tell lactating women what to eat, and later to supervise the transition from breast milk to other foods, was a licensed physician with modern science on his side.

By the 1790s a general professional agreement was evolving about the unique virtues of fresh cow's milk as a dietary mainstay of children from weaning through adolescence. By degrees, this consensus hardened into a nutritional dogma with few precedents. Using dairy animals' milk as a handy interim food for small children during weaning was not a new practice. But glorifying cow's milk as a superfood to be poured into juvenile bodies for years on end was one of those unaccountable aberrations that can, and in this case did, take on a life of their own. Eminent physicians who treated children offered much muddled advice on the issue in the name of science. As their budding discipline developed into one of the great branches of medicine in the British Isles and North America, it became more set in a belief that all children from weaning to puberty urgently needed to drink fresh cow's milk in copious amounts, and that it was also an incomparably healthful food for all adults.

This idea was probably one of the biggest mistakes in the history of modern nutrition, and certainly one of the most tenacious. On both sides of the Atlantic, one of its first and worst effects was to pump great profit incentives into a dawning commercial milk trade long before any means existed of publicly enforcing precautions against food-borne diseases (or indeed, of grasping how they could be transmitted). The explosive growth of both demand and supply spurred by the medical profession's endorsement of drinking-milk as the chief bulwark of child nutrition unfortunately went hand in hand with the spread of milk-borne contagions.

Medical insistence on the imperative duty of getting drinking-milk into every child would keep intensifying decade by decade, along with rapid urbanization or de-ruralization of the nations where adult lactase persistence was (unknown to anybody) a majority genetic condition. The resulting increase in the demand for fresh unfermented cow's milk among city families would expose its extraordinary talent for harboring the seeds of disease—not a completely unsuspected circumstance, but one that some privileged earlier milk-drinkers had been able to side-step. Pepys, in the late 1660s, had enjoyed the new milk of cows raised and milked in Hyde Park. Cheyne, on taking up his milk cure about forty years later, had not only drunk "*Cow-Milk* from the *Park*" but also "engag'd a Milk Woman, at a higher than ordinary price, to bring me every Day as much pure and unmix'd as might be sufficient for *Dinner* and *Breakfast*."[19] Both had had the means to pay for something as close as possible to milk on the hoof, not milk transported miles from the source and funneled through the hands of middlemen.

The rush to embrace unsoured drinking-milk would have proceeded more cautiously if early enthusiasts had thought seriously about the hindrances to moving large amounts of milk from cows to consumers in reliably fresh condition while the gap between city and country continued to widen. And it could never have been as unhesitating if child-care specialists had been in a position to understand that acidity could inhibit the growth of some pathogens.

THE ACID TEST

Unfortunately, scientific beliefs about the nature of acids were highly unsettled. The seventeenth-century pioneers of post-alchemy chemistry had made some headway in formulating distinctions between acids and bases; the crucial issues would come into sharper focus when later investigators like Antoine Lavoisier, Joseph Priestley, and Humphrey Davy studied the properties of hydrogen and oxygen. But leading-edge science had as much difficulty being translated into laypersons' language in the seventeenth and eighteenth centuries as Einstein's general theory of relativity in 1920. Scientific popularizers, and even stars of the medical profession, could only guess what really happened when a base was chemically converted into an acid. Should the process be understood as "fermentation," "corruption," and/or "putrefaction?" How seriously did the results endanger human health?

In 1689, during the first emergence of child care as a medical specialty, a prominent authority named Walter Harris had pronounced that children's delicate systems were inherently more acidic than those of adults, and that excess acidity was the root cause of all childhood diseases.[20] This dictum would have great staying power. William Cadogan's *An Essay upon Nursing* (1748), dealing with the management of children from birth to age three, reminded readers that "the first and general Cause of the Diseases that Infants are liable to is the acid Corruption of their Food."[21] What Cadogan had in mind was a prevalent theory that vegetable substances, much more heavily represented than meats in generally approved children's diets, tended to decompose into acid in the stomach while meat remained more alkaline. But advice-givers went on citing his remark about "acid corruption" for several generations, long after physiologists had pointed out that the stomach itself produced massive amounts of hydrochloric acid.

Negative associations with acidity meanwhile circulated widely. The celebrated American physician and scientific popularizer Samuel Latham Mitchill had decided that alkalis formed a heroic chemical shield against a deadly septic process through which "redundant acidity . . . otherwise would prevail and destroy the balance of powers in the natural world."[22] The interactions between acids and alkalis were familiar enough to English laypeople to furnish an offhand metaphor in Walter Scott's *The Heart of Mid-Lothian* (1818): when his Scottish heroine, the tactfully conciliating Jeanie Deans, proves able to keep the peace between her broadminded minister husband and her intolerant arch-Calvinist father, he describes her as "a mediating spirit, who endeavoured, by the alkaline smoothness of her own disposition, to neutralize the acidity of theological controversy."[23]

Milk fermentation could not have escaped being hauled into debates about undesirable acidity. Unsurprisingly, soured milk came under frequent (though never quite universal) suspicion as the drinking-milk trade grew. In 1799 a much-reprinted English translation of the German encyclopedist A. F. M. Willich's highly regarded *Lectures on Diet and Regimen* stated that "*sour milk* is unfit for use, on account of the chemical decomposition which has taken place in its constituent parts, and because it can hardly be digested by the most powerful stomach."[24] The idea that milk should reach tender juvenile systems only while perfectly "sweet" and uncorrupted soon crystallized into medical orthodoxy.

We can easily see why, as the spread of urban milk-borne epidemics accelerated in lockstep with the spread of milk-drinking, equating sourness with dangerous spoilage might have seemed logical. All appearances supported the commonsense idea of measuring milk's purity by freedom from fermentation. In England and North America, health advisers became increasingly committed to the belief that children should be fed great doses of "sweet" drinking-milk and strictly protected from touching sour milk. An occasional nay-sayer protested against such teachings. In 1798 Joseph Clarke, a young physician on the staff of a Dublin lying-in hospital, strongly questioned the Walter Harris doctrine of acidity as the underlying cause of childhood diseases while also casting doubt on opposition to sour milk: "History furnishes examples of whole nations using sour curdled milk as part of their daily food; we cannot suppose that such a practice would be continued if it were often followed by pernicious effects."[25] The Scottish political and agricultural writer Sir John Sinclair squeezed a speculative footnote on the subject into his *Code of Health and Longevity* (1807):

> It is a curious fact, that among the nations with whom milk constitutes a chief part of their diet, it is eaten in a state of acidity. The Tartars always ferment the milk of their mares. The Russians prefer their koumiss, which is reckoned a specific [remedy] for consumptions. The Caffres [Zulus] ferment their milk by keeping it in sheep-skins, which are never cleansed, in order to preserve the substance which ferments it. They expressed the utmost abhorrence on seeing Europeans drink some fresh milk, and said it was very unwholesome. Even among the poor people of Scotland, there is more milk eaten in an ascescent [in the process of souring], than in a fresh state.[26]

No scientific means existed for testing the validity of these remarks. Anyone who expressed reservations about the supreme virtues of fresh drinking-milk had as much chance of stemming the unstoppable tide of its rising commercial prospects as King Canute. If the nature of lactic acid fermentation had been deducible in the lifetimes of Clarke and Sinclair, the very concept of "pure" milk would have been differently framed. So would later arguments for milk pasteurization, starting in the 1880s.

The idea that milk touched by the least acidity was impure, or at least unfit to give to children, gained ground over the nineteenth century and looked like age-old truth to many by 1900. Sour milk and buttermilk had not entirely vanished from British or American kitchens. But they had scant practical value, except as food for hogs. Versions of sour milk or cream remained somewhat more visible in Scandinavia, the Baltic countries, Germany, the Netherlands, and northern France. In the English-speaking world, an old-fashioned taste for sour milk chiefly hung on among country folk in corners of Scotland, Ireland, and the American South, while the enlightened associations of unsoured drinking-milk steadily brightened along with its commercial prospects. Faith in what was considered pure milk and fear of impure milk would progress on parallel tracks throughout much of the nineteenth century, both in Old World centers of adult lactase persistence and in Great Britain's former North American colonies. The trade, as it *became* a trade, was headed for difficult and often disastrous growing pains.

4

SETTING THE STAGE
FOR PASTEURIZATION

N othing comes into being in a vacuum, and pasteurized milk was no exception. Its arrival depended on a long chain of other events that overtook all industrialized Western countries between the first and last years of the nineteenth century. Setting aside the swift march of science and technology, the most crucial shift was in *how societies viewed the role of government.*

At the national level, policy-setters began to treat food production as a vital underpinning of not just prosperity but power: an economic force to be purposefully steered and overseen along with food transportation and distribution. At the municipal level, lethal epidemics bred by unchecked urban growth helped to create an unprecedented sense that public health was the business of the entire community and that very young children—more disastrously affected than anyone else—were the members who deserved to be cared for first. In both cases, private interests had made scattered attempts to grapple with the issues before mid-century. But it took several generations for any kind of authority-wielding bureaucracy to materialize and compellingly address either farming or citizens' health. The most dramatic changes set in at around 1880, when would-be improvers of the status quo suddenly received reinforcement from diverse sources—among others, manufacturers pursuing advanced farm technologies, scientists bent on understanding microbes or the chemical makeup of food, medical educators determined to make infant and child care their top priority, and a widespread drive toward professionalization of all callings.

The pace at which knowledge could be swapped among interested parties increased sensationally once government agencies were creating or underwriting research initiatives. Opportunities for gathering and publishing specialized information expanded swiftly in all northwestern European countries. The French nation hailed (and remunerated) Louis Pasteur for having preserved such contributions to French greatness as winemaking, sheep farming, and the silk industry. Robert Koch was scarcely less honored in Germany. American emulators at first found little interest at major centers of learning. But they hoped to catch up soon in various fields of applied science, even as the United States raced ahead of everybody else as shaper of news and publicity.

This was the context in which cow's milk production, distribution, and consumption were being discussed when people on two continents began thinking about applying Pasteur's 1850s and 1860s heat treatment breakthroughs to milk. (Pasteur himself never experimented with what later came to be called milk pasteurization.) It was less than a century since prosperous parents had been told that paying whatever it took for the best new milk straight from the cow was the surest guarantee of a child's well-being. But as far as scientific and cultural attitudes were concerned, it might as well have been light-years. To understand how the first attempts at milk pasteurization came about, we must trace some shifting attitudes throughout the intervening decades. The path begins with cutting-edge practitioners plugging fresh drinking-milk as the latest panacea for well-born toddlers, and ends with a universal chorus of medical experts insisting that it was a permanent rock-bottom necessity for *all* children—especially the increasing numbers of new babies who, for reasons still debated by social historians, were not being breastfed.

MILK, CITIES, AND ILL-GOTTEN GAINS

After about 1800, the custom of using fresh unfermented cow's milk as the foundation of privileged children's diets began trickling down the social ladder—unfortunately, just as the terms on which an English or

North American dairy cow could earn her keep were being pitilessly rearranged. Grazing for cows on swathes of open ground within cities, a reality in George Cheyne's day as it had been in Pepys's, was being swallowed up by dense new tracts of housing. Exploiters rushed in to plant a new crop of city dairies close to crowded neighborhoods. Their strategy was to cram as many cows as possible into dank, unventilated sheds, feed the miserable animals any cut-rate substitute for grass, and pitch their output to urban families attracted by the new medical cachet of fresh drinking-milk. Though bad enough in London, such practices were soon taken to even worse extremes across the Atlantic in the former British colonies—most notoriously New York City, where the use of distillery wastes to feed cows was especially successful.

As pointed out in chapter 3, the milk that city consumers were in good faith lining up to buy for the sake of children's health—full-lactose drinking-milk, fresh from the cow—was both more welcoming to dangerous pathogens, and more upsetting to many people's stomachs, than any other form in which people had previously used milk. At the time, not even the wisest could have surmised that "sweet" milk was a better vector than soured milk for plague-carrying bacteria and that a great many people were genetically unfitted to digest it.

But there was no stopping the rush of what most experts considered progress, or the accompanying rise in child mortality fueled by milk-borne contagions. By the 1840s, the drinking-milk situation had become dire enough in London to provoke public alarm. It was still more appalling in New York City (that is, Manhattan) and Brooklyn, where enormous dairies mired in filth turned the dregs from next-door breweries or whiskey distilleries into the sole, unvaried diet of cows penned in tiny stalls.

It is at this juncture that histories of the milk industry routinely relate how dedicated public health pioneers and brilliant scientists came to the rescue by first working to shut down the perpetrators and later applying the resources of modern microbiology, refrigeration, and sanitation to ensure that drinking-milk could reach every child in safe condition. That version of the story is accurate as far as it goes. But it fails to recognize that the medical champions of milk-drinking had themselves triggered the emergency by creating an unprecedented demand, thus making a dangerously fragile form of milk into a cash cow too good for greedy opportunists not to exploit by cutting every possible corner.

By the early nineteenth century, the inexorable divide that had been opening up since the Middle Ages between the places where food was produced and consumed threatened to outrun available technological stopgaps. Butter and hard cheese, until then considered the surest bets for any farmer who raised cows, were relatively imperishable and could easily be carried from the countryside to the urban public markets. Fresh milk, however, was more disastrously affected than any other common food during the rapid growth of cities. The notion that children after weaning desperately needed it shot to the status of self-evident truth at breakneck speed, miraculously bypassing any attempt to weigh the idea as a theory to be proved or disproved. But the more rapidly demand increased, the greater became the difficulty of supplying it to city-dwellers without the awful stratagems of the mushrooming new urban dairies.

In the late 1830s the New York philanthropist and temperance advocate Robert Milham Hartley, a reform-minded Protestant chiefly known for exhorting the poor to lift themselves out of the gutter through teetotalism and other moral efforts, turned his attention to this horror story. He began writing exposés of the polluted city milk supply for newspapers and magazines. When the flickers of public interest that he had awakened petered out, he fiercely devoted himself to a book on the still-raging emergency. His *Historical, Scientific and Practical Essay on Milk as an Article of Human Sustenance*, published in 1842, may have been the most masterfully framed and executed tour de force of research and political advocacy ever produced on the subject for a lay audience.

The scope of Hartley's coverage is phenomenal. He spared no effort in setting forth the broadest possible framework for understanding fresh, clean cow's milk as the highest of the Creator's edible gifts. He examined milk in regard to the divine order of creation, prehistoric and Old Testament civilizations, and modern chemical knowledge before launching into a no-holds-barred account of the stranglehold that modern "slop dairies" had acquired on the urban milk supply, in defiance of plain reason:

> The manner of producing milk to supply the inhabitants of cities and other populous places, is so contrary to our knowledge of the laws which govern the animal economy, that from a bare statement of the facts, an intelligent mind might confidently anticipate the evils which actually result from it.[1]

His attention to detail extended to illustrating the anatomy of a healthy ruminant digestive system, the better to explain how lethally a grass-deprived diet of distillery leftovers wrecked the constitutions of animals subjected to it:

> They sometimes lose their feet at the navicular bones, or articulation of the first joint; their hoofs often become elongated several inches and curved upwards, and withal so tender as to produce lameness, and nearly deprive them of the power of locomotion.[2]

Hartley pointed to the unjust state of laws that at the time afforded the public some protection against the sale of diseased meat while allowing free rein to sellers of diseased milk.[3] He hurled deserved fury at the criminal insanity that allowed alcoholic poisoning of lactating cows to be reprised in children who drank the maltreated creatures' milk. He cited the confirming testimony of a former medical professor at the University of New York (the earlier name of New York University) who reported that distillery wastes passed into the animals' milk "with such rapidity, that we can smell and taste the identical slop still reeking, and fermenting from the infernal distillery; but in general, it is so colored, mixed, medicated and prepared, that it is well calculated to deceive the unsuspecting observer."[4]

Anyone venturing today on an historical survey of milk for a general readership must be awed by the clear-headed penetration with which Hartley identified and examined every aspect of the subject that a man with no understanding of either microbiology or lactose tolerance could conceivably have addressed. The chief remedy he proposed seemed to make eminent sense: opening up opportunities for suppliers of clean milk from healthy cows on real farms through the new blessings of rail and steamboat transportation between New York City and the countryside.

"Why should you not engage in this branch of business?" he asked farmers whose milk currently went into other dairy products. After all, sending pure milk to cities enjoyed every "pecuniary inducement" over the traditional uses: "The conversion of your milk into butter or cheese, with the loss of the labor of making it, will not pay more than two cents a quart, for which you may realize six cents [i.e., for drinking-milk] in these cities."[5] Along with fellow opponents of the distillery-milk racket, Hartley saw the prospect that farmers might find the genuinely fresh article *the most profitable form in which they could sell milk* as a moral victory.

He had no reason to question the premises behind thinking that fresh, unblemished milk was milk as intended by God. It was clear to him that he had modern chemical knowledge on his side. "Good milk is slightly *alkaline*," he announced, citing what he considered the up-to-the-minute evidence of litmus paper. His own observations had convinced him that "the alkaline property, in some degree, is essential to healthy milk . . . and is the unfailing characteristic of the fluid secreted by animals that are in healthy condition and properly kept," while the milk of animals kept in unnatural conditions "was as uniformly acid."[6] (It is now understood that even the most carefully manufactured litmus paper cannot accurately measure tiny variations in pH, and that fresh cow's milk as tested by the most sensitive methods is very slightly acid.)

Hartley had pointed to a possible solution of the "slop milk" problem but not one that could instantaneously take effect. A scattering of bona fide dairy farmers in the orbit of major metropolises did start giving up butter and cheese production in order to pursue the lucrative new opportunities of drinking-milk. But distilleries and breweries, affectionately leagued with next-door dairies that would convert waste into cash, had great political clout in Eastern Seaboard cities. Opponents of slop milk were a disorganized jumble of interests rather than a purposeful coalition. When city administrations mounted sanitary initiatives, they were short-term responses to yellow fever or other epidemic contagions that in time would go away and be temporarily forgotten. Any notion that local—much less state or federal—government should create some permanent agency empowered to take arms against a sea of health menaces was still in the formative stages.

The distillery-dairy partnership was too robust to be ended by mere exposés. In 1858, a struggling three-year-old weekly periodical named *Frank Leslie's Illustrated Newspaper* hit pay dirt with a long series of articles on what it called the "swill milk" business in Manhattan and Brooklyn. The first installment appeared on May 8, neatly timed to anticipate annual fears about the June-to-October season when milk-borne illness seemed to take its harshest toll on children. Leslie's well-orchestrated effort, preceded by adroit come-ons placed in other newspapers, promptly attracted advertisements from enterprises claiming that *their* milk was pure. (Two of these were very new manufacturers of something variously known as "concentrated" or "condensed" milk.)[7] The paper's team of crack illustrators captured dozens of swill-dairy scenes with an immediacy as shocking today as it was a hundred sixty years ago, while the reporters amassed enough documentation to trigger demands for prosecution from politicians who hadn't been bought off. Unfortunately, their efforts were easily defeated by kickback artists. Calls for an investigation led to an official whitewash that was universally denounced in the New York press but discouraged meaningful change until the aftermath of the Civil War.

The political grip of city distillers began to weaken during a series of affrays over federal excise taxes on liquor, first introduced as efforts to finance the war but continued afterward, that put many distilleries on the wrong side of the law and hampered their ability to intimidate local authorities. The most shameless excesses of the swill milk era (though not the last vestiges of the practice) faded from the picture by degrees during the 1870s and 1880s. Milk trains had already started appearing in the rural orbit of cities. But the immediate future was still clouded by milk-borne disease, which stubbornly refused to disappear along with the gradual elimination of swill dairies. The chief though yet unrecognized cause was a distribution system based on the retail sale of "loose milk."

The most common route from a farm to a city household began with the farmer, assisted by family members or hired hands, manually milking the cows into buckets, which were emptied into large cans (most often tin-plated forty-quart models sealed with lids or wooden plugs). These were hauled to the nearest railway depot, where they waited for the next milk train in sweltering or freezing weather. Any washing of hands, buckets, cans, lids, or the cow's udder was purely up to the farm personnel. Attempts at ice cooling in hot weather were widespread but not mandatory. (It was a far from negligible expense, since most ice was still seasonally harvested from frozen ponds and kept in insulated storage until the supply ran out rather than mechanically manufactured throughout the year.) Once the milk reached the city, it was usually transferred, in the original cans, to the delivery wagons of milkmen who carted it along routes supplying individual households. Large amounts also went to grocery stores where open cans sat on floors or shelves in the happy company of flies until the last drop had been emptied, when they were sent back to the farm rinsed or unrinsed. In either case, the milk was sold loose—i.e., dipped out of the can into a pitcher or other container belonging to the customer.

Neither farmers nor milkmen were always above eking out a given amount of milk with as much water—not to mention cocktails of other adulterants like plaster of Paris and molasses—as they could get away with. Most large cities had anti-adulteration laws. Some even tried to enforce them once in a while. But the perceived responsibility of city government didn't extend to doing the impossible: preventing milk from sickening or killing anyone. Physicians still lacked the knowledge that milk unprotected by souring and handled in a near-vacuum of hygienic protocols was an ideal breeding ground for pathogens, especially between late spring and early autumn. Every year brought the dreaded return of "summer complaint," marked by severe and often fatal diarrhea, among the very young. Children whose parents could afford to send them to the country before hot weather set in and see that they got plenty of milk straight from a live cow stood a good chance of avoiding summer complaint. The "cow with the iron tail" (water-pump handle) and milk transportation in unwashed vessels finished off many others.

CONCENTRATED ATTENTION

Hartley's assumptions about the benefits of replacing swill milk from city dairying operations with fresh milk from the countryside were not wholly borne out by immediate experience. Some entrepreneurs looked to the solution in preservation technology, which was gaining ground in all parts of industrial Northwest Europe and North America. At the time of the swill milk scandals, inventors everywhere were trying to extend the useful life of perishable foods by boiling them down into concentrates or extracts, or by putting them into hermetically sealed containers.[8] In the case of milk, assorted inventors hit on the bright idea of marrying the two attempts. But neither separately nor in tandem could the first milk preservation experiments become commercially viable without much floundering among unforeseen hazards through lack of bacteriological knowledge.

One of the things that made milk chemically tricky to work with as well as susceptible to dangerous spoilage was the complex role of water, which accounts for about 87 percent by weight of cow's milk. As I have explained in chapter 1, milk is a fat-in-water emulsion and a casein-in-water suspension, while also containing an intricate assortment of water-soluble substances. Simply boiling off the water was found to wreak havoc with the original milk flavors. Evaporation at temperatures well below the boiling point gave somewhat more acceptable results, but it was long, tedious, and sometimes spoilage-prone. The best defense against that problem was to ignore original flavors and add sugar as a preservative.

Various patents for "preserved," "concentrated," or "condensed" milk with sugar existed in 1849 when a middle-aged jack-of-many-trades named Gail Borden, Jr. began applying his restless wits toward inventing a form of preserved meat. Borden was one of the great American eccentrics: a tall, austere-looking scarecrow of a man with a monomaniacal faith in whatever notion he was currently hatching. He was fanatically devoted to a method he had devised for boiling down meat juices to a concentrate that could be worked together with flour and baked into "meat biscuits."[9] Like many kindred inventions of the period, Borden's Meat Biscuit was advertised as particularly suitable for explorers, members of military expeditions, and shipboard crews. While he waited for some scattered plaudits to translate into reliable sales, grand schemes for concentrating every food known to mankind into pill or extract form filled his imagination.

In 1851 Borden set out for the Crystal Palace Great Exhibition in London, hoping to win a medal for his immediate priority, the Meat Biscuit. The refreshment rooms happened to be offering the fruits of another medal-seeker's efforts: the Patent Concentrated Milk of Edward Duke Moore, which could be sampled by itself or in the form of cocoa or drinking-chocolate. Among other upshots of the exhibition, Borden went back to America with a gold Council Medal, while Moore's venture collected a less prestigious Prize Medal as well as an affiliation. The next year the firm of Moore and Buckley—I have been able to learn nothing about the latter—began advertising in various publications including *The Lancet*. Appended to descriptions of its line of concentrated-milk products was the brief claim: "Sole wholesale Agents for Borden's Patent Meat Biscuit, which received the Council Medal at the Great Exhibition."[10]

In his day job, Edward Moore was apothecary and physician to (among others) British royalty. But at his Staffordshire estate, Ranton Abbey, he also pursued a sideline in hopeful inventions. The Scottish writer James Caird, who had been commissioned by the *London Times* in 1850 to conduct a survey of English agriculture in rural counties, had observed the manufacture of the Patent Concentrated Milk. He reported that after four hours of being agitated at 110°F in "a long shallow copper pan" by "persons who walk slowly around the pan, stirring its contents with a flat piece of wood," the concentrate was filled into "small tin cases." The tinned product "supplies fresh milk every morning on board ship, and may be sent all over the world in this portable form."[11]

Later stories of Gail Borden's career left out the Moore connection. The most touching of several tall tales was that during a rough and grueling homeward voyage after the Great Exhibition, he had a humanitarian "Eureka!" moment on seeing babies about to perish because the two cows on board were too seasick to give milk. In fact, he returned to New York still filled with hopes for the Meat Biscuit but also starting to mull over ideas for preserving milk. Within two years he had worked out a modus operandi.

Realizing that any procedure dependent on stirring milk by hand in open vessels was an invitation to contaminating dust or debris, he painstakingly threshed out an alternative approach in which evaporation took place inside an enclosed vacuum chamber before the concentrated milk was filled into hermetically sealed cans. He did not know it, but he had solved or at least partly solved the problem of bacterial contamination from the open air. He also had managed to condense milk without added sugar. His method was a vast improvement over any previous attempt to preserve milk—in fact, a major technological breakthrough. The U.S. Patent Office, however, rejected his 1853 application on the grounds that his process was a mere rehash of earlier inventors' work.[12] Borden had to keep submitting successive applications for three years, doggedly dotting i's and crossing t's about exactly what he was or wasn't claiming as original innovations.

The patent application—which laid great stress on the fact that unlike rival products, the finished concentrate contained no added sugar—was finally approved in August 1856.[13] With that battle won, Borden struggled to gear up for production. It is doubtful that his underfunded effort would have survived for more than a few years if a lucky break had not occurred in 1857: Striking up a conversation with a seatmate on a train, Borden suddenly acquired a well-heeled partner named Jeremiah Milbank who was willing to give him something like carte blanche in building necessary equipment and driving contractual bargains with dairy farmers close to his first headquarters in Wolcottville, Connecticut.[14]

Within a few months the milk, put up in quart-sized cans, was being sold to steamship companies. In November a committee report for the New York Academy of Medicine declared that it offered to the citizens of New York "an article that for purity, durability, and economy, is hitherto unequaled in the annals of the milk trade."[15] The firm, now organized as the New York Condensed Milk Company, was soon ready to begin home deliveries in competition with existing city milkmen. An advertisement in the *Brooklyn Daily Eagle* on April 30, 1858, announced that Borden's Condensed Milk was available for delivery at 25 cents per quart, either in the form of "PURE MILK, from which when PERFECTLY FRESH, nearly all the water has been evaporated, and to which NOTHING is added" or as "Borden's Condensed Milk SUGARED, for Sea use and for long keeping on land." One quart, it was explained, could be diluted with water "until the taste is suited," with a ratio of 1 : 1½ producing the equivalent of two and a half quarts of cream, 1 : 4 five quarts of rich milk. At 6¼ cents a quart after dilution, it was not cheap by comparison with fluid cows' milk from other sources, which probably was between 3 and 5 cents a quart.[16]

By lucky coincidence, *Frank Leslie's Illustrated Newspaper* published the first installment of its sensational swill-milk exposé about a week after the *Daily Eagle* advertisement appeared, triggering a spate of ads by producers touting their own blameless milk. Borden joined the hopefuls with a small ad that appeared in the *Leslie's* issue containing the third installment (May 22). It pointed out that Borden's Condensed Milk was prepared in Litchfield County, Connecticut—far from the filthy horrors being documented on Sixteenth Street—and was free from "the admixture of sugar or some other substance" (the sugared version of the product goes unmentioned). The ad also appealed to economy by suggesting that using more water yielded "7 quarts good milk." But any success generated by this small publicity effort seems to have been modest at best.[17]

The real turnaround occurred several months after the outbreak of the Civil War, when the U.S. Army began placing large orders for the condensed milk. The war may have been the determining factor that led Borden—despite his original aim of patenting a "pure" concentrated product with no additives—to pay extra attention to the sweetened ver-sion. Not only was the preservative effect of sugar a decisive advantage for canned milk meant for use by armies in the field throughout all seasons, but men who wanted both milk and sugar in their coffee found presweetened milk a handy shortcut. Orders from Union quartermas-ters outstripped supply so fast that Borden could meet the demand only by opening more condenseries and licensing other manufacturers to produce milk by his patented process. A scattering of independent startups briefly got into the business, but the New York Condensed Milk Company ended the war with a commanding grip on the national con-densed milk market and survived to expand operations into the Mid-west before the founder's death in 1874. Ever the perfectionist, Borden kept fine-tuning his process with small (and duly patented) improve-ments. He did not live to see unsweetened canned milk undergo further refinements from other inventors during the 1880s and find a durable place beside his sugared version as "evaporated milk."

Gail Borden was an entirely self-taught engineer with no book learn-ing in chemistry, physics, or biology. When he started working with milk, he cannot ever have heard of a microbe. In 1871, the great Amer-ican dairy industry expert Xerxes A. Willard could only hazily relate a "theory" that some strange "fungi" had the power to spoil milk. But almost from the start, Borden had grasped that the condensing process magnified even the tiniest defect in the original milk—for instance, a speck of dirt from the farmyard or the cow's udder—so powerfully as to give the final product a nasty smell and taste. As he built his supply network of neighboring dairy farmers, he became increasingly fanati-cal about having each one agree to strict standards of animal care and milk handling. He ended up with a list of fifteen ironclad rules that he passed on to Willard, ranging from cleanliness in milking the cow and rapid cooling of the milk below a certain temperature to the cleansing of milk cans, pail, and strainers.[18] As my account of a slightly later model dairy will show, this kind of respect for sanitary precautions was in some respects a throwback to earlier practices that had been observed for cen-turies by diligent women dairyists on small mixed farms, and that long predated any knowledge of microbiology.

THE EXPANDING MANDATES
OF GOVERNMENT

An era of clean, safe non-preserved drinking-milk for everybody was on the horizon, though for at least another generation cleanliness and safety would most often be gauged by how much money retail custom-ers were able or willing to shell out for unregulated purchases. The idea that these blessings should be guaranteed by some elected or appointed authority didn't instantly win the hearts and minds of voters—certainly not American voters. Political will to enforce such notions slowly gath-ered before the mid-nineteenth century, but failed to reach a tipping point until three separate factors converged between about 1880 and 1890 to shake up relationships among federal, state, and city mandates. They were agricultural policy, the new sciences of food chemistry and microbiology, and public health initiatives.

The late eighteenth century saw a flurry of attempts to "improve" plants, livestock, and soils in all parts of northwestern Europe through new cultivation, breeding, and fertilizing practices. In the first years of independence, leading American farmers eagerly sought to build on progressive methods that had been spearheaded in Great Britain. (Washington and Jefferson, the prime Virginia examples, had the advantage of large slave crews to carry out their innovative plans.) Agricultural and horticultural societies appeared in all states, striving to spread useful information through regular meetings and ambitious journals. "Experiment" and "experimental" were among their favor-ite watchwords. Some wanted the federal government to take a role in promoting agricultural improvement, with a view to international commerce. But purposeful consideration of America's unprecedented challenges as a food-producing nation did not immediately materialize in Congress or the White House.

Regional boosters and the American version of rural gentry could encourage various aspects of agricultural progress. They could not yet formulate national policies matched to the stunning diversity of U.S. cli-mates and topographies as westward-racing frontiers brought new states into the Union. But when the divisions between free and slave states erupted into war, Congress and the Lincoln administration devoted serious thought to the nation's food supply. Perhaps the most famous result was the 1862 Pacific Railroad Act, meant to create a strategic coast-to-coast rail link for vital supplies including food. In the same year, Lincoln signed into law a bill establishing a U.S. Department of Agriculture and another, introduced by Representative Justin Morrill of Vermont, allocating substantial land grants to each non-seceding state while requiring it to found at least one agricultural college.[19]

The last two measures did not at once seem to be of earth-shaking concern. The mission of the state land grants and colleges that the Morrill Act was supposed to establish was foggily defined as "the Benefit of Agriculture and Mechanic Arts." The Agriculture Department was not considered important enough to warrant cabinet status, and was headed by a commissioner rather than a secretary. Its mandate as stated in the 1862 act was "to acquire and to diffuse among the people of the United States useful information on subjects connected with agriculture" and to "procure, propagate, and distribute among the people new and valuable seeds and plants." Animal husbandry went unmentioned—an easily remedied omission, since nobody had any trouble automatically lumping meat and milk production under "agriculture." Though by now drinking-milk had assumed great importance in children's diets, policy-setters had not yet started treating its producers and distributors as major contributors to the American agricultural economy. They were more occupied with makers of the sturdier (and exportable) products cheese and butter, which now were being displaced from the custody of farm wives and transferred to the commercial realm.

Far from eager to welcome troops of new Washington pencil-pushers, the existing community of agricultural advocates generally belittled Isaac Newton, the first USDA commissioner. Newton, a Pennsylvania dairy farmer who at one time had had an "ice cream and confectionery saloon" in Philadelphia making the most of his own milk and cream, nonetheless set to work with a will. Soon the department was putting together an agricultural library and museum, collecting meteorological data, compiling production statistics for major crops, and investigating sugar beets as a replacement for Southern-grown cane sugar. At the war's end it launched its own thirty-five-acre agricultural experiment farm for several thousand different plant cultivars on what is now the National Mall, close to the present USDA Farmers Market.[20]

REIMAGINING THE UPSCALE FARM

The infant USDA initially lacked the funding, staffing, or prestige to transform American food production. And as far as drinking-milk production was concerned, the ball remained decidedly in the court of private entrepreneurs addressing chosen clienteles, not government authorities trying to formulate large communal goals. Well-heeled farmers were still pursuing something like the prewar progressive agenda, though now aided by improved scientific understanding and statistical methods. An agricultural press led by the prolific publisher Orange Judd continued to champion these often lucrative efforts. *Farm Echoes*, a book issued by Judd in 1883, affords lively insights into an elite niche of the dairying scene in the first postwar decades, when most American dairy farmers were still concentrating on butter and cheese.[21]

The modest, attractively illustrated volume presented a glowing picture of enlightened practice on Echo Farm, which occupied several hundred bucolic acres in the Litchfield Hills of northwestern Connecticut. The author, F. Ratchford Starr, was nearing fifty when he discovered an unexpected talent for farming. In 1869 ill health had compelled him to give up a senior position at a Philadelphia insurance company and purchase a quiet summer home close to Litchfield. His energy was restored almost at once, and he rapidly fell in love with both the beautiful hill country and the work of bringing the land into useful order. The principal business of Echo Farm, he decided, was to be dairy farming. He set out to do the thing by the most advanced ways and means yet known.

By degrees, Starr created an operation handsome and polished enough to attract sightseers from miles around. He started from the assumption—unusual as late as the 1830s but rapidly becoming common wisdom—that since specialization was the key to success, no one should expect superior milk from anything but cows bred carefully and exclusively for dairy purposes. Starr's standard of excellence, eagerly touted by one wing of up-to-date dairying advisers, was high butterfat content, or the measure of how much cream you could get from skimming a given amount of milk. He chose to raise the newly fashionable Jerseys. The breed was known for remarkably creamy milk, and had acquired an enthusiastic following among American farmers after a few specimens were brought from the Isle of Jersey at around 1850. Visitors to Echo Farm marveled at the beauty of the sweet-faced animals and the comfort of the airy, well-lighted, scrupulously clean barns in which they were housed.

Starr's first and commercially unadventurous goal was buttermaking, an endeavor that until quite recently had belonged to farm women.

Since the Middle Ages the English word "dairy" had meant the farm building where—because plain fluid milk had no commercial value—women turned milk into butter and cheese. Properly managed dairies had long been proverbial for cleanliness. In 1615 Gervase Markham had declared, "Touching the well ordering of milke after it is come home to the Dairie, the main point belonging thereunto is the Hus-wifes cleanlinesse in the sweete and neate keeping of the Dairy house, where not the least moat of any filth may by any meanes appeare, but all things either to the eye or the nose so voide of sowernesse or sluttishnesse, that a Princes bed-chamber must not exceed it."[22] Two and a half centuries later Charles Dickens could write of an ex-navy officer's preternaturally scrubbed and orderly London living quarters that "his bath room was like a dairy."[23]

Farm dairy houses did not commonly acquire airs of "sluttishnesse" until after about 1850, when farmers began either supplying milk on a commercial scale to the many cheese factories that had appeared in North America or investigating the expanded market for drinking-milk. Men now furnished most or all of the labor. Slipshod dairying didn't result from a male lack of womanly talents for dealing with cows and milk. The difference was that previously the women of the household had carried out the entire hand-manufacturing processes for cheese or butter from raw material (their own cows' milk) through every step until the finished product left the farm to go to market. Strict care at every stage was crucial to the quality of the end result. In the new order of things, men milking much larger herds did nothing with their greater volumes of milk except collect it and ship it off the farm with or without any special attention to cleanliness.

Starr was one of the first commercial buttermakers to apply rigorous sanitary standards along with the use of modern machinery. Like Gail Borden, he understood that the traditional pursuit of immaculacy deserved to be observed detail by detail on a bigger scale. He experimented with increasingly complex, mechanized equipment as he got more serious about the enterprise. But from first to last, the facility he called the farm's Butter Department sparkled with cleanliness, aided by a plentiful supply of fresh water piped into the farm buildings from dammed-up cold springs a short distance uphill. By his orders, all equipment was to be kept spotless at all times. All milkers were required to wash their faces and hands and comb their hair before going into the milking room, and to use specially designed pails equipped with wire mesh-covered spouts (removable, for thorough cleaning), to strain out any visible dirt before the milk went through another triple-screen strainer.[24]

Echo Farm butter quickly earned a reputation as a carriage-trade article. Wrapped in muslin cloths and packed into one-pound cardboard boxes, it was shipped to Boston, Brooklyn, and New York City (meaning Manhattan) to be sold for the amazing retail price of $1 a box (close to $25 in 2023 dollars). An admiring writer in *Walllace's Monthly* assured readers that the butter's exquisite quality approached work-of-art status.[25]

By luck or good judgment, Starr had launched his butter business at a crucial moment in the decline of farmstead butter produced by dairy-women and the rise of commercial butter made on a larger scale. The latter was generally abominable. It reached grocery stores in sizable firkins, from which the grocer dug out and weighed required amounts of the unrefrigerated product in a heavily salted, often semi-rancid state. The technological wherewithal for producing very good butter in small factories known as "creameries" was starting to be developed, but at the moment Echo Farm was ahead of the curve.

Buoyed by his track record with butter, Starr turned his attention to an aim less assured of popular success. He had decided to try producing drinking-milk and cream for an upscale urban clientele. Health advisers were already horrified by the many opportunities the existing loose-milk system presented for dirt to get into the milk. The search was on for ways to replace large milk cans with some kind of securely sealed retail-size container, and again a few forward-thinking farmers like Starr were there at the right moment.

The Echo Farm milk operation, like its Butter Department, was designed to showcase state-of-the-art machinery and high sanitary standards. Demonstrating an awareness of European advances that were only inconsistently reaching American observers, Starr hired the Litchfield County medical examiner to look at the milk of each individual cow under a microscope.[26] All milk was poured into a custom-built tank cooled with an ice-water jacket, so that it could chill for several hours before being filled into quart containers. Cream, once skimmed, went into pint or half-pint containers. Starr initially used tin cans with tight-sealing lids. But he soon decided to go a more modern route.

Like many other branches of manufacturing, glass production had been getting better and cheaper since the Civil War. Glass not only permitted buyers to see any dirt that fell to the bottom but was more easily cleaned than most other materials. The first successful experiments in designing inexpensive and fairly durable bottles or jars for beer, milk, or fruit preserves occurred in 1878; within a year several manufacturers were marketing competing versions. In 1879 Starr switched to glass bottles made for the Philadelphia-based Cohansey firm. *Farm Echoes* proudly offered illustrations of his bottling apparatus, with a pipe running from the milk tank to fill twenty bottles at a time from as many spigots. The bottles themselves had swing-top caps fastened by wire clamps, and bore paper labels reading, "This bottle to be washed and returned to Echo Farm." Returned bottles received scrupulous further washing, both at the New York agency that distributed milk to customers and back at the farm.[27]

According to a brief 1880 notice in *The Cultivator and Country Gentleman*, "The amount of milk and cream that leaves the farm daily is upwards of 1,500 bottles."[28] The retail customers who ordered it in cities cannot have been the sort of people who had queued up, jug in hand, for swill milk at the height (or nadir) of its career. A quart of milk straight from the farm had then (according to John Mullaly's 1853 *The Milk Trade in New York and Vicinity*) sold for between 3 and 5 cents,[29] and retail prices did not increase greatly over the next half century. (In fact, after the 1870s milk dealers increasingly succeeded in forcing down wholesale prices paid to farmers in order to preserve profit margins while keeping retail prices steady.) But the German livestock husbandry researcher Martin Wilckens, who toured Echo Farm in 1890, reported that in New York (i.e., Manhattan) and Brooklyn a quart of Starr's milk or a half pint of cream fetched 10 cents.[30] As he pointed out, such a price excluded any buyers except city-dwellers who knew that their dime covered not just rich Jersey milk but carefully sealed clean bottles, overnight delivery, and (in hot weather) reliable ice cooling of the railroad cars that brought the milk to town.

Other well-to-do dairy farmers were venturing on similar experiments. One was the physician J. Cheston Morris. An Echo Farm admirer who grazed his own herd of prize Devon cows at his farm "Fernbank" in Chester County, Pennsylvania, he was eager to publicize the bottling approach. Nothing, he wrote in an 1884 article in the *Boston Medical and Surgical Journal*, could benefit humanity more than an unlimited supply of fresh, clean milk, since "no other article comes so near to being the universal food of man . . . Nor does any mode of preparation [i.e., processing into cheese or other forms] enhance its nutritive value. In by far the greater number of instances it is more wholesome and nutritious, more easily digested and more readily absorbed just as it comes from its source than in any other guise." Seeing the solution to milk-borne contagions in bottled milk, Morris predicted "that in the not distant future its cleanliness and superiority in every respect will put an end to the present milk-can system with all its dirt and liability to fraud and deception."[31]

Did men like Starr and Morris point toward the commercial future of drinking-milk? Certainly they put into effect ideas and principles that eventually would be the gospel of the mainstream industry. These began with systematic concentration on breeding cows for particular qualities, purposeful control of what they ate, and disciplined supervision of all farm employees. Well before any ironclad scientific consensus about the need for rigorous hygiene had reached all American physicians, members of this elite company not only zealously observed the sanitary protocols (straining, washing, chilling) for which the finest female cheesemakers and buttermakers of earlier eras had been renowned, but improved on them by creating a more ambitious infrastructure. They laid great stress on unlimited supplies of clean fresh water, elaborate piping systems, plentiful use of ice, apparatus for rapidly filling and sealing individual containers, and much more.

But to assume that these priorities were harbingers of a golden future for drinking-milk as a fixture on every American family table would be not 20/20 hindsight but severely astigmatic hindsight. If people like Starr and Morris presaged the future of dairying, they also harked back to the prewar days when research and development had been a scattershot affair supported by wealthy private parties in an overwhelmingly rural America. Post-Civil War farm production could neither go back to that model nor instantly start providing cheap food for millions in the nation's growing cities. Echo Farm and Fernbank were ambitious personal projects aimed at a small, affluent city-based market segment, not workable prototypes for the vast majority of dairy farmers.

More serious engines of change would eventually be put in motion with strategic shoves from the very young USDA. In the immediate postwar period it was not impressively funded or staffed, and the individual states had trouble formulating their own agricultural goals and establishing colleges in compliance with the Morrill Act. The long economic depression of the 1870s was a further hindrance to meaningful action.

An equal obstacle was mainstream American colleges' and universities' lack of enthusiasm for giving some promising scientific disciplines more than token representation in the curriculum. Their tepid attitude drove many bright young men (female scientists were the rarest of rare birds) to spend at least a few postgraduate years studying at French or German schools. In the 1870s the energetic Wilbur O. Atwater, a product of Yale, returned from Germany filled with admiration for the agricultural experiment stations at which that country was seeking to put rational, statistics-driven ideas of soil fertilization and crop management into practice for the benefit of farmers. For some years a fragmented band of Atwater allies at Yale and Wesleyan endeavored without great success to win over the state of Connecticut and the USDA to the idea. Their efforts did not lastingly pay off until the first administration of Grover Cleveland.[32]

In 1887, after years of wrangling, Congress passed a bill, sponsored by Representative William Hatch of Missouri, to establish a nationwide system of federal agricultural experiment stations under the direction of the USDA commissioner and the individual state land grant colleges. Their mission was to advance agricultural science through research on a multitude of subjects including plant and animal physiology, livestock rations, and "the scientific and economic questions involved in the production of butter and cheese"—still officially considered the most important branches of dairying.[33]

The Cleveland administration's final weeks (February 1889) also saw the passage of an act granting cabinet status to the USDA under a Secretary of Agriculture.[34] Incoming President Benjamin Harrison rapidly assigned the post to Jeremiah M. Rusk, an Ohio farm boy who had just completed six years as governor of his adoptive Wisconsin. The state was on the rebound from an unhappy love affair with soil-depleting wheat farms, and agricultural pundits had begun to lobby for dairying as a more sustainable alternative.

The Hatch Act did not instantly cast drinking-milk into a role large enough to eclipse butter and cheese in the calculations of leading agricultural authorities. But it and the companion act giving agriculture cabinet-level visibility did set in motion many cascades of change. First of all, they paved the way for the growth of a vast agricultural bureaucracy at both federal and state levels. They helped fill the land-grant schools with research-hungry faculty members convinced that their sovereign duty was to get knowledge flowing from experimental plots or chemistry laboratories to American farms, large and small, in every part of every state. The schools and experiment stations tried to keep up serious personal contact with real farmers and farm families, but were also expected to publish numerous bulletins. These ran a gamut from science-for-laymen advice aimed at rural Doubting Thomases to painstaking reports by specialists eager to share the details of experimental protocols with fellow researchers. The USDA publications, along with others issued by individual state land-grant schools, swiftly grew into a literature almost too massive to navigate even today with the aid of online indices and links. By no means was every listing in this monumental body of work a dazzling breakthrough. But the net effect was to let loose a flood of advances in all branches of agricultural science as well as other food-related questions.

Wilbur Atwater had already tutored a generation of converts to German nutritional theories that measured the net energy of food in terms of calories ingested and calories burned. Neither they nor any contemporary nutritionists suspected the existence of such things as vitamins, or could precisely calculate the mineral content of anything. But Atwater never tired of reiterating his belief, "Milk contains all the essential nutrients of food, and they are in the proportions needed to supply the needs of the body"—in contrast to meat, an American status symbol about which he had severe reservations.[35] In fact, late nineteenth-century food chemistry had enhanced drinking-milk's overall reputation with a modern scientific luster that delighted the up-to-date Pennsylvania farmer-physician J. Cheston Morris. Citing recent analyses listing the amounts of butter, casein, "salts" (a general rubric for minerals), and "lactin" (the initial term for lactose) in cow's milk, he concluded that the milk of the popular Shorthorn or "Durham" cows was deficient "in cream and sugar" (i.e., butterfat and "lactin"), while that of Jerseys was "poor in casein and sugar." His own preferred Devon cows, on the other hand, gave milk "nearly equal to the Jerseys in cream, and very rich in casein and sugar, and hence having the highest nutritive value." In a white population with a great preponderance of adult lactase persistence, it was easy to suppose that high lactose content contributed to milk's "nutritive value" for everybody.

But Morris had further concerns. It is hard to tell how far he subscribed to the new ideas about bacteriology coming from France and

Germany. He had, however, grasped that milk was apt "to be the carrier of the zymotic elements of disease." "Zymotic" was a term that medical authorities had adopted at around 1840, when many observers suspected contagions like cholera or typhus of being spread through a kind of miasmatic rot, and that still hung on as a conveniently vague synonym for "infectious" while the germ theory was gradually replacing earlier hypotheses. In 1884, Morris and many who thought like him were sounding an increasingly angry alarm about the terrible incidence of child mortality in cities. For the solution, he pointed to the example of concerned, intelligent farmers like himself who saw the importance of clean new technology (e.g., individual glass bottles instead of loose milk). But he did devote a sentence to one other promising force for change: "Systems of inspection under governmental authority have been largely resorted to, and with excellent effect; they should be increased and made more stringent."[36]

CHILDREN AND THE
PUBLIC HEALTH REVOLUTION

It is useless to try explaining how pasteurized milk replaced swill dairies without also following the path from municipal hand-wringing to purposeful attacks on the dreadful results of unmanaged urban growth. Decade by decade after the Civil War, major cities recorded increasing upticks in the number of children who did not live to see their fifth birthday. The reason was no great mystery. More and more native-born Americans were transplanting themselves from the dwindling countryside to the burgeoning cities just as waves of immigration from the poorest and most troubled regions of Europe further overwhelmed the capacities of urban housing. Well-meaning reformers might at one time have hoped the problem would go away if the undeserving poor could be taught to stop drinking and pull themselves up by their bootstraps. But even the most self-righteous moralizers now had to recognize that some kind of collective action was needed to prevent the filth and overcrowding of modern slums from becoming health menaces to everyone.

Cities in Great Britain and northwestern Europe where resources like clean water were no longer left to chance provided some examples. More immediately, the Civil War was a powerful stimulus to new ideas about "sanitary" management—"sanitary" at the time having a much broader meaning than it does today. It embraced anything related to furthering health and protecting against illness. From 1861, the hastily organized U.S. Sanitary Commission served as a semivoluntary relief agency bringing medical supplies and treatment to sick and wounded Union soldiers. The "sanitary fairs" held in many cities during the war were bazaars or exhibits meant to raise money for the perennially underfunded effort. By the late 1860s, both doctors and thoughtful laypeople recognized that the contagions prevalent in military hospitals could be prevented or at least checked by rational measures.

Not surprisingly, large cities were the first U.S. administrative entities to try applying these lessons to peacetime crises. City boards of health had existed here and there since the early nineteenth century, but they had been haphazard affairs with poorly defined and often temporary responsibilities. The Metropolitan Board of Health organized by New York City in 1866 was better conceived than any similarly named predecessor, and soon acquired powers not meant to be limited to the duration of one emergency. Counterparts were appearing in Boston, Philadelphia, and elsewhere. Unfortunately, they often found themselves in conflict with private physicians who saw them as illegitimate usurpers of authority bent on undermining the medical profession.

Decade by decade, city boards of health, municipal medical commissions, and the like, became more efficiently arranged while gaining prestige and political clout—though never with budgets to match their responsibilities. State boards or departments of health gradually came into being (and also tended to be meagerly funded). In 1872 a few dozen representatives of different agencies organized themselves into the American Public Health Association. As its constitution stated, "The objects of this Association shall be the advancement of sanitary science and the promotion of organizations and measures for the practical application of public hygiene."[37]

The trailblazing medical-social concept of "public health" struck a chord with civic-minded people everywhere. No belief of the pioneer organizers resonated more powerfully than their insistence that the protection of children's lives and health was a duty of society at large. It became axiomatic among them that statistics mattered, and that mortality rates among children under five were, in the words of one New York City official, "the most sensitive test of the sanitary condition of a community."[38] The spread of these convictions dovetailed with the growth of pediatrics as a medical specialty eventually boasting a recognized name of its own, as well as the rapid progress of the discipline variously called "bacteriology" or "microbiology."

The leader to whom American pediatrics owed virtually everything—even before most people had encountered that label—was the German-born, New York-based physician Abraham Jacobi (1830–1919). A student radical who was imprisoned during the failed uprisings of 1848, he came to America by way of England (where he made the acquaintance of Marx and Engels) and began a vigorous career as practitioner and educator. By 1861 he was teaching courses on childhood diseases at New York Medical College; by the early 1870s he was a recognized expert on children's diet.

Through the lens of his political convictions, Jacobi saw medical progress as an agent of the common good and children's health as the concern of society at large. Fifty years after his work on infant and child feeding had started to command respect, one of his pupils commented that "before 1872 the child had hardly been discovered."[39] No discoverer was more persistent than Jacobi. His first ideas were a far cry from twenty-first-century perspectives on child nutrition. But he ardently followed the innovations that multiplied throughout his career. By 1890, when he was considered the grand old man of American pediatrics, he and a generation of people trained by him had absorbed the new teachings of microbe investigators working in Europe. Up until then, American counterparts had been nowhere near the forefront of research.

Only in 1857 had Louis Pasteur begun the series of investigations that revealed the breathtaking importance of organisms invisible without a microscope. On both sides of the Atlantic, educated men and women who tried to follow the march of scientific progress learned that he had stopped some of these previously unknown life forms—certain yeast strains—from ruining wine or beer.

Swift improvements in instruments and data-collecting soon revealed both whole tribes of even smaller organisms and the fact that some of them were appallingly dangerous. The agents responsible for such diseases as scarlet fever and anthrax turned out to be unimaginably minute life forms whose very existence could never have been shown by anybody but a microscope-wielding scientist. Pasteur himself was among the first to suggest strict precautions against allowing disease-bearers to enter the human body. In the late 1860s, the Scottish-born physician Joseph Lister followed up this advice by devising a set of antiseptic protocols for surgeons and others dealing with open wounds. Ideas about washing hands and sterilizing equipment took some time to diffuse into general medical practice. It was the public health pioneers who recognized the importance of such antiseptic principles for every man, woman, and child and strove to spread the new knowledge through educational programs.

In a sense, belief in microbes was analogous to belief in the "evidence of things not seen" guaranteed to practicing Christians in St. Paul's epistles and Sunday sermons. Microbial "things not seen," however, could be lethal foes, and campaigns against them could achieve more immediate victories than anything in the New Testament. The microbiology story was bound up with the growth of a prestigious, mightily influential professional class trying to impose complete faith in teachings whose true rationale most laypeople could follow only in kindergarten versions prepared for nonscientists. The chief thing that many learners absorbed from the new creed was a fear much like that hammered into the devout by take-no-prisoners Victorian evangelicals warning backsliders to beware "Satan in the hairbrush" and other everyday lurking-places.

"FOSTER MOTHER'S" MILK

The young physicians who began practicing in the 1880s and 1890s were the first generation of medical advisers to have been systematically taught about either the correlations between visible disease and microscopic agents or the nutritional theories being expounded by Wilbur Atwater's food chemist colleagues. They worked under a strong sense of the responsibilities involved in putting new knowledge to use, especially where very young infants were concerned.

The rise of pediatrics as a specialty occurred just as most nations of the industrialized West were noting a steep decline in breastfeeding. This puzzling phenomenon cut across class lines and was anxiously discussed in conjunction with another source of bafflement, a general decrease in birth rates. The still-disputed reasons for the joint decreases are outside the scope of this book. What is certain is that fewer and fewer women nursed their babies. Working mothers—a mounting and generally hard-up category in cities—did not have the time to do so. Poor and well-off women alike often reported having insufficient breast milk. In another significant shift, it became common to wean children at six months or even younger, rather than a year or more.[40]

The use of wet nurses had fallen into disrepute in the past several generations. Medical advisers already disapproved of "hand feeding" or "artificial feeding" except in cases of desperate need, and the discovery of invisible new dangers reinforced their fears. Microbiologists had delivered the startling news that though human milk as directly absorbed by a baby at the breast was germ-free, cow's milk as transported from farm to city emphatically wasn't. (Later science has replaced "germ-free" with a much more complex picture, but it is still true that except in rare cases, breast milk delivered by the straight nipple-to-mouth route is free from pathogens.) With germs now in the picture, many physicians considered hand feeding the most lethal thing anyone could do to a baby short of strangling it. But clearly some way must be found to close the widening gap between infants' needs and the supply of mother's milk. The depth of public emotion now invested in what came to be called "the milk question" reflects a sense of collective emergency in which cow's milk seemed to be the only lifeline for otherwise doomed babies but was surrounded by its own deadly menaces.

Of course drinking-milk from cows had been steadily gaining ground throughout the nineteenth century—but as a wonder food for children anywhere between the age of weaning and puberty. Feeding it to infants almost from birth on as a direct substitute for mother's milk crossed some crucial cultural as well as medical bridge. At no earlier moment in modern Western history could anyone have proclaimed, "The cow is the foster mother of the human race. From the time of the ancient Hindoos to this time have the thoughts of men turned to this kindly and benef-icent creature as one of the chief sustaining forces of the human race." This tribute apparently began percolating in the brain of the dairy pub-lisher and one-time Wisconsin governor William Dempster Hoard at some point after 1885 and was circulated throughout the dairy industry by way of his seminal journal *Hoard's Dairyman*.[41] It was an inspired slo-gan for boosting the industrial-scale expansion of fluid milk production. It also foreshadows a mindset becoming more deeply entrenched among American consumers and voters at the same time that the nation's cities were developing something like a public conscience about the shame of infant mortality: an illogical conviction that an unlimited supply of pure, clean cow's milk should be as much every child's natural birth-right as mother love. "The human race through scores of thousands of years has developed a total dependency upon cattle for the rearing of its young," U.S. wartime Food Administrator Herbert Hoover would declare in 1918.[42]

The new crop of pediatricians soon began rethinking familiar medi-cal dictums about the deficiencies of hand feeding as opposed to breast-feeding. Recent research into food chemistry and infant digestion had shown that even the purest cow's milk was completely inadequate as a breast-milk substitute. Pediatric nutritionists, however, chose to view this fact as a challenge to be overcome by modern know-how.

The problem was the basic composition of cow's milk. It had both less lactose than breast milk and larger amounts of casein that formed a firm curd in the baby's stomach—too firm, the experts concluded, for easy digestion. Trying to bring cow's milk closer to the human counterpart, the new pioneers came up with various kinds of "modified" formulas. They began by mixing milk with water or cereal gruel, to cut back the proportion of casein. Dilution, of course, reduced the relative amounts of fat, sugar, and calcium. These were adjusted by adding cream, lactose or sucrose (in the form of cane sugar), and often "lime water" (a solution of slaked lime, or calcium hydroxide). The total amount and relative percentages could be adjusted to roughly correspond to the stages of maternal lactation along with the baby's growth.

The first man to hold an official professorship in infant care under the actual title of "pediatrics," Thomas M. Rotch of the Harvard Medical School, became obsessed with the fine-tuning of percentages for modified cow's milk. One school of the profession followed him in strict dedication to rigorous, baroquely complex mathematical formulas that mothers were supposed to replicate at home. Some thought it made more sense to have premixed formulas put up in bottles matching the baby's size and age. Abraham Jacobi led a wing of skeptics who found the whole idea of "percentage feeding" far-fetched and wanted modifications to be kept to the simplest possible outlines. All parties, however, agreed on the need for careful antiseptic measures under all circumstances. Jacobi championed the practice of boiling milk before feeding it to babies in any form.[43] Still other experts were looking to ideas coming from Europe.

THE SOXHLET TECHNIQUE

The lessons of microbiology were now reaching scientists who were not themselves trained in that field, including the first thinker to devise a systematic heat treatment of drinking-milk for protective purposes. He was the German agricultural chemist Franz Soxhlet, who had developed a keen interest in the chemical makeup of milk. An 1879 attempt to chemically separate milkfat from the solids in cheese led him to design a piece of laboratory equipment that still bears his name and that would prove invaluable in many other uses, the "Soxhlet extractor."[44]

Soxhlet was already celebrated for this breakthrough when in the 1880s he began pondering the dismal state of the cow's milk then reaching many thousands of nursing-age children in his adopted hometown, Munich. He started working on a method of "sterilizing" milk—the word "sterilize" was somewhat loosely understood, and "pasteurize" hadn't been coined—and unveiled it at a gathering of medical professionals early in 1886. He followed up this effort with a short two-part article in the *Münchener Medizinische Wochenschrift*. The idea rested on a home apparatus for heating individual infant-sized portions of milk—as fresh from the cow as possible, and modified according to a doctor's directions—in sealed glass bottles long enough to ensure that the contents would keep for three to four weeks at ordinary room temperature without souring. Each bottle held 150 cubic centimeters (5 fluid ounces) of milk and was fitted with a rubber nipple. The child's mother, or whoever was responsible for preparation, filled and sealed the bottles before arranging them in a holder that could be lifted in and out of a lidded cooking pot. This was filled with cold water up to the neck of the bottles and placed on a kitchen stove or other heat source until the water reached boiling point. The vessel, covered with a lid, remained over the heat for 35 to 40 minutes. The holder containing the bottles was then lifted out and the milk allowed to cool to room temperature. Before feeding it to the baby, mothers were instructed to place a bottle over hot water in a double-boiler arrangement and carefully rewarm it just to body temperature. Between uses, the bottles and equipment for filling them had to be painstakingly cleaned.[45]

Soxhlet's already substantial fame expanded dramatically, and he was awarded the Bavarian knightly title of "Ritter von Soxhlet." His milk-heating proposal was a milestone in drinking-milk technology, not so much for the particular details of his apparatus as for the excited conversations that he set going among pediatricians and public health authorities in Europe and America.

The main point of debate among those who liked the Soxhlet approach was how to avoid a boiled flavor and preserve some vestige of freshness while still arriving at the time-temperature combinations needed to reliably destroy particular pathogens. Meanwhile, physicians connected with public health programs began wondering how to carry out Soxhlet's home-oriented stratagem on a larger scale at approved facilities.

In the first decades after the Civil War, American cities coping with enormous public health challenges had begun setting up "dispensaries," which today probably would be called neighborhood clinics. Usually operating under some combination of public and private funding, they were often the only sources of medical care and actual medicines available to recent immigrants. In 1887 one such facility on New York's Lower East Side, the Eastern (soon to be renamed Good Samaritan) Dispensary, hired an attending physician named Henry Koplik to treat childhood diseases.

Koplik had received his medical training in the city and was just back from a round of post-internship studies at several European medical schools. Unhappy with the dispensary's routine responses to the seemingly endless gastrointestinal illnesses afflicting babies who for whatever reason could not be nursed by their mothers, he became convinced that their plight called for out-of-the-box thinking. In 1889 he began putting up the cleanest milk he could obtain in 3-ounce bottles and sterilizing it on a Soxhlet-like model, to be distributed by the dispensary's pharmacist after a consultation in which Koplik explained to the mother just how to feed it to the tiny patient with due precautions for extra cleanliness.[46] Milk carefully bottled in individual feeding portions was an astonishing novelty to the mothers of patients at the Good Samaritan. It also roused great curiosity in the burgeoning pediatric and public health communities.

Koplik had used state-of-the-art technology to create what would soon begin to be called a "milk depot," the first in the United States. But his was no isolated voice. At once he found sterilized milk being eagerly discussed among proponents, opponents, and the uncommitted. Among other reasons for this explosion of interest, the youthful U.S. Department of Agriculture now belatedly realized that unfermented drinking-milk was about to outstrip any other branch of the dairy sector in scale and cash returns. Butter producers still thrived. American-made cheese, however, was in a state of decline. The immediate future of commercial dairying clearly lay in supplying the cities with drinking-milk—but it would be necessary to address the threat of milk-borne disease more decisively than previous authorities. Educating farmers to the facts of microbiological life and a sense of their responsibilities was an urgent priority if fresh fluid milk were to fulfill its economic potential. At the same time, agricultural policy-shapers now agreed that the farm-to-consumer path also had to be made safer at the receiving end.

For the time being, many experts tried to use the general Soxhlet processing template as a guide, sometimes working out their own time-temperature combinations. Pediatricians in both private practice and dispensaries earnestly explained the germ theory to mothers as a paramount reason for committing themselves to endless rounds of conscientious bottle-washing in carrying out a prescribed number of feedings a day. The dispensary routines were equally labor-intensive for employees.

Some experts objected that milk depots at dispensaries could only worsen the deplorable falloff in breastfeeding. The reform-minded writer John Spargo, in *The Common Sense of the Milk Question* (1908), offered an unanswerable retort by "a working woman" with whom he had spoken at a depot: "The doctors as says that only guess what they'd do themselves if they was women."[47] What no naysayer could deny was a sizable decrease in reported cases of "summer complaint" and other gastrointestinal disorders wherever some Soxhlet-patterned procedure was adopted.

It would soon be obvious that home sterilization in individual baby bottles was not a promising model for the further expansion of the fluid milk trade. A major obstacle, as Koplik pointed out in an 1891 article, was "the simple reason of cost." The infant-sized glass bottles and other equipment needed for the scheme could not be cheaply manufactured, and the bottles also proved to be subject to cracking with repeated exposure to heat. Koplik foresaw that "future labors must lie in the furnishing of dairies with apparatus for sterilizing milk on the spot, and thus preventing decomposition in transportation."[48]

That idea received an unforeseen boost in 1892, when a wealthy New York businessman set out with his wife and children for their summer home at Saranac Lake in the Adirondacks. He had arranged to keep a cow "to be sure of having pure milk for my family." But when the animal "fell sick and died suddenly," the dismayed parents called in a veterinary surgeon and received the horrific news that her lungs were riddled with tuberculosis.[49] Luckily none of the children contracted the disease. But their father was appalled at what might have happened. He was Nathan Straus, the co-owner of Macy's department store and a man with a taste for righteous causes. The one with which he would be forever identified was milk pasteurization.

Straus happened to be politically connected as well as immensely rich. He was ideally situated to bridge the gap between an ambitious but underfunded public health bureaucracy and the enormous logistical demands of systematically furnishing clean drinking-milk to needy families on a large scale—large, at least, by comparison with anything that had been attempted to date.

5

PASTEURIZATION

The Game-Changing Years and Nathan Straus

SAFE MILK: FRAMING THE ISSUES

A history of milk pasteurization published in 1968 began by calling it "one of mankind's most thrilling stories of quest for truth; a triumph over the ignorance and superstition of past ages."[1] The authors would have been appalled to find many Americans of their grandchildren's generation ridiculing this idea and calling raw milk a miracle food. They well knew, however, that early campaigns for pasteurization had been filled with similar disputes.

By 1890 most physicians acknowledged that slipshod handling of milk invited invasion by the organisms responsible for diphtheria, scarlet fever, typhoid fever, and cholera, among other contributors to infant mortality. But we cannot assume in hindsight that all intelligent people promptly agreed on any one ideal measure against milk-borne pathogens, with only fools and knaves dissenting. Pro-pasteurization advocacy took some time to become a majority position. The germ theory in itself didn't support a single definitive conclusion to be drawn from the then-available evidence. The arguments that broke out over whose science was more scientific were not mere exercises in "ignorance and superstition."

To correct one widespread misconception: Pasteur himself never attempted to "pasteurize" milk. His original breakthrough in preventing harmful organisms from outcompeting the yeast strains needed for wine or beer production had been to heat the liquid to a certain temperature, *under the boiling point*, that was maintained for a certain length of time. Through repeated tries, he had found time-temperature combinations that killed undesirable organisms while leaving useful ones intact. Other researchers subsequently sought to apply the same principle elsewhere. But none of their targets posed challenges as difficult as drinking-milk. A major factor was that no food was more entangled with cultural assumptions and political dogfights.

In the United States, heating milk by some scientifically approved protocol met much resistance in what S. Josephine Baker of the New York City Bureau of Child Hygiene called the public's "unhappy prejudice against 'cooked' milk."[2] It was a stubborn cultural barrier. True, people from some parts of Eastern Europe often brought milk to a boil before using it; true, some American pediatricians echoed Abraham Jacobi's urgent plea never to give unboiled milk to children. But great numbers of consumers were instinctively repelled by the thought—not to mention the taste—of cooked milk. And a sizable wing of pediatricians insisted that any heating procedure robbed milk of crucial nutrients (though ideas of what these might be remained rudimentary). Meanwhile, millions of laypeople assumed that milk in unchanged straight-from-the-cow condition should be the standard for judging all forms of drinking-milk.

Dairyists' experiments with controlled heat treatments had started in Germany and Denmark. The original idea was not to rid drinking-milk of pathogens but to ensure more predictable conditions for large-scale butter and cheese manufacture. Albert Fesca & Co., a Berlin-based industrial engineering firm that had explored centrifuging techniques for separating butterfat from skim milk without agitating milk or cream in churns, got in the first recorded claim with an 1882 patent for a device that heated milk to temperatures between 158°F and 176°F (70°C and 80°C), probably as part of a buttermaking process. The Danish dairy scientist Niels Johannes Fjord shortly introduced a rival invention expressly meant for use in conjunction with butterfat separators.[3] Appliances like these, though not directly intended to process drinking-milk, were important as the first means of commercially heat-treating large amounts of milk or cream at once, as distinguished from Soxhlet-style arrangements that had mothers heating and cooling formulas in individual baby bottles. Danish manufacturers soon led the world in producing equipment.

By 1890 the field of heat treatments was crowded enough to inspire a detailed survey in an article by Heinrich Bitter, titled "Versuche über das Pasteurisiren der Milch" ("Experiments on the Pasteurizing of Milk") and chiefly focused on drinking-milk. Bitter, a researcher at the University of Breslau's Institute of Hygienic Medicine, may have been the first writer to unequivocally argue that for the sake of public hygiene some form of heat treatment should be mandatory for commercially sold milk, either as a direct requirement or through regulatory limits on bacterial counts. Choosing the term "pasteurizing" (*das Pasteurisiren*) as a general rubric for all current approaches, he systematically evaluated the advantages and drawbacks of different procedures.[4] They fell into two broad groups. Those on the Fesca or Fjord model were rapid methods—soon to be dubbed "flash pasteurization"—involving a continuous flow of milk over a heated metal surface. The others called for a batch of milk to be pumped into a vat, gradually brought to a prescribed temperature, and held for a certain length of time before being drained into another vessel for rapid chilling. In English-speaking countries, these would be collectively called "batch," "holding," or "bulk" methods. The perceived drawbacks were their slowness compared to continuous methods, and the extra expense of rinsing out and thoroughly cleansing the vat between batches. On the upside, they could be more carefully controlled and monitored than existing flash pasteurizers, which were still fairly crude.

Until about 1910 American commentators hesitated among terms including "sterilization," "purification," and "Pasteurization" before finally coming around to "pasteurization." Whatever the label, the entire idea promptly invited controversy. Among other reasons, researchers were learning to use bacterial counts as practical indicators of any pathogen-killing measure's success. They found that boiling milk in a pan on a home stove produced haphazard and short-lived results.

Flash-pasteurized milk also fared badly under the microscope. Public health authorities were thus appalled to realize that untrained dealers were eagerly importing Danish pasteurizers and processing milk through them with the aim of getting sloppily handled or aging milk to pass as raw before it could go bad—i.e., sour. (Others held off souring with such additives as borax, salicylic acid, and formaldehyde.) In a retrospective several decades later, the eminent public health officer Charles E. North wrote that this unauthorized hocussing had been "practised in secret and the milk marketed without any label" to record that it had been done because of "the strong sentiment against pasteurization by the dealer."[5]

These shady operators lent fuel to anti-pasteurizers who claimed that heat treatments were mere camouflages for filth. On occasion, farmers themselves were known to secretly pasteurize questionable milk and sell it as raw. Unsurprisingly, within a few years pasteurization advocates had to defend the very word against implications of chicanery.

"Fraud and pasteurization entered the milk business together, and so far there has been only indifferent success in divorcing them," a 1910 article in *Pearson's Magazine* charged. Thanks to flash pasteurization, "even the oldest and filthiest milk could be prevented from turning bad for several days. In fact, it never soured once it had 'flashed' through the machine. It merely rotted." The author, Arno Dosch, was no enemy to "real pasteurization" using the batch method. But by his estimate, "At least nine-tenths of the pasteurized milk sold today is a snare and a delusion. It has not killed off the germs it pretends to have rendered harmless. Instead, it has frequently made it particularly easy for the worst germs of all to grow."[6] In 1907 an editorial in the *New York Medical Journal* sternly questioned proposals for compulsory pasteurization of all milk sold in New York City. Might not such measures put the "progressive" dairyman who had invested heavily in sanitary precautions on the same level as the "slipshod" counterpart who ignored them, simply "because the city had decided to attempt covering up the impurities or other dangerous qualities of the milk by pasteurization?"[7]

Through all the cacophony, city health officials struggled to make bacterial counts a part of routine supervision and distinguish reliable pasteurization methods from cheap dodges. Bacteriologists patiently experimented with the parameters of effective heat treatments: What was the "thermal death point" at which any individual pathogen was rendered harmless? How long must that reading be maintained? At what time-temperature combination could the undesirable "cooked" flavor be avoided without compromising safety?

Medical defenders of pasteurization were obliged to admit that some opponents had perfectly rational arguments bolstered by the advancing adoption of bacterial counts during the 1890s. If the goal was milk free of known pathogens, it could be almost certainly guaranteed by culturing a sample on gelatin or agar plates, then examining it under a microscope and calculating numbers of bacteria per cubic centimeter without trying to identify individual kinds. The overall total furnished a rough but useful idea of how long ago the milking had been done and what ambient temperatures the milk had been exposed to (a danger sign in summer). Though debate over different ways of performing standard plate counts soon arose, their net effect was to raise awareness of how basic sanitary principles might inhibit germs from multiplying.

Bacteriologists had at first assured medical authorities that milk was perfectly sterile inside a cow's udder, picking up bacteria only when it entered the outer world. Here, starting with the touch of a milker's hands, it encountered conditions that ranged from conscientiously scrubbed to filthy. Echo Farm and other farm dairy operations supplying milk to elite urban clienteles might pursue the cleanliness once associated with diligent dairymaids. But most milk still entering the general supply was of a very different sort. Its producers were thousands of people on small family farms widely removed from either the Jeffersonian ideal of an American yeomanry or the new, improved models being touted by agriculture school professors and the rising agricultural bureaucracy. Often called "dirt farmers," they raised a smattering of produce and livestock for their own use and contracted with dealers to sell various items that brought in only modest returns per farm but collectively could contribute a fair amount to a regional supply. Milk from a few cows was often part of the mix—cows that might live for years with no farmer or hired hand thinking to wash their begrimed flanks and udders before milking them into equally uncleaned pails. Such was a good deal of the "country milk" that found its way into pooled milk for the cities with little or no oversight by any public health authority.

Despite the urgings of Abraham Jacobi, Henry Koplik, and some allies, pediatricians were among the leading anti-pasteurizers. The lesson that many of them drew from horror stories about dirty-handed ignoramuses doing the day's milking a few feet away from manure piles was that modern preventive bacteriology had to be applied *at the source*. In 1890 a New Jersey pediatrician named Henry Leber Coit began asking how to rid the drinking-milk trade of contagions like those that had killed his small son. Over the next few years he worked out a system through which individual dairy farms agreed to comply with demanding sanitary requirements for the milking process, while also allowing their premises to be inspected and their milk to undergo frequent bacterial counts. In return, their raw milk would be certified as pure by "medical milk commissions" that eventually coalesced into a national organization, the American Association of Medical Milk Commissions.[8]

It is important to recognize that Coit never pictured throwbacks to some pre-industrial fantasy with happy cows presenting nature's unspoiled bounty to rosy-cheeked babies in daisy-studded meadows. To him, raw milk was a practical resource that too often had delivered disaster to the consuming public but that could now be made safe by reinforcing painstaking sanitary precautions with cutting-edge technology. The most effective new tools were numerical tallies of multiplying bacteria and efficient chilling through the miracle of improved ice manufacturing and refrigeration. Together with thousands of other scientific observers, Coit had grasped that maintaining milk below a certain maximum temperature limit (then usually set at about 50°F/10°C) at every critical stage from milking to point of consumption made an impressive difference between pathogens under control and pathogens let loose. (That it also hampered any anti-pathogenic action of lactic acid bacteria in the milk was the last thing that proponents of raw or pasteurized drinking-milk were thinking about.) His certifying program was meant to apply such rigorous science-supported standards toward the goal of freedom from bacterial contamination.

Microbiological researchers had now identified a large handful of major pathogens that invaded raw milk and were working to determine how they got there. Almost all the chief bacterial menaces shared one signal feature: they found their way into milk once it left the reportedly germ-free confines of the udder and encountered an outside environment where befouled barns, pails rinsed perfunctorily if at all, and other microbial hazards lay in wait between cow and consumer. Pro-pasteurization bacteriologists tried to zero in on the different production and distribution stages at which the germs causing diphtheria, scarlet fever, and the rest were able to infiltrate milk. Armed with this knowledge, they were confident that they could determine time and temperature specifications at which each individual threat would be effectually knocked out. (The New York physician Rowland Godfrey Freeman, writing in 1892, had persuasively argued that maintaining milk in baby bottles at a temperature of between 158°F and 176°F/ 70°C and 80°C for half an hour reliably killed all the major bacterial threats with less damage to the milk's intrinsic qualities than more aggressive heating.)[9] On the other side, the certified-milk party wanted to eliminate the same pathogens but believed that the solution lay in identifying their favorite lurking spots and keeping them from getting a foothold in the first place.

THE WHITE PLAGUE

It was not impossible for vigorously disagreeing pro- and anti-pasteurizers to conduct rational conversations about microbial invaders with a strong sense of common ground as members of a clean-milk movement—at least, not at first. Mutual mistrust and scorn along with luridly polarizing media partisanship would gradually set the two groups at loggerheads as bacteriologists learned more about one ancient menace that defied usual generalities. Medical observers had puzzled over its symptoms and possible causes for centuries while calling it "phthisis" or "consumption." The deathly pallor of patients in advanced stages caused it to be popularly dubbed the "White Peril" or "White Plague."

The germ theory of communicable diseases had allowed late-nineteenth-century public health authorities to improve on earlier interpretations of "epidemics," or contagions that could readily be disseminated among people. Agricultural authorities were meanwhile studying patterns of bacterial transmission in the animal equivalents, "epizootics." The scourge most difficult for either group to make sense of was consumption, now officially renamed "tuberculosis," and the only common illness then known to be both an epidemic and an epizootic disease. As researchers gradually put together bits of a difficult puzzle, at least some concluded that TB also belonged to another alarming category that had recently been dubbed "zoonoses," meaning infections that could travel from animals to humans. One means of transmission was milk, and the route by which it could spread TB was completely unlike those that had been traced for diphtheria and the rest.

Mycobacterium tuberculosis, the bacillus responsible for the human form of the disease, belongs to a clan of closely related organisms whose origin and genetic links are still under debate. Students of microbial genomics now agree that for millennia *M. tuberculosis* has been an intimate fellow traveler with human beings. Along the way, apparently step-by-step with domestication of some animals and exploitation of others in the wild, it evolved into a number of other mycobacteria tailored to the immune systems of specific nonhuman hosts. One of this versatile tribe's great talents is to silently coexist for years or decades with a host instead of killing it outright. In the words of one modern study, a *Mycobacterium* bacillus "acts as both a pathogen and a symbiont"[10]—meaning that it is equally able to launch devastating attacks on the host system or live harmlessly and indefinitely within the system.

The nearest genetic relative of *M. tuberculosis* is a pathogen that infects cattle and a number of other animals, *M. bovis*. Like many other bovine victims, Nathan Straus's doomed cow seemed to be in excellent health almost up to the time of her death (see chapter 4). And like many human TB patients, she was a prime example of how successfully mycobacteria have shadowed humanity and its animal companions during every historical twist and turn. Ramped-up urbanization in Western countries throughout the late nineteenth century crowded huge numbers of people into airless tenements that were ideal breeding grounds for *M. tuberculosis*; during the same decades, the enormous growth of the city drinking-milk market created localized populations of dairy cows that became perfect targets for *M. bovis*.

Unequipped to penetrate TB's genetic mysteries, microbiologists of the day took some time to work out its usual modes of transmission. It never struck like influenza or other epidemic diseases that quickly manifested as acute illnesses and swept through a population leaving so many corpses and survivors. It never spread in the same way as milk-borne plagues that seized their opportunity when milk was exposed to surrounding conditions like dirty vessels or July heat *after leaving* the udder. Care and cleanliness didn't seem to be the issue. In fact, the assumption that all milk was perfectly germ-free when secreted looked more and more dubious. A few observers began to suggest that not only could cow's milk be invaded by bovine tuberculosis bacilli *while still in* the udder, but the bovine disease was a zoonosis capable of being transmitted to humans in raw milk regardless of all sanitary precautions in handling.

This startling hypothesis turned out to be accurate. But though it lent strength to the pasteurization movement, it wasn't solidly proved until 1911 and didn't completely quash vociferous opposition until the eve of World War II. By then microbiologists had long known that *M. bovis* could cross the species barrier to infect people as alarmingly as *M. tuberculosis*—and on occasion vice versa. Children could get the bovine version from cow's milk; cows living next to sanatoriums sometimes acquired human TB from eating grass on which patients had spat.[11] Interspecies transmission was rarer than the human-to-human and cow-to-cow routes, but still frequent enough to be a real public health concern.

The chief finding at autopsy of a bovine or human TB victim would be "tubercles," or small hard nodules enclosing a cheesy-looking mass of dead cells and infectious matter, that (with people) usually appeared first in the lungs. But tubercles might show up in other organs or tissues, causing different symptoms from pulmonary TB. In cases where children had become infected with *M. bovis*, the most common site was lymph nodes, usually in the neck or abdomen.

The great microbiologist Robert Koch shone some light on the subject when he announced in 1890 that a substance he had isolated from tubercles and named "tuberculin" could furnish a test for distinguishing cows or people who harbored the disease from those who didn't. Unfortunately, he also added to the general confusion by first declaring that bovine and human TB were identical but switching course in 1901 and mistakenly claiming that they differed enough to make transmission from cows to humans virtually impossible.[12] Polemicists on both sides of the pasteurization question seized the opportunity to invoke Koch in support of their own arguments while denouncing each other's bad science.

Meanwhile, pediatricians' and public health authorities' usual discussions of milk-borne TB focused on two main angles of attack: either pasteurization carefully carried out at temperatures already proved to kill bovine mycobacteria, or tuberculin testing of cows to ensure that these organisms hadn't invaded the milk when it was secreted in the udder. Each of these proposed measures touched off furious battles involving anybody with a stake in the drinking-milk enterprise: country-based producers, city-based retail customers, representatives of municipal councils and health boards, and a growing class of dealers who not only hauled and distributed milk between the points of origin and consumption but were finding a new source of profit in bottling it for retail sale with or without prior pasteurization.

An additional problem was the obstinately persisting "loose milk" business described in chapter 4. Public health advocates denounced unrefrigerated milk dipped out of forty-quart cans in neighborhood grocery stores as a menace, but—tuberculosis, diphtheria, and typhoid fever notwithstanding—thousands of city-dwellers had nothing better or more convenient. Legal remedies were slow in coming. It took New York's Board of Health until 1896 to start requiring permits for people who wanted to sell milk in the city, and the first offender arrested for violating the new regulation fought the case through the state and federal judicial systems until the U.S. Supreme Court ruled against him in 1905.[13]

In a vexed and uncertain regulatory climate, several inconvenient questions surrounded both milk pasteurization and tuberculin testing.

Did anyone propose to make either of these new-fangled measures mandatory, and if so, on what legal basis? Who would be punishable for noncompliance? And most contentious, who would shoulder the cost of the necessary infrastructure?

British and European examples didn't suggest practical solutions. *M. bovis* was far more endemic in the Old World than the New, probably because regions with large beef or dairy cattle herds contained deeper and more ancient environmental reservoirs of the disease (for instance, soil and decaying vegetation) than anything in North America. Britons and Europeans put up long, stubborn resistance to either pasteurization or cattle testing, while Americans tried to thresh out their own measures in a climate of mounting acrimony. Many small farmers and milk dealers denounced all pasteurization requirements as pernicious and costly pseudoscience, while some urban zealots wanted state health departments to oversee tuberculin testing and destroy all animals that tested positive. That idea was routinely blocked in states with active dairy farm lobbies.

The first municipal ordinance involving milk pasteurization was enacted in 1908 as part of a political straddling act hastily performed by Chicago after the Illinois state legislature had defeated a bill requiring tuberculin testing of dairy cows. Scrambling to salvage what it could from a bad situation, the city council decreed on July 13 that all milk, cream, buttermilk, and ice cream sold in Chicago from January 1909 to January 1914 must come from tuberculin-tested cows. An exception was made for cows whose milk was pasteurized to municipal standards— standards that weren't spelled out because at the moment nobody had gotten around to it.[14] Nearly all present-day accounts of the episode either exalt technicality over accuracy by stating without qualification that Chicago was the first large city to require pasteurization of the milk supply, or somehow reverse the emphasis to make pasteurization the default condition and tuberculin testing the exception. In any case, the state legislature soon blocked the testing requirement under pressure from the farm lobby, and the pasteurization requirement also had to endure several years of challenges.

But the Chicago donnybrook lay well in the future in 1893, when Nathan Straus leapt into a roiling cauldron of competing interests and still-ambiguous evidence.

BIRTH OF A MISSIONARY

The sheer voltage of Straus's personality can be grasped from an obituarist's possibly bogus claim that he became betrothed to his wife the day after first meeting her during a business visit to Germany.[15] He was a man of impassioned beliefs, white-hot energy in pursuing them, and unbounded generosity. In his hunger to do good on earth, he was a force of nature. He was also an obsessive glory-hound and egoist who never tired of singing his own praises, or hearing them being sung by others. He could enter no controversy without hammering home a messianic conviction that the party in shining armor was Nathan Straus and any opponent was leagued with powers of darkness. His career of holy wars was punctuated by at least two psychiatric crises that the family explained as "nervous breakdowns" brought on by overwork. No single human being did more to inject partisan animus into the already vexed question of milk pasteurization, or to ensure that it would permanently distort all future debates of the issue.

The Strauses were a German Jewish family who had originally come to New York as founders of a china business before acquiring both a stake in R. H. Macy's department store and a number of political connections. Nathan, born in 1848, was the only one of three brothers who never achieved any especially prestigious public office. Isidor, the oldest and Nathan's partner at Macy's, was elected in 1893 to fill out a predecessor's unexpired term in the House of Representatives, while Oscar, the youngest, served as American minister to the Ottoman Empire and later became Theodore Roosevelt's secretary of commerce and labor. But there are conspicuous signs that after 1890 Nathan hoped to make a political bid of his own.

He was an enthusiastic, skilled perennial star of the harness races that at the time were a fashionable urban street sport. Through a shared love of racing and racehorses, he had forged a lifelong friendship with the rising Tammany-backed Democratic politician Hugh J. Grant, who won consecutive two-year mayoral terms in 1889 and 1891. In 1890 Grant appointed Straus to the municipal Park Commission, where he remained until 1895.[16]

In American society at large, the start of the 1890s saw remarkable links being forged among medicine, politics, and philanthropy. Andrew Carnegie's 1889 essay "Wealth" or "The Gospel of Wealth" had electrified a wide audience with its message that making a fortune should be only a preface to giving away every cent in altruistic causes before the end of the fortune-maker's life.[17] From his Park Commission niche, Nathan Straus began to ponder such teachings.

Troubling fiscal omens had been on the horizon for a year or two when economic disaster crashed over the nation: the Panic of 1893, which would be slow to relax its grip. The most terrible depression in American history to that point, it wiped out railroad companies, stockbrokers, and banks while sending the labor market into a tailspin. Unemployment rates had reached 20 to 25 percent by the start of the year. New York families shivered in unheated tenements, while thousands of homeless and jobless men slept on city streets. Many affluent citizens were galvanized into charitable action. Among these, Straus earned approving newspaper coverage for distributing coal to the poor at cost, establishing a grocery depot where bread, flour, and other necessities were sold at a pittance, and setting up all-but-free lodging houses for the homeless.[18]

The hottest season of the year called for other priorities. Everybody knew that May and June heralded a long stretch of "summer complaint" accompanied by grim child mortality statistics. The new advances in bacteriology had made the cause frighteningly plain to public health authorities: a rogues' gallery of pathogens in drinking-milk that had traveled from farm to neighborhood grocery without refrigeration or other measures against warm-weather proliferation of microbes. Here and there, some poverty-stricken families had access to dispensaries where physicians like Henry Koplik and Rowland Freeman were overseeing small "milk depots." But many more were dependent on loose raw milk transported from the farm in already dubious condition and ladled out of unwashed cans in flyspecked grocery stores.

Seeking a summer complement to his winter projects, Straus decided that no concern was more urgent than clean milk for poor children. He was not present at the actual launch of the effort, since it was his custom to spend several months of nearly every year in Europe on buying expeditions for Macy's and visits to German relatives. With Lina, his wife, he sailed from New York at the start of May, leaving the most arduous preparations to be carried out by his private secretary, Alexander L. Kinkead, who had administered the coal program and other relief efforts.[19] (The Strauses probably had more reason than usual to want an interval away from the city: Their oldest son had died of pneumonia less than three months earlier, a few days before his sixteenth birthday.)

Straus, Kinkead, or both had had a splendid idea perhaps sparked by Straus's Park Commission service. For a summer milk depot they had chosen a spot that offered some relief from the stifling New York heat and for which the city dock commissioners were granting rent-free use: a pier on the East River at the foot of Third Street, usually favored with fresh sea breezes. Here they wanted New Yorkers not to visit a baldly utilitarian facility where milk was processed and dispensed at nominal prices, but to enjoy a pleasant spot provided with seats and awnings—a well-judged invitation for families to treat themselves to a little coolness and leisure.

Strange though it sounds in light of Straus's later reputation, the new venture offered raw milk under the vague designations of "pure," "fresh," or "natural," along with heat-treated milk. Kinkead had visited some upstate dairy farms to evaluate the cleanliness of the operations, taking along a city Board of Health veterinarian to inspect the cows. To ensure that the milk would be kept on ice and protected from dirt on its way to the city, he had enlisted the distributor who sold milk to Macy's in-house restaurant.[20]

Kinkead had consulted with public health officials and pediatricians before deciding on the forms in which milk was to be dispensed and the best sanitary protocols. Mothers of babies could buy six- or eight-ounce bottles of milk modified according to a formula suggested by Rowland Freeman (lime water, lactose, and a little water) and prepared onsite by his heat treatment method. Both pasteurized ("sterilized" or "purified") and raw ("pure," etc.) milk were available in quart or pint glass bottles, the raw being cheaper. Loose milk was also dipped out into customers' pails or other containers in the old way—but with the difference that the milk had been handled under conscientious sanitary precautions (including ice chilling) from milking to point of sale. The "pure" milk could be consumed onsite, for a penny a glass.

The Straus milk depot opened on June 1, 1893, with Kinkead supervising all logistics, and was an instant hit. Newspapers commented admiringly on the enjoyable atmosphere and smooth professionalism of the operation, and Kinkead's picture appeared twice in the *New York World*'s front-page story.[21] The depot remained open until the end of October. That cutting-off point made sense, since summer complaint always declined with cooler weather. So did milk yields; most farmers still let cows dry off after breeding them at the end of summer.

The winter of 1893–1894 found Straus returning to coal distribution and other relief efforts while planning to expand the milk program. His motives, while certainly generous, may also have included more than a little self-interest. In May 1894, he published an article in the venerable *North American Review* titled "Helping People to Help Themselves," strongly suggesting that he was using humanitarian uplift to position himself as a bidder for political office.[22] He dwelt movingly on the injustices and humiliations of poverty. But at the same time, he managed to claim some implicit moral superiority for his own ideas of how to aid the victims of the ongoing depression. In his capable hands, relief efforts free of undemocratic, condescending *noblesse oblige* would place the relieved on a footing of equal dignity with relievers, making them sharers in practical transactions rather than passive recipients of charity.

That summer he dramatically heightened the visibility of the milk program by increasing the number of depots to six and adding several lesser stations in city parks where milk was to be had by the glass as a refreshing summer beverage. There is no telling how much—if at all—the approaching city mayoral election weighed in his calculations. But by August or September at the very latest, he must have been discussing it with the Tammany stalwarts Hugh Grant (who had declined to seek a third term), Thomas Gilroy (the current mayor), and "Boss" Richard Croker (another horse-racing chum of Straus's, and at the moment the undisputed head of the Tammany machine). In October the New York State Democratic Party nominated Straus as its candidate for mayor of New York City.

He promptly accepted, not realizing that the climate was disastrous. A firestorm of protests against outrageous corruption was sweeping over the city. A reform wing of Democrats, newly emboldened to buck the machine, refused to support the ticket. Several newspapers opposed Straus as a Tammany tool trying to capitalize on his charitable activities. In little more than a week he was forced to withdraw from the race.[23] The party, now in something approaching complete disarray, was unable to field any more plausible replacement than Grant, who went down to ignominious defeat against the reform-trumpeting Republican William Strong. As a further humiliation, the new administration instantly began pouncing on people who had worked under Grant and Gilroy with a great flurry of indictments based more on headline-chasing than legal evidence. In April 1895, Straus was indicted for supposed irregularities in the awarding of Park Commission contracts and—along with various other Democratic appointees guilty of nothing but party affiliation—speedily exonerated.[24]

Many later accounts airbrushed this incident into a tale of self-sacrifice in which Straus, though offered the mayoral nomination, had magnanimously declined in order to focus on his charitable interests. That indeed he did. Never again seeking elective office, he threw himself into the milk cause with new zeal and a remarkable change of direction.

For the first two seasons of his milk depots, he had offered pasteurized milk (both in modified form in infant-sized bottles and in its own right) as well as raw milk, without expressing any special fear of the latter. But from the start of the 1895 season, he seems to have suddenly appointed himself a national spokesman for pasteurized milk. He had now built a pasteurizing and bottling plant on Avenue C to serve as headquarters of the milk operation, and named it Nathan Straus Pasteurization Laboratories. This facility (later moved to East 32nd Street) opened while the indictment episode was playing out and sent pasteurized milk to all his milk depots and booths by wagon and eventually automobile. The large stenciled images of his flowing signature on every vehicle soon made "Nathan Straus" into one of the city's most instantly recognizable logos. Early in June, he composed a manifesto about "pure" milk—now using the word in a sense that hadn't occurred to him before—and dispatched copies to mayors of all large U.S. cities.[25] The message, he explained, was meant to answer a tremendous nationwide outpouring of queries about his work with pasteurization, and he wanted to share the benefits of his experience. Two years later he followed up this communiqué with a much longer, more detailed letter to major city health boards.[26]

Straus was one of those who always thoroughly believe whatever they are saying at the moment. "I have long held," he told the nation's mayors with more sincerity than accuracy, "that the day is not far distant when it will be regarded as a piece of criminal neglect to feed young children on milk that has not been sterilized." For his part, "I have addressed myself during the last two years to the task of placing within the reach of every poor family absolutely pure forms of infant diet. These [meaning milk for babies] have been either milk carefully sterilized without admixture, or in combination with barley water and a little sugar."[27] From then on, Straus was an impassioned missionary for pasteurization and increasingly opposed to raw milk. Facile parallels with today's pasteurization wars are distorting, since controversy then primarily revolved around feeding infants who were not receiving breast milk.

What it took to dramatically thrust the cause to national and international attention was just what Straus commanded: fervent conviction, philanthropic zeal, and a vast fortune—all ready to be set in motion through the formidable circuitry of his personal and political connections. He was a close friend of the powerful editor Arthur Brisbane (of Hearst's *New York Journal* and later the *Evening Journal*), and had enough of a relationship with the journalist William Wirt Mills (a reporter for various newspapers) to deploy him as a publicist on

critical occasions. He stoutly kept up his alliances with Tammany Democrats, who returned to power after a short hiatus. Still more important: the first two seasons of the milk depot program had earned him
the undying gratitude of the municipal Board of Health and every local
pediatrician who favored milk pasteurization—above all Jacobi, who
had been campaigning against raw milk for decades.

At the time, cities were barely starting to frame regulatory barriers
to the sale of pathogen-infested milk, and public health agencies had
neither the money nor the legal authority to tackle the problem. Straus
had the means to privately fund more and more depots and supply them
with milk—raw milk that was first certified as clean according to Coit's
exacting standards, then pasteurized through increasingly refined and
inexpensive versions of Freeman's method and sold (bottled) for infants'
use by either Freeman's formula or another devised by Jacobi. It was the
first demonstration that pasteurization could be carried out on a scale
large enough to affect infant mortality statistics, and it made a deep
impact on public health authorities everywhere. So did Straus's well-jus-
tified attempts to publicize the fact that the goal was "too great to be
adequately met by private efforts" like his own.[28] For all his compulsive
self-glorification, his letters to the nation's mayors and health boards
dramatized a real need for municipal oversight that no public official
could have made politically palatable. (It should be noted that because of
the state of tax laws during his career, elaborate nonprofit organization
machinery didn't figure in the plans of Straus and contemporary philan-
thropists. He never claimed a cent in tax breaks.)

His milk depots' impact on the dairy industry was also tremendous.
Of course, the volume of milk that Straus handled was tiny in proportion
to nationwide milk production. But it made a modest, much-noted contribution to the overall New York City milk supply. The farmers whom
he dealt with, like those who supplied Coit's certification program and
milk condenseries on the Gail Borden model, were a lesson to others
that milk produced with special regard to cleanliness could command
higher farm prices than carelessly handled milk.

In 1895 he began making sure that at least one of his depots would
furnish pasteurized milk throughout the year, not only in the usual

June-through-October season. It was a powerful incentive for some dairymen in the city's orbit to abandon the old practice of drying off all the cows in a herd after breeding at the end of summer, thus making year-round milk production a norm rather than an exception. Progress-minded instructors at agriculture schools had been talking about a twelve-month flow of milk for some years on the grounds that the usual interruption represented anything from four to seven months' lost income. But most farmers had not immediately rushed to embrace staggered breeding schedules. Straus's successful program helped to solidify expectations of a uniform yearly supply not affected by season—a serious cultural shift for city customers (who understood less and less about bovine reproduction) as well as rural producers (who increasingly forgot that they were rearranging a formerly season-bound cycle). Again, he had contributed to a change with profound future implications for the nationwide industry.

The scientific breakthrough that made year-round milk production feasible was silage: grasses and other fodder plants harvested green, packed into a cylindrical structure called a silo, covered, and left to ferment through the action of naturally occurring bacteria. Partly preserved by fermentation, it could see cattle through the winter more reliably than untreated hay. The idea had been introduced by crop scientists in the 1870s but did not start winning over dairy farmers until they saw significant growth in year-round demand for milk.[29] Silage never completely ironed out seasonal differences in cows' lactation cycles, but it helped to transform farmers' business models. In a few years all of the Straus milk depots supplied milk on a twelve-month schedule.

Straus's name became more widely known and respected year by year as his pasteurization work earned him golden opinions in the press. He basked in the spotlight of public favor, traveling tirelessly in both the United States and Europe, speaking at medical congresses, visiting eminent public health authorities, and incessantly proclaiming the gospel of milk pasteurization. He zealously collected statistics showing a steady year-by-year decline in New York City infant deaths among the poor since the founding of his first depot. He shared information about pasteurizing equipment with concerned officials in other cities, and patented a home-pasteurizing apparatus adapted from one devised by Freeman, to be sold at cost to families. Between about 1905 and 1909 his pleadings became sharply focused on milk-borne tuberculosis, which he correctly saw as a more compelling argument for universal pasteurization than any other infectious disease. His criticisms of raw milk relied more and more on emotion-laden rhetoric about endangered infants— "The babies, who cannot protect themselves from infected milk, need a pure milk law"; "I might appeal for the lives of the babies"; "I am asking for nothing for myself, but I do ask, for the defenceless babies, that they be shielded from the milk that kills."[30]

In Germany, where he had been born and which he regarded as his second home, he did battle against a dairying situation even worse than that in America. He went so far as to set up a second Straus Pasteurization Laboratories headquarters in Heidelberg for the manufacture of the home pasteurizer. In 1908 he delivered a weighty address at the University of Heidelberg, placing great stress on measures for combating the spread of bovine tuberculosis to human victims and sounding a call for greater governmental participation in the cause.[31] At the moment, he seemed to be at a peak of popularity and influence on two continents, with newspapers reliably showering epithets like "noble" and "benevolent" on his every action. The Heidelberg speech conveyed an aura of statesmanlike dignity.

But within a year Straus had begun receiving unwonted criticism on two fronts. One was the affair of the Lakewood Preventorium.

Much earlier he had created a sensation in Lakewood, New Jersey, by setting up a hotel in competition with another that notoriously excluded Jews. *His* establishment, he proudly declared, welcomed people of all creeds and races. In 1909 he chose Lakewood as the site of a charitable experiment rooted in his growing concern with tuberculosis. He had been struck by the story of a Canadian facility called a "preventatorium" or "preventorium," where poor children exposed to TB by family members in cramped city tenements could be removed to the countryside and housed in conditions—fresh air, exercise, plenty of milk—meant to restore them to blooming health after a several months' sojourn.

In no time, Straus was blindsided by furious opposition. The year-round residents and the tourism interests of Lakewood banded together to denounce a New York Jew who had already brought undesirable elements into their midst and who now, they wrongly claimed, planned to expose the entire community to the worst killer disease of the age. With his usual attention to high-minded goals rather than details, he had first tried to put up children in a wing of the hotel (which raised protests from paying guests), then moved them to a nearby cottage that didn't actually belong to him. In a prolonged storm of recriminations and (on his part) hysterical counter-recriminations, he suffered a mental breakdown so severe that by January 1910, Lina Straus could write to the superintendent of the New York pasteurization laboratory that "he will never be allowed to undertake serious work again."[32]

The doctors forbade the family to discuss business affairs or the milk program with him. As soon as weather permitted, Lina took him to Europe, accompanied by nurses, for consultation with a Heidelberg specialist followed by a lengthy period of recuperation. (His perennial press ally Arthur Brisbane of the *Evening Journal* had quietly solved the Preventorium mess by paying to have the operation reinstalled at a site several miles from Lakewood.) Eventually he began to recover. But by then—still under doctors' care and supposedly ordered to avoid stress—he had also become enmeshed in an imbroglio created by the brazenly unconscionable publisher of the *New York Herald*, James Gordon Bennett, Jr.

REVENGE BY NEWSPAPER

Bennett, the son of the founding publisher, loved nothing more than a bruising and, whenever possible, dirty fight. His home base was Paris, to which he had had to decamp some thirty years earlier after a drunken escapade had caused him to be blackballed by New York society. He ruled the *Herald* with a whim of iron, aided by a transatlantic cable that he had helped pay for in the interest of supervising every operational detail in the New York office. In an age of yellow journalism, he was master of every fire-and-brimstone shade.

When not in Paris, Bennett could usually be found aboard a yacht fitted up with every amenity, including cows to provide fresh milk, cream, and butter for his well-furnished table. He was cruising in British waters early in 1908 when he decided to put into a nearby port and stay for some time. Not knowing that he was running afoul of stringent new regulations, he began arranging to have his three shipboard cows put out to pasture for the duration. In a trice, health inspectors showed up asking whether the animals had been tuberculin-tested and, when told that they hadn't, insisting on administering the test. All three tested positive and were summarily slaughtered.

Bennett's appetite for vendettas was legendary, but he couldn't retaliate against the local authorities. Instead he reportedly cabled the *Herald* offices in New York ordering his subordinates to "give the tuberculin test hell."[33]

American opponents of the test were still trying to destroy its scientific credibility in 1908. From May on, the flagship newspaper in New York joined in with front-page articles denouncing individual states' attempts to enact mandatory tuberculin testing and hailing dissenters as the voice of sanity. The London and Paris *Herald* editions that Bennett had founded took up a similar party line.

"Tuberculin Cast Aside as Fad In New Hampshire," proclaimed a typically polemical headline in the New York paper. The article went on to praise the state's governor, a farmer named Nahum J. Batchelder, for having "fought tuberculin with all his energy. In the face of the strongest opposition from the faddists and the veterinarians who sought employment, no matter what the cost to the farmers, he won, and to-day New Hampshire uses less tuberculin than any State in the Union." According to Batchelder, "No State has a right to wage a wholesale tuberculin testing campaign. None has any right to go beyond a physical examination of cattle . . . When The HERALD describes tuberculin as a useless medical fad it is not very far out of the way."[34]

(In fairness to Batchelder, it should be said that at the time tuberculin tests often produced inconsistent or inaccurate results. To anticipate much later events: An iron-fisted 1930s federal program for testing all dairy herds by more reliable methods and slaughtering tuberculin-positive cows would finally eradicate bovine TB from the U.S. milk supply before 1940.)

Nathan Straus, who had been calling more and more insistently for tuberculin testing, shortly ended up in the *Herald's* crosshairs. Bennett had a reputation for disliking Jews, but until now his reporters had chimed in with the usual automatic praise of Straus's pasteurization work. Having grown accustomed to seeing himself taken at his own very high valuation in virtually all newspapers, Straus was affronted to find an extremely popular one making him the butt of virulent public scorn as Bennett's campaign expanded to include milk pasteurization.

In the summer of 1908 Bennett began waging war on the pasteurization cause, and on Straus personally, through the New York and overseas branches of the *Herald*. The seething Straus responded that autumn by pulling Macy's advertising from the hometown paper.[35] This tactical error didn't materially affect advertising revenues. It did, however, give Bennett an opportunity to play the independence-of-the-press card in fine style, while mocking Straus's well-known habit of endlessly pointing out his own wisdom and magnanimity. He kept up the attack for about two years, during which Straus was also being plagued by the Preventorium debacle.

The *Herald* reporters had no difficulty finding medical authorities who opposed pasteurization or lifting out-of-context data from others who didn't oppose it at all. Some of the more lurid claims were reprinted in newspapers throughout the United States (and have been approvingly cited by anti-pasteurizers of today). "Pasteurization is a recourse to palm upon a credulous public milk unfit for food," asserted the New York pediatrician Joseph E. Winters. In his opinion, "The zealot of pasteurization is as arbitrary to the law of nature, which is the law of the creator, as is the anarchist to the law of government." As proof: "In a downtown dispensary where pasteurized milk was used for years by the physician in charge, his successor reported that 98 per cent of the children had rickets."[36]

Bennett's hired guns also managed to torture the work of the eminent researcher Milton J. Rosenau into supposed proof that raw milk has an important germicidal action. *The Milk Reporter*, a dairy industry publication, helpfully recycled some figures lifted from Rosenau by the *Herald*, showing that in one cubic centimeter of very clean raw milk carefully drawn from one sample cow, total bacterial counts two hours and four hours after milking were respectively 430 and 100.[37] In fact, the *Herald* had ignored Rosenau's painstaking examinations of much other data as well as his scruples about applying the term "germicidal" to what he considered a weak and transient inhibiting effect on the multiplication of bacteria—scarcely relevant to a commercial scene where no urban household could hope to enjoy milk drawn as little as four hours earlier.[38]

Printers' Ink, the advertising trade organ, backed Bennett as a champion of journalistic integrity in the matter of the Macy's ads. By its lights, the *Herald* had rightly put principle over profit in frankly reporting on "scientific drawbacks to the pasteurization idea. It declined, further, to publish commendatory notices of Mr. Straus's work." *Printers' Ink* approvingly quoted one of Bennett's editorials defending the paper's stance: "Mr. Straus, for reasons best known to himself, has come forward as a sort of Lohengrin of pasteurized milk. As the scientific world questions the value of the pasteurization process the Herald, as a duty to its readers and the general public, could not support Mr. Straus's project . . . If he thinks milk and water lectures made in Germany praising pasteurization—and incidentally Mr. Straus—can be foisted upon the American people as news, he is woefully behind the times."[39]

Straus's family and friends must literally have feared for his sanity as the American, English, and French branches of the *Herald* kept up the barrage of jeers and purported exposés. In August 1910, the New York paper announced that three scientists whom it had retained to look into milk safety had discovered shocking numbers of bacteria in some of the milk sold in the city.

By chance or design, this investigation coincided with a new effort by the Board of Health to stamp out the trade in loose milk, whether raw or pasteurized. It was no surprise to microbe sleuths that pasteurized milk was as vulnerable as raw milk—if not more so—to invasion by pathogens. Bennett's reporters managed to manipulate the facts so as to imply that the Board of Health supported the *Herald*'s opposition to pasteurized milk.

The paper had started its investigations in July, about a month before it broke the story in several lengthy front-page articles naming places where contaminated milk had been found and tabulating the three experts' bacterial counts. By now the local Straus operation had expanded to include seventeen milk depots as well as booths in public parks where milk was poured from large cans into chilled tanks and sold by the glass. The *Herald* was now giving hell to the park booths as sources of dirty milk. They were described as operating in a manner that "greatly resembles a public function"—that is, freeloading on the city by being granted park space, water for washing the equipment, and some police presence "to maintain order and keep the customers in line." In addition, the paper claimed that the booths offered unreliably refrigerated milk transferred from cans to open tanks and filled into sloppily rinsed glasses. The *Herald*'s experts stated that some of the bacterial counts were scandalously high. They had not tried to identify individual pathogens, but did report that the milk contained excessive amounts of "liquefying" bacteria, meaning varieties capable of dissolving a solid culture medium like gelatin or agar. As a class they were often considered highly dangerous or in the *Herald*'s language, "putrefactive."[40]

The Board of Health, after reviewing the evils of loose milk sold in grubby grocery stores, had recently issued an advisory that whether raw or pasteurized, it should be boiled before home use. In the reporters' spin, the board "has again called attention to the futility of pasteurization, especially when conducted in a commercial way," and implicitly endorsed the *Herald*'s own view that pasteurized milk was "biologically weakened."[41] One of the experts, the first article announced, had "demonstrated in his laboratory for the HERALD that normal bacteria where milk is relatively good destroy what objectionable germs may have been present." (Some raw-milk activists still cling to this muddled belief, which the *Herald* didn't bother to back up with specific details. The truth is more complicated; see chapters 6 and 10.) In fact, the board's action "is looked on by many persons who are interested in sanitary reform, as meaning the death knell of commercial pasteurization."[42]

The *Herald*'s coverage sometimes distinguished between the batch ("scientific") and flash ("commercial") methods of pasteurization, but more often blithely lumped all pasteurization together as a menace. Nor did it offer more than a hasty acknowledgment that the bottled pasteurized milk for babies at the Straus outlets was remarkably clean.

The Strauses were in Berlin when the New York office of the paper cabled an abbreviated version of the exposé to its Paris sibling and waited for the news to be picked up in other cities. In a few days all editions of the *Herald* were chortling over Nathan Straus's discomfiture. About two weeks later, world capitals on every continent were rocked by the announcement that he had decided to shut down his New York milk pasteurization enterprise.[43]

THE TURNING POINT

It seems unlikely that Straus was merely trying to call the paper's bluff. Given the severity of his recent breakdown and Lina's fears that he would have to give up work permanently, his family and personal physicians must have at least discussed persuading him to withdraw from further ordeals inflicted by Bennett's hatchet men. His official explanation, as published in the *New York American*, was: "I have come to this decision in order that I may not stand in the way of the further progress of the pasteurization movement, which is being hurt by personal attacks on me." To the *New York Times*, another paper in his camp, he declared that his enemies had "waited until I went away sick before they began their attacks." Annie Nason, the superintendent of the pasteurization laboratory, told the *Times* that she had learned of people buying milk at the park booths under suspicious circumstances before the *Herald*'s first article was published, apparently with the intention of doctoring test results.[44]

Straus was fond of poses struck for dramatic effect, but the decision to abandon his New York milk stations probably wasn't one of them. His bombshell announcement had come from Berlin on August 24; he stepped off the boat in New York on September 4 maintaining that he was not to be talked out of his resolve. He was perfectly willing to continue funding pasteurization efforts abroad and in other states, but his work in the hometown of the *New York Herald* was at a declared end.

The city's public health hierarchy was thrown into consternation, and for good reason. At a time when the Board of Health's entire annual budget amounted to about $2,750,000, Straus's publicist William Wirt Mills estimated that his boss was spending $250,000 a year on supplying clean milk to New York families.[45] Straus himself had been saying for years that the task really belonged in municipal hands. One inadvertent effect of James Gordon Bennett's machinations was to bring together various private and public champions of clean (not necessarily pasteurized) milk for poor children into a strong coalition united in outrage at the *Herald*'s attacks on Straus. Another was to goad the Board of Health—in defiance of the *Herald*'s rhetoric about the "death knell" of pasteurization—into taking the question of municipal responsibility for affordable safe milk more seriously.

Prominent authorities rushed to Straus's defense amid near-universal condemnation of the *Herald*'s calumnies. Dr. Ernst Lederle, the New York Health Commissioner, told the *Brooklyn Daily Eagle*, "We need more milk stations of the kind Nathan Straus has established."[46] The nation's most famous public health officer, Dr. Harvey Washington Wiley, the architect of the 1906 Pure Food and Drug Act, declared that Straus "deserves much credit for his work in the protection of humanity."[47]

Public sentiment culminated on October 8 in a great assembly at Cooper Union. Arthur Brisbane read a cablegram in which William Randolph Hearst "bitterly denounced The New York Herald and James Gordon Bennett, its owner, for their attitude toward the Straus philanthropy." A prominent rabbi summed up the meaning of Straus's work as "We are our brother's keeper, and also the keeper of our brother's baby." The organizers presented a resolution thanking Straus for having made clear to "the citizenship as a body, and Governments, municipal, State, and National . . . their duty toward the children" and for inspiring them all to carry forward his work "at the public expense, and on the widest possible scale." And, they continued in something like bended-knee desperation, "we respectfully urge and request him, even at great personal sacrifice, to continue his work."[48]

Straus relented a few weeks later, though not without reminding well-wishers who wanted to give a banquet in his honor, "I have been under the care of physicians since last winter, and have promised them and my family to accept no engagements that might involve any degree of excitement, a full year of quietude having been declared essential to the restoration of my health, which was seriously shattered by twenty years of unceasing efforts to stop the slaughter of the babies."[49] (The actual figure was seventeen.) Of course he was finally talked into attending the proposed banquet, which took place on January 31,1911, at Café Boulevard, a German-Hungarian restaurant on Second Avenue. It was not so much a vindication as a consecration.

The five hundred guests included John D. Rockefeller, John Jacob Astor, Cornelius Vanderbilt, and the Turkish ambassador. Hearst and the new governor of New York State offered congratulations in person, President Taft by telegram ("His work in improving the condition and alleviating the suffering of those less fortunate should make it a pleasure for all to unite in offering him this banquet"). The city controller recited "Build thee more stately mansions, O my soul!" Abraham Jacobi declared, "Nathan Straus did not say: 'Let the little children come to me,' but he went to the little children himself, and he has been successful in his way."[50]

Straus's speech of thanks underscored the nobility of his own work by sounding his favorite refrain as often as possible:

> I beg of you, for the sake of the babies, to sustain every effort that is being made to extend this work, for in so doing you will help to stop the killing of the babies. They can't defend themselves against the milk that kills. We can defend them by seeing that they have the milk that saves . . .
>
> I often think of the saying, 'The world is my country; to do good is my religion.' This has often been an inspiration to me. I might say, 'Humanity is my country; to save the babies is my religion.'
>
> Forget me; remember the babies.[51]

Bennett and the *Herald* had by now retired from the battlefield with only a few parting shots. The victory belonged to Straus—and more lastingly, to milk pasteurization as part of a public health agenda that members of municipal and state medical bureaucracies were finally summoning the will to carry out. The very shamelessness of Bennett's attacks had backfired, finally confirming the intended target in the role of fearless truth-teller. In fact, a few days before the Café Boulevard banquet Health Commissioner Lederle was already announcing plans for the city to open fifteen new publicly funded pasteurized-milk depots.[52]

In the next few years New York and other big cities began to enact and enforce more serious regulations requiring pasteurization of most milk sold in their jurisdictions. According to an article published in the *Journal of the American Medical Association* in 1913, roughly 5 percent of the New York milk supply had been pasteurized in 1903. The estimate for 1912 was 40 percent. A 1916 USDA bulletin put the current figure at 88 percent.[53] Though it's hard to gauge the exact reliability of these figures, the trend is clear. The first decade of Straus's milk distribution program had made about as much difference in the amount of pasteurized milk reaching the city as one man's efforts could, but something beyond private efforts had materialized and dramatically expanded thereafter.

Public health and medical spokespeople now formed a somewhat coherent body of opinion inclined to agree that the disadvantages of raw milk far outweighed any reported benefits. Sleazy, unreliable flash pasteurization was starting to fade from the picture as batch methods became more precise. Straus himself had always insisted on using certified raw milk for anything pasteurized in his laboratories, as double insurance against dirt. Popular opinion in the nation's major cities was swinging toward pasteurization as consumers came to associate it with start-to-finish maintenance of high sanitary standards.

The shift was much slower in smaller cities and towns, while states uniformly declined to enact mandatory pasteurization laws. What would eventually clinch the argument was not medical opinion but inexorable demographic change. 1920 was the first year in which the U.S. census recorded a larger number of people living in urban than rural areas, 51.4 percent to 48.6 percent.[54] The power of cities to shape public health policy beyond their own borders grew decade by decade. Raw milk consumption still thrived among farm families and in rural towns, but more and more people lived in jurisdictions where pasteurization was compulsory.

After about 1910 experts calling pasteurized milk a menace to a bamboozled public were in retreat in all large and many mid-sized population centers. The majority opinion was now that of Straus and his firm ally Jacobi: it was raw milk that deserved to be considered guilty until proved innocent—or rather, guilty *instead* of proved innocent. After Straus's triumph in the *New York Herald* affair, his attacks became still more histrionic and vehement, as well as more unquestioningly revered by the public at large.

For his part, Henry Leber Coit was just as exasperatingly obstinate in refusing to admit any rational excuse for pasteurization, even when done carefully by the best batch methods. Coit and the Medical Milk Commissions were already watching the price of certified raw milk drive away potential buyers. Rosenau had observed in 1912, "The extra price paid for certified milk is one of the cheapest forms of insurance against disease"—but the bottom line was "Pasteurization is the cheapest form of life insurance the consumer can take out." Rosenau gave the average price of certified milk as "about sixteen cents a quart," though capable of varying from twelve to twenty cents.[55] In 1916, the average price of milk (generally pasteurized) in New York City was nine cents a quart.[56]

The market share of certified raw milk was understandably tiny and waning fast when in 1914, cows in the herd of a New Jersey certified operation, the Fairfield Dairy Company, reacted positively to the tuberculin test. It was a mortifying blot on the certification program's record. The company, an Essex County-based star of the program, had been the very first dairy to produce raw milk to Coit's specifications in 1894. Still more discomfiting, Coit happened at the moment to be opposing a recommendation of pasteurized milk at a meeting of the American Association for the Study and Prevention of Infant Mortality.[57]

Alfred W. McCann, a muckraking reporter for the *New York Globe and Commercial Advertiser* who had gotten himself named the paper's "pure food expert," launched a sensational raw milk exposé.[58] Coit and the Essex County Medical Milk Commission quickly opened their own investigation, recruiting a committee of three independent and highly respected veterinarians to subject the dairy's premises and records to careful scrutiny. The committee's final conclusion was that Fairfield Dairy's owner, eager to expand the size of the operation, had bought too many cows too fast and inadvertently introduced new herd members with dubious tuberculin-test records. (An initial test could itself cause an animal to show false negatives in subsequent tests for weeks or months, so that through either guile or ignorance dealers sometimes sold cows that were only apparently nonreactive.) The new arrivals had soon gotten shifted round into different barns where they had infected healthy neighbors. The only solution—after rigorously testing the entire herd and ridding it of infected cows—was to increase the size of the herd gradually rather than hastily: by breeding unquestionably tuberculosis-free cows from the existing stock rather than buying others with possibly unreliable credentials.[59]

No actual human cases of bovine TB were traced to Fairfield Dairy's milk. Straus, however, had rushed in with guns blazing the minute he heard of the infected herd.

The *New York Herald* affair, coming after years of increasing visibility in the pasteurization cause, had helped to propel him to a place among the popular ranks of greatest living Americans. His utterances on the subject of pasteurized milk had acquired the prestige befitting scientific pronouncements, a circumstance that did not lessen his already glowing self-esteem. Scorning any pretense of fair-mindedness, he took righteous pride in damning the raw milk cause as nefarious error and its leader, Coit, as a false prophet.

On learning of the Fairfield Dairy episode, he promptly shared his shock and horror with the president of the AASPIM: "I do hope that the Association was not misled by Dr. Coit, who has long posed as the 'father of certified milk,' but who was thoroughly discredited last month. That he should cast a shadow over your Association and deliberately mar your splendid work for the babies is inexpressibly wicked." Castigating Coit's mistaken actions in prematurely reinstating Fairfield raw milk's certification after what proved to be an incomplete count of the infected animals, he raged, "*I hold that it is murder to give tuberculous milk to a baby. I am at a loss for terms to describe the crime of certifying that tuberculous milk is free from tuberculosis.*"[60]

After he had begun focusing on TB and especially during his fight with Bennett, Straus had increasingly managed to hack away any common ground that might have existed between clean-milk advocates who wanted to stop milk-borne disease through rigorous sanitary or testing protocols for raw milk and counterparts who thought pasteurization was the best solution. General discussions of raw and pasteurized milk never recovered any approach to civility or evenhandedness after about 1910 or 1915. Lost in the rancorous shuffle was the fact, clearly noted by such observers as Rosenau and North, that Coit and the certified raw milk party had made giant strides in establishing the importance of sanitary measures—rigorous cleansing of cows, milking barns, hands, equipment, and vessels; scrupulously maintained refrigeration—for *all* commercially handled milk. When Straus began distributing pasteurized milk, his original depots had worked with the best and purest starting material: raw milk produced according to Coit's certification standards. The double insurance policy that he had insisted on— approved by authorities like Jacobi, Freeman, North, and Rosenau— would become accepted operating policy for future dairy farms and milk-processing plants, though with Coit's contribution largely forgotten or (as it was by Straus) actively maligned. In fact, Straus and his medical allies soon began recommending triple insurance, as tuberculin testing and pasteurization came to be seen as mutual reinforcements instead of alternatives.

But by the time of the Fairfield scandal, Straus had already decided that the pasteurization campaign could succeed without his full-time participation and was devoting much of his energy to another cause. Always keenly interested in the Jewish homeland, he had become an ardent Zionist who hoped to see the Holy Land become a model of religious tolerance and brotherhood for Jews, Christians, and Muslims. He and Lina began diverting more and more of their remaining fortune to projects in Palestine, where the city of Netanya would eventually be named for Nathan. His emotional investment in the cause became as intense as his earlier championship of milk pasteurization.

Gradually he began to withdraw from his many pro-pasteurization involvements. In 1919 he announced that he planned to give up the remaining Straus milk depots, believing that they could now be safely turned over to municipal authorities.[61] He died in January 1931 at eighty-three, hailed by numberless admirers as compassionate humanitarianism incarnate.

Arriving in New York to deliver the principal eulogy, the Yale professor William Lyon Phelps got into a taxicab, gave the driver the address of the synagogue where the funeral was being held, and was promptly told, "He was the world's best man." Rabbi David de Sola Pool, a close Straus friend who wrote the obituary for the *American Jewish Yearbook*, quoted President Taft as having said, "Dear old Nathan Straus is a great Jew and the greatest Christian of us all." In short, he was remembered just as he wished to have been.[62]

Few if any public health allies of Straus's pasteurization ventures figured in the ranks of notable pallbearers and praise-givers who marked his passing—probably because much changing of the guard had taken place since those stirring campaigns. But his advocacy of pasteurized milk was not forgotten. He had become too deeply identified with the cause for that. Some thirty-eight years after his first milk depot opened, he remained the best-remembered public face and patron saint of milk pasteurization in America, the hero of a saga about lives snatched from the grim reaper's clutches.

LEGACY OF THE PASTEURIZATION CRUSADE: IFS, ANDS, OR BUTS

Did Straus and his pasteurization mission save millions of lives, as many accounts claimed at the time and have claimed since? The question itself contains a certain buried "When did you stop beating your wife?" fallacy.

In 1908 the popular socialist writer John Spargo, a well-known campaigner against child labor and other infamies of the era, had examined the many dimensions of the milk supply in *The Common Sense of the Milk Question*, a book dedicated to Straus "with the author's profound admiration and gratitude." It was a worthy successor to Robert Hartley's 1842 *Essay on Milk*. There was scarcely an imaginable aspect of "the milk question" that Spargo did not try to probe. He examined a deepened public awareness that children's lives *mattered*, a puzzling decline in breastfeeding and birth rates, the reasons for adopting modified cow's milk as an admittedly imperfect substitute for human milk, the scandalous conditions under which much milk was collected on farms and transported to cities, the growing field of dairy bacteriology, and much more.

Wrestling intelligently and at length with the competing claims of raw and pasteurized milk, Spargo described supporters of pasteurization as "opportunists"—meaning pragmatists—and their opponents as "radicals"—i.e., idealists. He viewed "opportunists" as quite willing to understand the "radical" point of view: "The advocates of pasteurization have no attack to make upon their rivals of the clean milk school, their only criticism being that they are holding out an ideal that is unattainable within any computable time." (This claim makes one wonder just how well Spargo really knew Nathan Straus.) On the other hand, the radicals supplied the "bulk of the criticism" and "have placed the advocates of pasteurization on the defensive" with hard-hitting objections that Spargo summarized in detail but respectfully rejected.

He urged both sides to put aside differences and focus on their common goal: eliminating the invisible but horribly concrete menaces in the milk then reaching households. "As I see it, the present situation may be likened to an outbreak of typhoid in a city, which has been traced to the water supply." The doctors surveying the situation split into the "radical" camp demanding that the city "put an end to the pollution of the water supply" and the "opportunists" who protested, "But that will take five years to accomplish," and wanted people to be instructed to boil water in the meanwhile. "In such a situation, the obvious thing to do is to adopt both plans—to urge boiling the water while the fundamental reform is being carried out." With this joining of forces, "There would be no fear that pasteurization would be regarded as a solution; no fear that the movement for better inspection [i.e., of raw milk] would be retarded."[63]

The fallacy in the comparison is also the fallacy in the "Did Straus save lives?" question. There is no universal lifelong need for milk, while the ineluctable need for H2O is something that we share with other life forms, from paramecia to redwood trees. Even limiting the focus to *Homo sapiens*, it is illogical to equate all humans' dependence on at least a minimum daily amount of water with some human infants' temporary dependence on cow's milk that they have been fed because of flawed medical reasoning.

There is no straightforward "Yes" or "No" answer to the question about saving lives because the question itself rests on skewed assumptions about the unique life-giving qualities of cow's milk. These beliefs had gotten built into thinking about child care in advanced Western societies between the beginning and end of the nineteenth century, by shaky scientific rationales. Experts telling people to instantly start boiling a city's typhoid-contaminated water would have been addressing a plain and immediate threat to every resident. Experts demanding mandatory pasteurization of all cow's milk sold in a city were addressing a complex, contradictory situation created by several generations of manufactured dietary theory that had exalted unfermented cow's milk to unprecedented economic importance and made the cow the supposed "foster mother of the human race." Placing the question in historical context: Straus and milk pasteurization saved vast numbers of lives that wouldn't have been endangered in the first place if a long succession of influential authorities hadn't decreed that fresh cow's milk was an unquestionable necessity for children. "Fresh" was taken to mean "unsoured"—that is, as we now know, full-lactose, and especially vulnerable to invasion by pathogens.

But another scenario was beginning to unfold. While urbanized America went on discovering new reasons to embrace full-lactose drinking-milk surrounded with precautions against any and all bacteria, milk in areas of settled or nomadic dairying throughout much of Asia (where people usually couldn't digest appreciable amounts of lactose) continued to display its normal behavior: It went sour under just the same bacterial conditions that had been exploited in prehistoric times.

Wherever dairy herds were untouched by modern scientific teaching, milk drawn from cows', goats', ewes', or water buffaloes' udders throughout the warmest months speedily fermented through the action of lactic acid bacteria. A substantial replacement of lactose by lactic acid would occur spontaneously at favorable ambient temperatures. But dairying peoples knew how to help it along and give the most useful bacteria a fighting chance by saving a little of one batch to inoculate freshly drawn milk, which they most often boiled before cooling to the temperature that experience had taught them best encouraged the desired fermentation.

Throughout Nathan Straus's campaigns for pasteurization, full-lactose milk's readiness to sour had been treated as a terrible liability by many laypeople and medical authorities. But curiously enough, the most recent researchers in dairy microbiology and the biochemistry of digestion (especially infant digestion) were starting to discover unforeseen virtues in lactic acid fermentation. They were developing a new respect for the fact that as noted by Sir John Sinclair in 1807, "among the nations with whom milk constitutes a chief part of their diet, it is eaten in a state of acidity" (chapter 3). In fact, sour milk was about to undergo a certain return to scientific favor. The path toward this rehabilitation had been paved by a scattering of less than scientific nineteenth-century medical reports brought back to the West by travelers in Asia.

6

SOUR MILK, BRIEFLY RETHOUGHT

After Nathan Straus had donated a model pasteurization plant to Washington, DC, as part of his campaign to bring cities on board with the cause, the district chamber of commerce commissioned a report on the state of the municipal milk supply. Published by the Government Printing Office in 1911, it presented an exhaustive survey of all the issues that American cities were then wrestling with in trying to get safe drinking-milk to consumers. One small aside in the discussion of bacterial menaces in raw milk mentioned a recently discovered fact:

> It is a matter of curious interest why sour milk and its products are considered a safe food to be consumed raw, when stale sweet milk is looked upon with suspicion. This apparent anomaly may be explained by the circumstance that, for a long time after milk is drawn, all the bacteria in it increase in number, this increase being more or less rapid and depending chiefly on the temperature at which the milk is kept, and some of these bacteria may be the kinds that produce disease. Finally, however, when milk sours the harmless lactic acid bacteria and the lactic acid which they produce tend to destroy the other microorganisms, including the disease-producing bacteria, so that by the time the milk is sour it is practically free from harmful germs.[1]

The authors of the report never returned to this throwaway comment. But that they felt obliged to mention sour milk at all shows that students of dairy chemistry and microbiology had recently come across some major surprises.

In fact, modern science was taking notice of a few exotic vogues that had begun drifting into Western Europe toward the start of what historians call the "long" nineteenth century, loosely denoting the interval between the French Revolution and World War I. The most colorful of these supposed novelties was actually a contribution of nomadic tribes on the Great Steppe of Eurasia, where it had been around for millennia.

THE KOUMISS CURE

Educated Westerners who had read the classical Greek historians recalled that more than two thousand years ago Herodotus described a strange drink prepared from mare's milk as the most treasured food of Scythian horsemen. It may have been the first fermented food to leap to fame in modern industrial societies through publicity about rediscovering primitive wisdom. The tribes of horse-raising nomads still living along the Great Steppe between the former Scythia and imperial Russia's Central Asian provinces were loosely lumped together as "Tartars" (modern spelling "Tatars"). Their chief dietary mainstay remained mare's milk, fermented much as it had been in Herodotus's time to make a prized beverage known to modern Russians as *kumys*.

At about 1779 the Scottish-born physician John Grieve took up a post as medical officer with a Russian army division. He returned to Scotland in 1784 with fervid convictions about the powers of "a wine, called by the Tartars KOUMISS," and in 1788 submitted a paper on his discovery to the Royal Society of Edinburgh.

Grieve marveled to see an elixir that "had escaped the observation of men the most skilled in chemistry" improbably being "taught us by a horde of Tartars, whose rank in society is not above that of Barbarians."[2] His Russian colleagues seemed perfectly ignorant of it. Finding little but errors in descriptions by earlier writers, he had decided to dispatch a patient from the headquarters of his division to the closest source of real information: the country of the Bashkir Tatars, on the Great Steppe just north of today's western Kazakhstan.

The chosen guinea pig, a twenty-six-year-old Russian nobleman doubly stricken by a venereal infection and a series of devastating mercury treatments, was too ill to get into his carriage unaided. He returned six weeks later in the pink of health, declaring that after just a few days of exposure to the koumiss made by his Tatar hosts, all of his symptoms had begun to melt away and "he felt as if his vessels had been distended with a fresh cooling liquor."[3] He had also managed to bring back a detailed description of how the Tatars made the astonishing substance. Grieve soon concluded that it promised to cure most ailments known to medical science.

Russian observers belatedly got around to noticing this neglected miracle drink on the empire's doorstep. Nobody else's claims quite matched the extravagance of Grieve's. But by mid-century a number of experts began pinning their hopes on koumiss as the long-sought answer to pulmonary tuberculosis. In 1858 the Russian physician N. V. Postnikov, who had seen a consumptive patient make a remarkable improvement after drinking koumiss among the Tatars, founded a sanatorium near Samara in the same general region, where the Volga River winds through steppeland on its way to the Caspian Sea.[4]

Other institutions soon sprang up nearby. Enthusiasts sought to export the vogue to Moscow and St. Petersburg, but the road was rocky. Proprietors of southern sanatoriums argued that lengthy stays in the pure air of the steppes were essential for full recovery. Hopeful entrepreneurs close to the northern cities found that Tatar mares not only were unsuited to the local climate but repelled attempts by non-Tatars to milk them like dairy cows. Even under the best conditions, they gave milk in incredibly tiny amounts compared to cows or goats. And like the cows pictured with calves in Egyptian tomb paintings or Sumerian wall friezes, they refused to give it at all unless the foal were there to take a first drink and stimulate the letdown reflex.

Then there was the matter of milk chemistry, still only half-understood. Mare's milk contains much less casein and fat than that of cows and other ruminants. In fact, it is useless for making cheese or butter. On the other hand, it has far more lactose—so much that in the unfermented state, it causes even more digestive distress than usual dairy animals' milk to people who undergo the usual shutdown of lactase production during childhood. In fact, some people who can easily tolerate the lactose in cow's milk find mare's milk strongly laxative. (This is also true of ass's milk, notwithstanding the fact that for centuries it was thought to be especially digestible.) But when mare's milk is allowed to sit for any length of time in summer heat, the extra lactose also has the effect of encouraging fermentation by sugar-digesting yeasts along with the lactic acid bacteria that ferment other kinds of soured milk, giving koumiss enough alcohol and carbon dioxide to sustain comparisons (by quixotic enthusiasts) with sparkling wine.

Since producing true koumiss was impossible anywhere other than the Tatar grasslands, attempts to concoct simulations from modified cow's milk blossomed in Russia and soon spread elsewhere. News of koumiss's extraordinary properties traveled back to other parts of Europe and into the American medical press. In 1871 Dr. Victor Jagielski, a German subject living in London, obtained both British and U.S. patents for an ersatz koumiss made from cow's milk: after removing the butterfat and diluting the casein content with either water or whey, he added yeast and cane sugar or "grape sugar" (glucose) and let the mixture ferment until effervescent. He began manufacturing it in several bottled versions differing in degree of effervescence (those with the most CO_2 had to be sold in champagne bottles and uncorked with great care) while promoting the product through both reports to medical societies and advertisements placed in medical journals. By his account, koumiss was one of the sovereign elixirs yet discovered—a sure remedy for pulmonary tuberculosis but also excellent for various ailments from scurvy to "nervous debility." It was particularly to be recommended in cases of "wasting" diseases, meaning those accompanied by drastic weight loss.[5]

THE WHITE HOUSE PUBLICITY BOOST

In a few years American medical journals had picked up reports on Jagielski's cure-all from publications such as *The Lancet*, and scattered experiments with marketable cow's milk koumiss were being made by American physicians and druggists. Their golden opportunity began on the morning of July 2, 1881, not quite four months into President James A. Garfield's first and only term.

Garfield had just walked into the Baltimore and Potomac train station in Washington, DC, meaning to travel to western Massachusetts and the New Jersey shore. A few minutes later, two shots from a pocket revolver blasted through the station noise and Garfield lay bleeding on the floor with a bullet lodged close to his spine. All members of the presidential party rushed to his aid until a handful of physicians could be summoned. The deranged shooter, Charles L. Guiteau, was seized while trying to escape. Garfield was carried back to the White House.[6]

By now Pasteur's and Lister's warnings about preventing germs from entering open wounds had received considerable coverage in American medical literature. But the team attending Garfield had only half-absorbed any principles of germ theory or antisepsis. The first doctor on the scene started probing the site of the wound with unwashed hands. The colleague who officiously took charge of the case, Dr. Doctor (his given name) Wilbur Bliss, supervised an endless series of semibotched operations to search for the lodged bullet, insert drainage tubes, and remove bone fragments with only fitful, inconsistent attention to a measure or two like putting carbolic acid on dressings. His patient, or victim, rallied remarkably until late July, when signs of massive systemic infection (initially waved off by Bliss) developed and inexorably progressed for nearly two months. Garfield died on September 19. Guiteau, a frustrated office-seeker who soon found himself convicted of murder, was not alone in avouching that the doctors bore at least as much blame as the bullet.

During part of his long ordeal Garfield was given the newfangled remedy koumiss. We know this because scores of newspaper reporters converged on the White House immediately after the shooting and started asking for reports on the president's condition. The Bliss team set up a schedule of news bulletins including such data as the patient's temperature and pulse at certain hours of the day, the medicines most recently administered, and what food or drink he had been able to take. On July 27, three and a half weeks after the assault, "four ounces of koumiss" appeared in the official briefing.[7]

The timing is significant. From the beginning Garfield had suffered frequent nausea and vomiting. But he had mostly been free of fever, and though rapidly losing weight had been able to eat some solid food. On July 22 and 23, his temperature spiked and the doctors tried switching to a mostly liquid diet. At least one of the team must have been following reports of koumiss's efficacy against fever and inflammation, excessive vomiting, and emaciation. Garfield was fed several ounces of koumiss—undoubtedly some cow's-milk version from a pharmacist—once or more a day from July 27 to August 23, when it was clear that no treatment was working.

No amount of the supposed cure-all could have saved anyone from catastrophic septicemia. But for thousands of newspaper readers, the effect of seeing the word "koumiss" in print every day for nearly four weeks was galvanizing. Even before Garfield had mercifully been released, *The Scientific American* felt obliged to publish some account of the suddenly famous remedy. The brief description concluded, "A few days since the news was flashed over the country that koumiss had been recommended in President Garfield's case, and that a supply of it had been forwarded for his use. Koumiss has accordingly become a subject of extensive inquiry, and thus has originated the present article."[8]

Garfield's doctors had helped give koumiss the aura of an ancient, exotic restorative scientifically validated by modern experts—the first form of fermented milk to acquire such a reputation in the United States. Drugstores hastened to announce that they could supply it. Newspapers printed formulas for making and bottling it at home. The undertaking was fraught with surprises, given the powerful pressure of CO_2 that built up in the bottles during fermentation. One who cautiously took up the challenge in February 1882 was the Reverend Joseph Hopkins Twichell, a close friend and neighbor of Mark Twain's. Twichell had procured a bottle of koumiss for his sick wife to try and wrote to Twain that she had enjoyed it—"i.e. *the little of it we succeeded in saving.* The most of it is on the wall, and in [Twichell's four-year-old son] Burton's hair—who, or which happened to get in the way." The Twichells were in the midst of trying to make up a fresh batch. Twain, apparently familiar with the erupting-bottle problem, advised, "Now there is no sense in *all* people being idiots: take a big 2-quart pickle-jar, up-end your Koomis [*sic*] bottle, & uncork *downwards* into that. Then you'll save it all."[9]

Within a few years American cookbook authors were presenting recipes for koumiss (or "koumys" or "kumis") as either an addition to an invalid diet or a beverage of general interest. The usual idea was to combine fresh cow's milk with a little pre-dissolved yeast and sugar and fill the mixture into bottles before setting it away to ferment in a cool place for several days. As Mary F. Henderson's *Diet for the Sick* (1885) explained in eight painstaking pages with detailed line drawings, there was more to the story, "for if one's life or the roof of the house is regarded of value, a bottle of koumiss should not be opened without a champagne-tap."[10] Fannie Farmer provided a perfunctory formula in *The Boston Cooking-School Cook Book* (1896); a slightly more systematic version in her *Food and Cookery for the Sick and Convalescent* (1904) observed, "Koumiss is often retained by those suffering from severe gastric trouble and gives variety for fever patients."[11]

The American infatuation with koumiss was short-lived. But it points to a gradual reshuffling of medical thinking about fermented foods—and the marketing opportunities they might present—during the late nineteenth-century rise of microbiology. At the outset, scientists of the generation directly taught by Pasteur and Koch were still wrestling with the relationship between bacteria and enzymes like those in the digestive tract, which some people still loosely called "ferments." (It took some time to establish that fermenting bacteria worked by secreting their own enzymes to break down complex molecules.) But researchers were making rapid strides in both studying the chemical makeup of foods and differentiating the kinds of harmful or useful organisms that colonized them. Sensing a more favorable climate, emigrants from the Middle East and southeastern Europe began vigorously promoting their own versions of fermented milk in the West, especially the United States and France. These novelties had the advantage of having originally been made with ruminants' milk instead of the virtually unobtainable horse's milk. Today they collectively go by the name "yogurt" in the industrialized West.

THE ARRIVAL OF YOGURT

Members of the yogurt clan can be broadly distinguished from North European versions of sour "buttermilk" or sour cream by the temperature preferences of the fermenting lactic acid bacteria. Typical daytime summer temperatures in most of the area that I think of as Yogurtistan commonly reach 95°F–115°F/35°C–46°C. But until the recent acceleration of global warming, the shorter summers of the Baltic and North Sea countries rarely got much hotter than 80°F/27°C. Roughly speaking, the usual fermenting organisms that naturally frequent places in the latitudes of Baghdad or Riyadh are classified as *thermophilic*, meaning that they work best in the range of 104°F–113°F/40°C–45°C, compared with 70°F–85°F/21°C–29°C for their *mesophilic* counterparts in northerly latitudes. Thermophiles act more quickly than mesophiles and produce stronger acidity. Though there are regions where the two overlap, the first English travelers to encounter yogurt in Turkey or the Arab lands would have found the flavor unfamiliar.

A solitary seventeenth-century English mention of the word occurs in "The Grand Signiors Serraglio: written by Master Robert Withers," which takes up some eighty pages in *Hakluytus Posthumus*, Samuel Purchas's vast 1625 collection of travelers' narratives. The otherwise unknown Withers notes that the Turks of Constantinople scarcely eat milk "except it bee made sower, which they call Yoghurd, for that it being so turned sower it doth quench the thirst; and of that both they and the Christians doe eate a great quantitie."[12]

Somewhat later a lively stream of books and illustrated magazines fed a more modern British and American appetite for accounts of exotic travel, sparking interest in the same substance. Western visitors to Turkey and neighboring fiefdoms of the Ottoman Empire had already happily taken to *yaourt* or the Arab equivalent, *laban* or *leban*. In 1799 William Eton, a former British consul in several Middle Eastern posts, tried to convey an idea of how people prepared it by inoculating milk with a bit of an old batch. "In a few hours, more or less, according to the temperature of the air, it becomes curdled of a uniform consistence, and of a most pleasant acid." It could also be dried out and reconstituted with water to make "a fine cooling food or drink, of excellent service in fevers of the inflammatory or putrid kind . . . Fresh yaourt is a great article of food among the natives, and Europeans soon become fond of it . . . [Local people] give no rational account how it was first made; some of them told me an angel taught Abraham how to make it, and others, that an angel brought a pot of it to Hagar, which was the first yaourt (or leban)." Eton was enthusiastic enough to provide a recipe in a footnote.[13]

(Here I should note that "yaourt" certainly is a better way of spelling the Turkish word *yoğurt* in English than "yogurt" pronounced with a hard "g." In the modern Turkish alphabet, the "ğ" in "yoğurt" is silent but indicates that the preceding vowel is prolonged, producing something close to "yawwhhrt." Incidentally, when Withers and Eton encountered the ubiquitous sour milk in Constantinople, they would have been trying to transliterate the word from the Arabic alphabet, since the revised Latin alphabet introduced by Kemal Atatürk wasn't officially adopted until 1929.)

The English physician J. Griffiths, who in 1805 published an account of a long excursion made some twenty years earlier, had found yaourt a blessing: "In travelling, it frequently happens that no other [food] can be procured; and after being accustomed to it for a little time, Europeans eat it with great pleasure; it has often been my only support for many days together."[14] Later English sightseers regularly described it as deliciously thirst-quenching. A section about practical preliminaries in an 1840 handbook for English tourists in "the East" observed, "*Yaourt*, a thick sour milk, will be found refreshing after a journey. It is sold in all the towns and villages."[15] Though its pathogen-inhibiting effects were still to be recognized, it also undoubtedly was much safer to drink or eat than the fresh unfermented milk that English people often expected when Middle Eastern tourism became more programmed to their wants. An 1895 travel guide from the same London publisher explained that milk from some dairy animal or other might have to be ordered in advance, and that "the native custom is to boil it as soon as procured," before offering lukewarm recommendations of the fermented alternatives.[16]

Inspired by the koumiss vogue, entrepreneurs from the lands of yogurt began producing it (though not under that name) in the United States. Armenians from the Ottoman Empire got in the first claims, with Dr. Markar Gevork Dadirrian (who some years earlier had earned a medical degree in New York) a nose ahead of the competition. He settled permanently in New York in 1884, while koumiss was still going strong. In 1885 he began manufacturing and selling *matzoon* or *madzoon*, a word utterly unknown to non-Armenians, as a remedy of vast powers. His public relations launch began with a speech to the New York Academy of Medicine describing matzoon as "fermented cow's milk," universally known in all Eastern regions. "It is made in every house, and ordinary milk is not at all used as an article of diet." Its virtues included being "highly nutritious," "an antidote for all kinds of poisoning," "a prophylactic during every epidemic," "a panacea in all acute febrile diseases," and useful against "impaired digestion and for chest troubles." As an added sales advantage, it was "more savory than koumiss."[17]

Dadirrian produced the marvelous remedy for retail sale in bottles, as well as supplying the starter ferment to druggists who could then make up orders for customers. By 1890 he had progressed to claiming that matzoon was not only effective against anything from "Cholera Infantum" (i.e., "summer complaint") and diabetes to nervous exhaustion and seasickness, but "both more palatable and effective than *Kumyss*."[18] The only flies in the ointment were other Armenians who had started selling rival versions. A series of court battles began in 1895, centering on the exact meaning of the term "matzoon" and whether Dadirrian had the exclusive right to use it as a trade name. After an unfavorable verdict in the federal courts, he dodged the problem by registering "Zoolak" as a trade name prominently displayed on his matzoon labels. Later, however, he got the New York state courts to enjoin competitors from calling their product "matzoon" when a judge—not burdened with any knowledge of Armenian, and apparently too busy to question anyone else who spoke the language—bought Dadirrian's argument that the name was "a fanciful designation," coined by his own imaginative flair with only an airy nod to any vaguely similar word in his native tongue.[19]

The judicial dupe had stumbled over one of the greatest barriers to the understanding of cultured sour milk in the modern West: a Babel of unintelligible names. All the non-European regions where fermented milk has been at home since the Late Stone Age used some non-Latin alphabet—chiefly Arabic, but among others Amharic, Armenian, Cyrillic, Georgian, and Sanskrit—that can be only clumsily transliterated for English-speakers. Koumiss, first "discovered" by Western enthusiasts who had lived in imperial Russia and published English-language tributes, had gotten a half-accidental American visa through the case of President Garfield and had been doctored into something far removed from the essential staple of horse-riding steppe nomads.

Some people conflated it with another Russian or "Oriental" mystery called "kefir" or "kephir." The misunderstanding remains to this day. The active agent of true kefir is a "SCOBY," or "symbiotic culture of bacteria and yeasts," that forms whitish or light beige clumps faintly resembling misshapen cauliflower florets; it ferments milk into a sour, slightly alcoholic, slightly carbonated beverage with a great vogue among Russians. But since there is no federal standard of identity requiring the use of specifically named fermenting organisms in any commercial version of cultured milk, products cultured by any sort of lactic acid bacteria or yeasts can be labeled "koumiss" or "kefir" without penalties for misrepresentation.

The combination of foreign concepts and foreign writing systems left various kinds of sour milk open to limitless misinterpretations. "Matzoon" was the commonest way of transliterating the Armenian word for a product that was indeed "made in every house" in the old country. But it could also be rendered as "madzoon," "maadzoon," "matsoun," and other permutations. Similar versions of the "laban" universally known throughout all Arabic-speaking countries might be marketed under the transliterations "leben," "lebben," and so forth. In fact, Dadirrian had originally claimed to be making this along with matzoon, without explaining how the two differed; one defendant whom he tried to sue for trade name infringement quickly renamed his matzoon "lebben."[20]

American consumers who tried the exotic new sour milk products don't seem to have exclaimed over the delicious, refreshing qualities that converted Western travelers in the Middle East. Of course, thirsty tourists might have found any offered beverage an answer to prayer after all-day treks through arid regions. But in all probability much of their pleasure in yaourt and its near relatives reflected the fact that it came from extremely flavorful milk. The unimproved local dairy animals, which had little if any access to lush green meadows, gave milk that was scanty but concentrated, untouched by the management practices that were gaining favor with Western dairy farmers. Another advantage lay in the source of milk fermentation throughout Turkey, Persia, and the Arab lands: large, intricate, diverse communities of microorganisms that thrived in very hot weather and produced subtle complexities of flavor. Transplanting southeast European and Middle Eastern yogurt traditions to other regions—convincing Western consumers that it would taste good on its own regardless of health food publicity and without copious doses of added sugar—is hampered even today by the difficulty of reproducing such conditions.

THE STUDY OF "BACTERIOLOGICAL STRUGGLES"

Dubious medical claims or out-and-out quackery powered the early growth of koumiss and matzoon/laban in the modern West. At the same time, genuine research on milk-fermenting bacteria was taking shape in European and U.S. laboratories. Advances in microscopes and imaging techniques rapidly gave bacteriologists the tools to identify various microorganisms that could live in milk and pick out ones that caused it to sour.

Despite the new fermented milk fads, the most zealous proponents of safe drinking-milk (whether raw or pasteurized) still viewed ordinary milk that went sour in time-honored fashion as a menace. But in 1901 two bacteriologists at the Storrs, Connecticut, Agricultural Experiment Station published the results of a yearlong study that stood that assumption on its head. Herbert W. Conn and William M. Esten had been growing curious about exactly what set off the souring process. They described milk drawn from the cow into the outside world as the site of "an intense bacteriological struggle"[21]—a penetrating Darwinian insight that was also occurring to French and German counterparts. Researchers were learning to view populations of different bacteria as competitors in perpetual battles for existence. Like herds of different animal species moving into new terrains, the organisms that invaded raw milk had to adjust to the conditions in which it was being held and start reproducing in competition with each other.

Through repeated experiments, Conn and Esten found that lactic acid bacteria (LAB) in raw milk consistently got the upper hand from a fairly early stage and continued growing in numbers until they had virtually crowded out other communities. In the authors' opinion, "the lactic bacteria, so far from being a detriment to the wholesomeness of the milk, are really advantageous. It is true that they cause the milk to sour if they become too abundant; but the acid that they produce in milk protects the milk from other fermentations which are probably more injurious." In fact, "much of the diarrhoeal disturbance in children is due to the putrefactive fermentation of milk" during digestion, and "the milk is protected from the action of putrefactive bacteria by the rapid development of the lactic bacteria."[22]

The article attracted little notice from the chief parties in the pasteurization wars—pediatricians, public health policy wonks, and the mainstream drinking-milk industry. But the logic of the idea was quickly convincing dairy bacteriologists without political axes to grind. The *New York Herald*'s comments on "normal" bacteria in raw milk being able to destroy "objectionable germs" (chapter 5) probably were a garbled version of the main argument being advanced by Conn and Esten along with many colleagues. The paragraph about the "apparent anomaly" of safe soured raw milk in the 1911 District of Columbia report more accurately reflects a scientific consensus that still broadly holds more than a century later: raw milk's propensity for souring at middling or warm ambient temperatures offers a generally strong protection against many agents of milk-borne disease. (As will be discussed in chapter 9, raw milk that is kept from souring through refrigeration is another story.)

The study of LAB expanded astonishingly, with discoveries of new species being announced every year. Here I should note that family-genus-species taxonomy according to the eighteenth-century Linnaean system presented messy obstacles for classifying microorganisms, especially as microscopy became more sophisticated and variant strains were added to family trees. For this reason, the official scientific names of all organisms mentioned in this chapter were eventually revised or discarded; replacements will be introduced as necessary.

THE INTESTINAL MICROFLORA: A NEW FIELD OF EXPLORATION

While LAB in milk came under new scrutiny, the complementary discipline of intestinal microbiology was providing unforeseen insights into infant digestion of milk. Nobody as yet suspected the role that widespread differences between infant and adult lactase production played in the case. But researchers were combing through the contents of human digestive tracts like '49ers panning for gold.

In 1885 the Austrian Theodor Escherich began publishing his findings on a microorganism so ubiquitous at the far end of the gut that he dubbed it *Bacillus coli communis* or *Bacterium coli commune*, the common bacillus (or bacterium) of the colon. In fact, it would become the most versatile, most useful of all bacteria for laboratory research. It proved to have so many variant strains—both harmless and virulent—that after it had been renamed in his honor decades later, a pair of genetic researchers wisecracked, "It is a truth universally acknowledged that there are only two types of bacteria. One is *Escherichia coli*, the others are not."[23]

Escherich was both an experimental bacteriologist and a practicing pediatrician at a time when not many original researchers combined those specialties. He was able to demonstrate that his "common" bacillus formed large (in fact, dominating) populations in infants' colons. He had grasped that these colonies were bound up with the physiology of digestion as food underwent its final breakdown before leaving the system. He was also interested in the effect of diet on children's digestions, and—a century before anybody coined the term "microbiome"— had developed a strong belief that plain breast milk produced a very different bacteriological flora in the gut of a nursing infant from formulas based on cow's milk.[24]

This perception was soon borne out in the work of Ernst Moro, another pediatrician-bacteriologist whose path had crossed Escherich's at the University of Graz (Austria). In 1899 he isolated a strange bacillus from the stools of breastfed babies and pointed to the even stranger fact that he hadn't found it in the stools of either their formula-fed counterparts or adults. It could be propagated in the laboratory, but only in a culture medium replicating the strongly acidic conditions of the colon. In recognition of this distinctive preference, he named it *Bacillus acidophilus*.[25] Moro's research was published in time for the Frenchman Henry Tissier, then working at the Pasteur Institute in Paris, to note the *B. acidophilus* discovery and add that he had concomitantly found what he considered a second, more important organism unique to the stools of infants fed only on breast milk. He had named it *Bacillus bifidus*, from its characteristic forked shape.[26]

Moro and Tissier did not at once know it, but they had stumbled on the foundations of something long afterward labeled probiotic therapy.

Continuing his work with infant digestion, Tissier decided that the presence of *B. bifidus* was the distinguishing mark of a healthy baby's colonic flora. A few years after his paper identifying *B. bifidus*, he proposed that digestive disturbances like severe diarrhea in infants might indicate that the gut flora had been overwhelmed by an occupying army of pathogens and needed to be restored to their proper bacteriological balance. His suggested treatment was to stop any feeding of cow's milk and give the patient nothing but a clear liquid diet containing carbohydrates like glucose or lactose, while also administering a pure culture of another LAB that Pasteur Institute researchers knew as *Bacillus acidiparalactici* or *B. paralacticus*. He suspected that some other undetected organism had suppressed *B. bifidus* in the colon, as indicated by its absence in the stools. As he had hoped, the second LAB counteracted the invader. *B bifidus* reappeared after a week or so of the therapeutic regimen, signaling renewed gut health.[27]

Tissier's suggestion that enteric pathogens could derange the system fitted well with a much-discussed theory of "autointoxication," or self-poisoning, recently introduced by the French pathologist Charles Bouchard. The gist of the idea was that when the digestive system—specifically, the colon—didn't do a proper job of eliminating the waste products of digestion, these were attacked by putrefying bacteria and released a slow but eventually threatening flow of dangerous toxins into the bloodstream. Any organ from the kidneys to the brain might be slowly poisoned by this process.[28]

One of those who had been greatly struck by Bouchard's autointoxication theory was the deputy director of the Pasteur Institute, Élie (Ilya) Metchnikoff or Metchnikov, a researcher of many interests. Among other achievements, he had conducted groundbreaking experiments on what we now call immune responses in a number of different species. Musing about autointoxication and digestive anatomy, Metchnikoff had been drawn to a recent theory that the mammalian colon with its toxic potential was a terrible evolutionary error. He estimated that it slashed optimal human life expectancy by some seventy or more years.

Metchnikoff, who came from the Ukrainian-Belorussian region formerly known as "Little Russia" and called himself a "son of the steppes,"[29] was gradually evolving a set of beliefs linking the diet of some hardy Old World peoples with popular reports of their great longevity. One thing these communities seemed to have in common was a pronounced fondness for versions of sour milk. Tissier's use of a lactic acid bacillus to fight an infection in a baby's colon dovetailed neatly with Metchnikoff's growing conviction that the way to repel life-shortening enteric pathogens was to maintain strongly acidic conditions in the lower digestive tract.

Léon Massol, a colleague who had moved from the Pasteur Institute to a Swiss medical laboratory, put him in touch with a younger Bulgarian-born subordinate named Stamen Grigoroff or Grigorov, who had brought some sour milk from home and studied it under his microscope in Geneva. Grigorov's findings appeared in the *Revue médicale de la Suisse romande* as "Study of an edible fermented milk: The 'Kissélo-mléko' [sour milk] of Bulgaria" (*Étude sur un lait fermenté comestible. Le 'Kissélo-mléko' de Bulgarie*). He found this mainstay of Bulgarian peasants to be teeming with different kinds of organisms. Eventually he was able to isolate and culture three, each of which seemed capable of fermenting sterile milk (sterility was important to avoid accidentally introducing extraneous microbes) to pronounced sourness and thickness. He didn't try to assign them scientific names beyond the loose generic pigeonholes of "Bacillus A," "Micrococcus B," and "Streptobacillus C."[30]

Metchnikoff probably had access to Grigorov's research before it was published in 1905. But it is difficult to sort out what happened next from a tangle of later fictions. The one certainty is that Massol managed to procure some of Grigorov's Bulgarian sour milk for Metchnikoff. Analyzing it in his laboratory at the Pasteur Institute, Metchnikoff decided that "Bacillus A" was the crucial fermenting principle. He named it "bacille bulgaire" or *Bacillus bulgaricus*, in honor of the discoverer as well as rural Bulgaria's reported track record in the longevity department.[31]

Metchnikoff's arguments about extending the human life span, sprinkled with startling extrapolations from his genuinely pioneering immunological research, had already received sensational coverage in newspapers on every continent. By 1900, he had become a bona fide celebrity, notwithstanding his discomfort with some journalistic maulings of his scientific beliefs. *B. bulgaricus* promptly got dragged into the spotlight. Metchnikoff propagated a pure culture of it in the laboratory, used this to inoculate milk, and declared to the news media in 1905 that the resulting ferment offered useful protection against life-shortening autointoxication.

For some reason he decided to ignore the Bulgarian name and call his scientifically fermented milk "yahourthe," a phonetic French transcription of the Turkish name. He also insisted on starting with pasteurized milk, partly in order to avoid accidental brushes with rival bacteria but also because his dietary beliefs included a fanatical opposition to eating or even touching any kind of raw food.[32]. His new brainchild at once achieved cult status in France. After a brief flirtation with "yaghurt," British and American writers began spelling the name (respectively) "yoghurt" and "yogurt."

Many minds naturally raced ahead to the advertising opportunities of a food promising something like Old Testament life spans. Metchnikoff, to his credit, always tried to play down the more preposterous claims for yogurt's powers. He was content to argue that great longevity was a fact among some hardy, plain-living mountain and steppe tribes who used sour milk as an everyday staple, and that a major reason must be the therapeutic effect of *B. bulgaricus* in occupying the colon and driving out toxin-producing microbes. But he did agree to endorse a hopeful startup calling itself "La Société Le Ferment" that soon began selling a version of milk soured with *B. bulgaricus* as "Lactobacilline." (Dairy bacteriologists were already thinking about regrouping a few dozen LAB under the genus "Lactobacillus.") The culture could be furnished to pharmacists, but the company also sold it as desiccated starters in tablet or powder form that retail customers could order for making their own yogurt.[33]

Le Ferment rapidly established overseas branches in England and the United States (where the product became "Bacillac"). Rivals immediately claimed their own slices of the pie. In New York, the ever-ambitious Markar Dadirrian began advertising his Zoolak with the magic words, "Claimed by Prof. Metchnikoff to be the ELIXIR OF LIFE and that by drinking freely of this nourishing beverage life will be greatly prolonged."[34] Newspaper coverage soon spread from coast to coast, with eager attention to the fabled longevity of Bulgarian peasants.

It now dawned on many bacteriologists that peoples from Persia to Mongolia, South Africa to India had long been exploiting bacterially soured milk to an extent only narrowly reflected in Bulgarian kissélo mléko, matzoon, laban, and yogurt. Searches for information became broader as well as more carefully focused. Western-trained scientists in many parts of the non-Western world began analyzing specimens of their own local favorites under the microscope and preparing scientific papers on the fermenting organisms.

The growth of knowledge, however, was hampered by an understandable tendency to think that the most important organisms were the ones easiest to identify and grow in the laboratory, like useful crops being spotted and rescued from patches of weeds for intensive cultivation. This was indeed the quickest means of preparing articles for commercial sale—though as researchers would eventually understand, a superficial means liable to misunderstandings. With the best of intentions, Metchnikoff had made some large blunders.

Colleagues might have raised objections to his *B. bulgaricus* theory sooner if he hadn't been chosen to share the 1908 Nobel Prize in the category "physiology or medicine." The achievement for which he was cited was his much earlier work on immune defenses and phagocytes (which belong to the general category of scavenger cells). To the lay public the prize seemed to confirm that Metchnikoff knew what he was talking about when he exhorted people to eat Bulgarian yogurt. But in fact, he had never done original research on milk fermentation or LAB, and had been over-quick to seize on what he thought was the only really crucial agent in Grigorov's sour milk.

His most mistaken idea was that *B. bulgaricus* taken by mouth could get past chemical barriers in the stomach and small intestine, travel to the colon, and form sizable permanent communities there. Students of digestive microbiology repeatedly failed to find evidence backing up this claim and launched serious challenges to it after Metchnikoff's death in 1916. Leo F. Rettger, a bacteriologist at Yale University, had addressed himself to the question several times before teaming up with his Yale colleague Walter L. Kulp in 1924 to write an article decisively proving that *B. bulgaricus* was knocked out by digestive acids in the foregut and never became established in the colon.[35]

This finding took much of the shine off *B. bulgaricus's* stardom. But Rettger was ready with a successor. He successfully demonstrated that *B. acidophilus*, which Moro had discovered in infants' stools, could make its way from mouth to colon as Metchnikoff had claimed for

B. bulgaricus. So, indeed, could Tissier's *B. bifidus*—but Rettger saw more potential in the Moro discovery. In the early 1920s he began trumpeting the virtues of "acidophilus milk" as a cure for both constipation and diarrhea.[36]

Neither Metchnikoff nor Rettger had any interest in the *taste* of a supposedly therapeutic sour milk. For both of them, the point was simply to find an organism that would keep a highly acidic environment going in the colon. Stamen Grigorov, however, had actually grown up eating kissélo mléko. He described how Bulgarian peasants fermented it from *podkvassa* (home-prepared starter) and wrapped the inoculating pot in furs to protect it from cold. He had worked carefully to ascertain that each of the three organisms he had isolated took a shorter or longer time to coagulate milk at a given temperature, showed a greater or lesser ability to tolerate certain maximum temperatures, and created greater or lesser acidity in fermentation. All three, with their individual qualities, participated in composing the final kissélo mléko. Metchnikoff had chosen "Bacillus A" for his bacterial poster child simply because Grigorov had found it to go on producing acid longer than the others—in fact, it made milk inedibly sour when allowed to ferment for four days.[37]

Grigorov knew that the flavor of milk soured only by one or another of his three organisms was respectively less or more acid than real kissélo mléko made from a true podkvassa. Metchnikoff and Rettger, however, were unequipped to think of sour milk as a pleasurable food in its own right instead of a remedy for some presumed physical failure. Consequently, neither Metchnikoff's Bulgarian yogurt nor acidophilus milk prepared by Rettger's standards was anything like the real Bulgarian kissélo mléko, the delightfully refreshing yaourt praised by earlier Western travelers in Turkey, or matzoon and laban as known in Armenia and the Arab lands. The traditional fermented foods had a mellow balance of flavors resulting from interactions among many different bacteria. The two scientists' purported cures were uncompromisingly sour; when Metchnikoff's longevity-promising "yaghurt" made it to the United States in 1905, a quip in various newspapers announced that someone who had tasted it "says he would prefer to die young."[38]

Manufacturers who actually knew something about the sour milks of the Balkans and points east soon understood that the broad principle behind authentic versions was feedback between different organisms that fermented lactose in subtly different ways, rather than the unaided operation of *B. bulgaricus*. Today the process of ordinary commercial yogurt fermentation begins with the bacterial twosome now officially known *as Lactobacillus delbrueckii* subsp. *bulgaricus* (Grigorov's "Bacillus A," Metchnikoff's *B. bulgaricus*) and *Streptococcus salivarius* subsp. *thermophilus* (almost certainly Grigorov's "Micrococcus B"). Most people streamline the names to *L. bulgaricus* and *S. thermophilus*. The usual procedure is to heat milk to about 180°F/82°C and allow it to cool to 108°F–110°F/42°C–43°C. It is then inoculated with pure cultures of the two organisms and maintained for some hours at the inoculating temperature. Microbial lactase directly secreted by *L. bulgaricus* and *S. thermophilus* is responsible for converting large amounts of the original lactose to lactic acid.

S. *thermophilus* gets to work first, soon producing enough lactic acid to create conditions inhibiting to its own further growth and more friendly to *L. bulgaricus*, which now grows vigorously and continues to lower the pH until it has used up most of the lactose. When they operate together, *S. thermophilus* contributes some of the more delicate aromatic notes of yogurt, *L. bulgaricus* a pleasant, clean, non-overwhelming acidity.[39] There is another wrinkle that was recognized much later: though fermentation of commercial yogurt stops before all of the original lactose has been converted to lactic acid, enough of the two LAB survive transit through the stomach and duodenum to digest most of the remaining lactose in the small intestine. For this reason, all but a tiny fraction of lactose-intolerant people can easily digest yogurt containing live *S. thermophilus* and *L. bulgaricus* cultures.[40]

This two-bacteria scenario produces a far more enjoyable yogurt than the medically oriented monocultures of Metchnikoff and Rettger. Still, it is the product of a mentality that expects pure cultures propagated under strict laboratory conditions to yield uniform results time after time. The trouble with this assumption is that pure cultures of particular organisms don't exist in nature, where any one species is constantly engaged in Conn and Esten's "intense bacteriological struggle."

Trying to keep any one kind of microbe pure is a high-tech effort that involves maintaining it in solitary confinement while keeping watch against both submicroscopic enemies and chance mutations. Clearly these precautions are desirable in producing cultures for many medical uses. And where commercially fermented foods are concerned, undeviatingly uniform results from laboratory-propagated bacteria have the advantage of supporting brand names' market stability. But cultures like those that once populated the podkvassa in Bulgarian peasants' households, as well as kindred starters in millions of households from the Balkans to Mongolia, are quite another proposition. For stability over time amid perpetual bacteriological contests, they depend on the opposite of solitary confinement.

A hundred-plus years after the first post-Metchnikoff flowering of LAB research, bacteriologists recognize that the numbers of identifiable microbes living on this planet are beyond computing. The great majority stubbornly resist being cultured, visualized, and counted in laboratory conditions—meaning that they exist but decline to be interviewed and registered by census-takers. (Genome sequencing is only now starting to fill in some of the gaps in taxonomy based on standard plate counts.) The same would be true even if we limited the field to microbes on a few square inches of human skin—or on one of the carefully wrapped-up handkerchiefs that women coming to the United States from yogurt bastions like the Balkans, Turkey, Syria, or Armenia used to pack with their belongings. They were living legacies.

Before starting on the journey, a housewife would thoroughly soak the handkerchief in a batch of yogurt and dry it out for carrying in safety. Once the new kitchen was set up, the cloth would be soaked in milk to revitalize the family equivalent of podkvassa—a unique starter culture, an irreproducible microbial community with hundreds of times more members than could be fully identified even today with the aid of advanced genomic technology. No one home starter was identical to another. Each harbored humble cousins of pure laboratory-propagated *S. thermophilus* and *L. bulgaricus* strains that maintained their identity not in spite of but *because of* living alongside hundreds of other LAB species—probably also including some stray yeasts and unrelated organisms—in a complex bacteriological ecosystem that was kept in balance by its very diversity. Each had its own flavor nuances that could be recognized and knowledgeably praised or criticized by neighbors and family members in yogurt-making, yogurt-eating societies.[41]

In fact, the podkvassa that Grigorov knew in Bulgaria undoubtedly contained an astonishing multitude of different organisms. That he was able to isolate and culture only three meant not that only three existed but that the vast majority were undetectable by extant technology (many probably still are).

Contemporary fans of homemade yogurt who begin by using a little of some commercial brand as their starter usually find that it can be cycled through only a few batches before its action weakens. The reason is the absence of "weeds," in the form of many nameless LAB and hangers-on. Pure cultured strains of organisms like *S. thermophilus* and *L. bulgaricus* are hothouse flowers that fail to grow when transplanted to the outside world. But—to vary the metaphor—"unpedigreed" strains of the same microbes can thrive for decades as part of a large mixed community. Standing together as a diverse population can shield them in bacteriological struggles for a long time. This is the reason for the current mystique surrounding "heirloom" yogurt starters—though unfortunately, anything can be advertised as an heirloom starter with no guarantee of really being anything but an ad hoc combination of a few commercial strains.

Rettger's acidophilus milk was the third twentieth-century attempt to exalt an individual LAB species as a star health promoter. But *B. acidophilus*—eventually renamed *Lactobacillus acidophilus*—was radically different from any other bacterium that had previously been used to sour milk. No one had ever used it for that purpose, and for good reason: it seldom or never occurs in in milk, or any other natural food source. The preferred habitat in which *L. acidophilus* thrives is the digestive tract of mammals, particularly young ones being nursed on mother's milk. Moro had discovered it in babies' stools; bacteriologists had subsequently learned to propagate it in the laboratory. After about

1925 it edged into the popular role of colonic policeman that Metch-nikoff's *B. bulgaricus* had been demoted from. Its fondness for highly acidic conditions, and its ability to create them by fermenting lactose into lactic acid more thoroughly than any of the common LAB, seemed to promise a strong defense against putrefactive filth at the far end of the viscera. Acidophilus milk soon became a marketable specialty among the offerings of commercial dairies.[42]

Much rethinking of the classifications *L. acidophilus* and *B. bifidus* has taken place over the last century; Tissier's single species has now become an array of species in the genus *Bifidobacteria*. But time has only confirmed the most important fact to emerge from early studies: breastfeeding and weaning powerfully affect the makeup of the colonic microflora. Various *Bifidobacteria* achieve a dominant presence in the colons of breastfed infants several days after birth and retain it until weaning begins, at which point they start losing some importance to other bacteria. They dwindle into a smaller percentage of the normal bacterial population in toddlers by the age of three. In infants fed on cow's milk formulas, organisms characteristic of breastfed infants are far less prominent.

Some *Lactobacilli* including *L. acidophilus* also appear to help regu-late the balance of organisms in the colon, though their activity isn't as striking as that of the *Bifidobacteria*. *L. acidophilus* had the luck to be found and named before the rest, and to be commercially sold for sup-posed medical purposes before any of the other true colonic bacteria. During the 1920s and 1930s, Rettger's advocacy helped acidophilus milk succeed to the market segment of the debunked Bulgarian yogurt before it too faded from stardom.

But well before that, the entire idea of fermented milk had started to be restored to scientific respectability. Looking back on swings in medical opinion throughout her career, the veteran public health officer S. Josephine Baker, longtime head of the New York City Bureau of Child Hygiene, noted in 1940, "Many doctors today are using types of sour milk such as buttermilk and koumiss for baby feeding," while forty years earlier, "Sour milk was supposed to be lethal poison—for babies anyway."[43] As early as 1907, one New York physician began openly criticizing the city health department for blanket statements about sour milk being a germ-ridden menace. He was Henry G. Piffard, a well-known dermatologist with a spare-time interest in documentary photography (he had contributed many photos to his friend Jacob Riis's *How the Other Half Lives*), as well as a microphotographer experienced at capturing informative images of bacteria under high magnification.

In an article published in the *New York Medical Journal*, Piffard directly interjected fermented milk into the public debate over mandatory pasteurization of city milk supplies—this at a time when pasteurization had not yet shed unsavory associations with fly-by-night operators. Reviewing the many dangers posed by unclean milk, he firmly sided with authorities who still found pasteurized drinking-milk suspect from some medical standpoint and pointed to sour milk, "the favorite beverage in the hay and harvest fields of my youth," as a perfectly viable alternative.[44] He quickly returned to the attack in a more detailed piece titled "A Study of Sour Milks," illustrated with his own magnified photographs of microorganisms.[45]

Piffard, a spirited contrarian, had decided that it was time for someone to show up the obsolescence of the anti-sour-milk position and its irrelevance to public health. He was at best cool toward pasteurization, and didn't treat "the defenceless babies" over whom Nathan Straus had emoted as the be-all and end-all of milk policy. Instead, he pleaded for the general rediscovery of fermented raw milk as a sound, healthful, flavorful tradition belonging to peoples in many parts of the globe and dating back at least to the lifetime of the patriarch Abraham.

He had chosen to analyze a large handful of the many fermented milk products arriving on the market. With the help of several scientists at the city health department's bacteriological laboratory, he subjected cultures of the fermenting organisms in Bacillac, Zoolak, kefir, and other preparations to microscopic examination, along with samples of the actual commercial products. In many cases, he regretfully noted the presence of unauthorized organisms that signaled lax quality control rather than careful attention to laboratory conditions. As for the "alleged buttermilk" sold in New York, Piffard found a combination of skim milk, a household "potato yeast" starter meant for bread, and some whole milk being churned into a ridiculous travesty of the country buttermilk that he remembered being churned from sour cream in his boyhood. The manufacturer blamed this sad expedient on an illogical Board of Health regulation.[46]

Piffard saw a bright future for the general field if manufacturers could strictly ride herd on the makeup of their cultures. He was, however, bothered by the high prices that manufacturers charged for their proprietary versions of sour milk—a serious barrier to the wider adoption of a "wholesome and nutritious" resource. The usual retail prices he cited were scarcely ever "less than twenty cents a pint," at a time when 15 cents a quart put highest-quality drinking-milk almost "out of the question" for ordinary consumers who might bridle at anything over 8 or 9 cents. Luckily, he was able to recommend a splendid solution known to many German immigrants and Ashkenazic Jews. It had been passed on to him by "another Abraham"—i.e., the medical patriarch Jacobi, who related that in summer he liked to put some fresh milk in a deep soup plate, cover it, and let it stand in a warm place. The next day it would be ready to eat sprinkled with a little nutmeg or cinnamon.[47] (This informal suggestion brings home just how intensely focused on save-the-babies priorities the pasteurized milk movement was: its greatest pediatric proponent didn't hesitate to treat himself to an old-fashioned unpasteurized milk dish.)

As the lead article in the *New York Medical Journal*'s first 1908 issue, Piffard's study attracted wide notice. A lively and timely contribution, it was reprinted or commented on in other professional journals and received a prominent mention in the *New York Times* "Topics of the Times" feature.[48] Piffard had boldly jumped into the raw milk debates with concrete examples of how useful milk became through both managed and spontaneous fermentation, rapped the knuckles of public health officials who ascribed imaginary dangers to sour milk, and shown how to at least start demystifying some of the fermented products on the market.

Piffard was not a peddler of inflated health claims for sour milk, though he had occasionally used it in his own dermatology practice and found some of Metchnikoff's arguments convincing. Nor did he aspire to any special fame. In these respects, he was a far cry from a Battle Creek, Michigan, colleague who had been kind enough to send him some authentic Bulgarian cultures from Sofia to help in his research on "Maadzoun" and "Yoghourt."

THE AMERICAN PROPHET OF AUTOINTOXICATION

John Harvey Kellogg (1852–1943) was the George Cheyne of his age, a medico-religious go-getter who knew how to endear himself to celebrity patients. Like Cheyne, he incurred much scorn among fellow physicians who thought him a charlatan or a crank. But his worst enemy could not have denied that he was one of the finest surgeons of his era, as well as a hardworking practitioner who zealously kept up with a range of medical innovations throughout his sixty-plus years at Battle Creek. He had personally met Pasteur and corresponded with people like Pavlov. Facts, theories, opinions, speculations, and *idées fixes* coursed through his fertile brain at impetuous speed, making any clear summary of his thinking next to impossible. The dozens of books he wrote abundantly prove that he could leap from one fervent medical conviction to its opposite with no more embarrassment than Walt Whitman about con-tradicting himself. Milk, both fresh and fermented, occasioned some of his most startling swerves.

Kellogg was a birthright member of the Seventh Day Adventist Church. In his teens he had been picked by a founder of the sect, Ellen G. White, to receive a first-rate medical education so that he might become director of the establishment that she and her husband, James Springer White, had set up in the town of Battle Creek, the Western Health Reform Institute. Starting in 1876, he and a browbeaten busi-ness manager (his brother Will, who eventually decamped to start a rival career) spent more than twenty-five years building it up from a small health resort treating handfuls of patients on humble Adventist principles into something like a luxury hotel for sufferers from almost any noncommunicable ailment. No religious affiliation was required. By 1906–1907 the Battle Creek "Sanitarium" (a name coined by John Kellogg) was the most famous medical establishment in the United States. It boasted thirty-two buildings and a staff of between eight hundred and a thousand. Throughout a calendar year, the handsome portals of the "San" welcomed more than seven thousand patients—though Kellogg now often preferred to call them "guests."[49]

Unfortunately, his theological opinions had already gotten him into hot water with his co-religionists and especially the Whites. The publication of his book *The Living Temple* in 1903 touched off one of the bitterest controversies in the history of Adventism.

The Living Temple was a grand philosophical attempt to weave together all knowledge pertaining to health and well-being in the context of both modern medicine and the divine creation, from blood corpuscles to solar systems. To Ellen White, Kellogg's flights of thought seemed to replace belief in the doctrinal Christian God with pseudo-religious rationalizations about God being the sum of Nature, or vice versa. After a period of mounting tensions, the church declared him excommunicated, or in Adventist terminology "disfellowshipped." By a fluke of timing, the break came at the very moment in the autumn of 1907 when he was hoping to announce a new wonder food to the San and his sizable national following.[50]

Earlier that year he had been traveling in Europe and had spent some time in Paris, where he encountered Metchnikoff's and Tissier's work on intestinal microbiology. He returned to Battle Creek radically converted to the beliefs of Metchnikoff and several other European autointoxication theorists, and ready for some compromises with Adventist dietary principles in the meals offered by the San's ambitious kitchens. These were the province of his wife, Ella Eaton Kellogg, who had immersed herself in Adventist doctrines regarding food as well as medical teachings about proper regimens for different conditions, in order to present wide-ranging menu choices to patients being treated for anything from diabetes to anemia.

The Whites had strictly enjoined believers from eating meat and only grudgingly sanctioned small amounts of animal-derived foods like milk or eggs. In 1899 the San's magazine *The Gospel of Health* (co-edited by John and Ella Kellogg) had replied to a reader's question on some matters of diet with the standard Adventist answer that "we do not consider any of the milk foods very desirable." Though fresh buttermilk was more acceptable than the rest, "Fruits, grains, and nuts form the ideal diet for adults whether sick or well."[51] But while John Kellogg was preparing himself for the disfellowshipping crisis, he was also preparing subscribers to the magazine—now renamed *Good Health*—for a new emphasis on intestinal well-being in an article headed "A Remarkable Discovery."

The discovery in question was Metchnikoff's supposedly scientific revelation—corroborated by other authors whom Kellogg was eagerly reading—that the physical ravages of old age resulting from chronic autointoxication through the slow release of bacterial toxins into the blood could be counteracted by "a new lactic-acid-forming ferment which excelled all other lactic-acid-forming ferments." Its "great activity in the formation of acids" allowed it to "flourish in the colon" and combat poison-forming germs, heading off the causes of autointoxication at the pass. A "milk preparation containing the ferment" had wide currency "in the orient generally," but Kellogg hinted that it could be troublesome to prepare properly. Luckily, "a concentrated preparation of the ferment has been devised" and "introduced into small capsules" that could be conveniently swallowed with or after meals. The article concluded: "The new ferment in concentrated form is furnished in this country under the name of 'Yogurt.'" The supplier, the Yogurt Company of Battle Creek, had also placed advertisements with mail-order information in *Good Health*.[52]

Another ad printed in the *New York Times* at the same time as the *Good Health* article gives a clue as to Kellogg's ambitions for the product and the name. Under the caption "FRIENDLY GERMS FOR SALE BY MAIL," it began, "Whoever heard of such a thing? Well, if you haven't heard about the friendly germs which feed upon and destroy disease germs in the intestinal tract, then you are way behind the times." The heart of the matter was: "These friendly germs can be purchased by mail in capsules—50 million in a capsule—four dozen capsules in a box sent to any address upon receipt of one dollar. They are sold only under the trade name of YOGURT."[53]

If the ad's attempt to pass off "Yogurt" as a proprietary trade name now looks as brazen as Dr. Dadirrian's grab for first dibs on "matzoon," its talk of recruiting bacteria to fight other bacteria had the editors of *Collier's* magazine in stitches. Picturing "a force of benevolent bacilli who will keep the wicked germs too busy dodging uppercuts and left leads to have any leisure for their characteristic cussedness," they wondered whether we might in time expect "the bacterial training quarters" to start charging different rates for "Ordinary friendly germs," "Domesticated germs that will purr and eat out of your hand," and "Old Dog Tray selected germs, warranted ever faithful."

"Such quackery as this of the Yogurt Company," in the magazine's opinion, could be traced to "the avid appetite for scientific sensationalism which pervades the public and is catered to by careless editors."[54] Kellogg, who was equally impervious to well-informed or (as in this case) ignorant criticism, had meanwhile embarked on some serious reconsideration of milk.

Since his arrival he had steadily expanded the scope of the San's various therapies to a depth and breadth unmatched by any other medical facility in the nation. At the same time, he had remained devoted to most of the core Adventist priorities—for instance, the "water cure," or hydropathy. This had been the central focus of the Whites' original "health reform institute." It was a practice founded on the belief that large amounts of water administered in different forms flushed pollution out of the system. No hydration cheerleader of today could have equaled hydropathists' faith in the powers of clean, pure water liberally applied to the human exterior or interior.

The water-cure mania had emerged earlier in the nineteenth century as a modified remnant of previous medical theories holding that undigested residues clogging the alimentary canal and the bloodstream with corrupting matter were the source of most chronic diseases. Cheyne had been eloquent on this point. So was the twenty-four-year-old Kellogg when, during his first season as director of the institute, he published

a book titled *The Uses of Water in Health and Disease.*[55] It was remarkably free of some baggage that later came to be indelibly associated with
Kellogg—notably, a fervent interest in the state of everyone's bowels.

This increasing obsession probably was strengthened by Kellogg's
simultaneous preoccupation with ever-more complicated gadgets and
paraphernalia meant to assist in hydrotherapy (including a range of
different enemas) and other therapies. It received a boost from discussions of autointoxication with Metchnikoff during his 1907 visit
to Paris. As he and the San weathered the break with Adventist lead-
ership, he decided that some milk products (though never ripened
cheeses, which he thought pernicious) deserved more of a place on the
Battle Creek table.

The coming change of direction can be glimpsed in *The Battle Creek
Sanitarium System*, published the year after the disfellowshipping crisis
and reissued in an expanded version in 1913. Meant to implicitly establish himself as the official voice of the San, it mentioned a "Milk Diet"
as one of the institution's accepted dietary therapies and spent much
time citing autointoxication as the root cause of many conditions being
treated by his staff, from neurasthenia (shades of Dr. Cheyne's "nervous
complaints") to insomnia, migraine, and "rheumatic gout," or rheuma-
toid arthritis. This last was said to respond well to one or two enemas a
day. But virtually all could be countered by Metchnikoff's friendly germ
in various forms offered to San patients—"yogurt buttermilk," "yogurt
cheese" (drained of whey until nearly solid) and the remaining "yogurt
whey," and yogurt-bacilli capsules for those who balked at swallowing
actual yogurt. Ordinary buttermilk was available for those who disliked
yogurt, plain milk for holdouts who disliked both. Cottage cheese was
a new possibility. Overall milk consumption at the San had increased
enough to require the milk of five hundred cows.[56]

At this point Kellogg firmly believed in pasteurizing all fresh milk
used in the San, with the possible exception of certified raw milk for
patients who claimed to have trouble digesting anything else. In the next
few years, however, he would develop an equal faith in raw milk. His
bacteriological reasoning was that raw milk was capable of being fermented to a helpful acidity in the colon while pasteurized milk merely

putrefied, releasing colonic toxins as hideous as those produced by meat (which Kellogg always abhorred).

Soon the San's new X-ray and fluoroscopy equipment allowed him to actually *see* the colon with a bismuth or barium meal moving along it, redoubling his appetite for the struggle against systemic poisoning. His maturing convictions were broached in *Colon Hygiene* (1915) and more fully developed in *Autointoxication or Intestinal Toxemia* (1918). With a conscientious nod to his earlier Adventist distrust of cow's milk as an animal product not fully adaptable to human physiology, he nonetheless extolled its capacity (when raw) to deliver aid to the besieged colon.[57] The factors that were supposed to accomplish this were LAB and lactose itself, which Kellogg considered a tremendous boost to digestion. He thought that if enough of it reached the colon undigested, it would furnish a rich food source for any LAB that had made it through the upper digestive tract, helping to discourage harmful organisms by adding to the acidity of the colonic environment.[58]

He was now wedded to a belief that the bowel habits of the higher apes and primitive humans (on which he had interrogated zookeepers and missionary physicians living among supposedly uncivilized peoples) should be a model for victims of modern civilization's errors.[59] One bowel movement a day was tantamount to constipation; three at least should be the norm. A vegetarian diet rich in fibrous vegetables, together with bulk-promoting supplements like bran and Japanese agar and some assistance from mineral oil, should produce the desired result. When cases of advanced autointoxication didn't respond satisfactorily, other therapies might be necessary. *Autointoxication or Intestinal Toxemia* especially recommended "the Milk Regimen," which might last as little as two or as much as ten days. It was intended to flush out the entire digestive tract, from mouth to colon, with a constant stream of milk. Whether fresh or soured, it certainly should be raw. Each day's ration was to total between six and twelve pints (three and six quarts), depending on the patient's size, and to be portioned out at half-hour intervals between morning and night. Kellogg assumed that this saturation tactic would send copious amounts of beneficial lactose flooding all the way through the stomach and small intestine into the colon.

To be sure of complete cleansing, he followed up the orally administered deluge of milk with water enemas and a rectal "injection" of whey cultured with *B. bulgaricus*.[60]

By now, however, his faith in Metchnikoff had been somewhat shaken. That visionary had disappointed trusters in yogurt-stoked Abrahamic life spans by dying in 1916 at a mere seventy-one. Kellogg attributed this failure to Metchnikoff's stubborn continuance in the fatal habit of meat-eating, the surest recipe for a colon full of putrefying bacteria. He was also starting to note the complaints of researchers who were showing that *B. bulgaricus* could not establish itself in the colon and paying more attention to the organisms championed by Tissier (*B. bifidus)* and Rettger (*B. acidophilus*) as demonstrating true colonic activity.

Kellogg's ever-churning brain soon spun away to embrace new causes. One was a wonder plant called the soybean, which he and Henry Ford—a perennial San guest and in many ways a Kellogg soul-mate—seem to have become enraptured with at the same time. In 1918 an article in *Good Health* celebrated its dazzling possibilities, citing a recent discovery by University of Wisconsin home economists that "the protein of the soy bean appears to be as valuable as the casein of milk." By the time Kellogg sang its praises at greater length in *The New Dietetics* (1921), he had combed through enough of the growing soybean literature to learn that soy milk might be a good substitute for cow's milk and "tou fu" for dairy cheese.[61] Over the next decade or so he somehow discovered how to connect the dots between his growing faith in soy milk and his equally ardent conversion to belief in *B. acidophilus* as the body's best hope against putrefying colonic bacteria.[62]

Soy milk must have looked like a heaven-sent gift to Kellogg. He could embrace it without any cost to the most fundamental Adventist principles, few of which he had really broken with despite his 1907 disfellowshipping. For years he had allowed a doctrinally questionable animal product to be widely consumed at the San for the sake of anti-autointoxication imperatives. Now any qualms of conscience could be put to rest as he introduced a pure vegetarian replacement. Furthermore, he had found that *B. acidophilus*, unlike the discredited *B. bulgaricus*, was easy to culture in soy milk. And it produced an extra jolt of lactic acid when dosed at the outset with a small percentage of lactose, a method for which he obtained a patent in 1934.[63]

The infallible Kellogg nose for publicity shortly sent him into action, armed with his new patent, when he learned that one of Canada's relentlessly exploited miracle babies, the Dionne quintuplets, was very ill with a bowel infection. As documented in William Shurtleff and Akiko Aoyagi's monumental history of soy foods, he promptly volunteered to send the quints' doctor, Allan Roy Dafoe, a supply of his soy acidophilus milk. The frail little girl made a remarkable recovery. Soon Dafoe was giving soy acidophilus milk from Battle Creek to all five babies. (Kellogg made every effort to turn this uplifting story to profitable account by getting permission to use images of the quints on labels of his lifesaving milk, but never was able to talk an unimpressed Ontario minister of health into going along with the scheme.[64])

Kellogg died in 1943 aged ninety-one, having partly outlived his fame. The peak of his career probably was the period between about 1910 and the 1930s, when the San attracted a nonstop stream of health-seekers from every part of the United States and the guest list was spangled with names like John D. Rockefeller, Upton Sinclair, Amelia Earhart, and Calvin Coolidge. In his heyday he had the power to start national fads or encourage existing ones. Some of his pet beliefs, like "race betterment" to free humanity from the inferior genetic legacy of dark-skinned minorities, had already attracted a wide following before he joined the bandwagon. Others—the value of celibate marriage comes to mind—understandably failed to catch on.

Where food and diet were concerned, Kellogg was destined to be both justly and unjustly remembered as something of a crank. Certainly he brought more prestigious scientific credentials to the vegetarian movement than any predecessor. But the mainstream American public would not be ready to treat vegetarianism as anything but a fringe fad until the 1970s. His championship of nondairy milk substitutes—Ellen White's followers at Battle Creek were interested in peanut milk, almond milk, and other variations on the theme—was too stubbornly enmeshed in his own *sui generis* amalgam of Adventist vegetarian doctrine and scientific rationalizations to be seen as a direct inspiration of today's more highly processed "alternative" milks. (The real soy milk story, as related in Jia-Chen Fu's fascinating *The Other Milk*, begins in Paris shortly before 1910, with the expatriate anarchist Li Shizeng deciding that with proper processing *dou jiang*, the strained-out soybean slurry that is the precursor to coagulated bean curd, would make a splendidly cheap and nutritious substitute for cow's milk in modern Chinese diets.[65]) Nor did he give fermented milk a serious and lasting commercial boost commensurate with the first-class insight that concludes his survey of different societies' versions: "It thus appears that the use of lactic acid ferments is a practice known to widely scattered nations and from the most ancient times. The great care which is taken by the most primitive people to preserve the purity of the particular ferment which they employ, and the high value which they place upon it in the treatment of many diseases, leads one to wonder that civilized people should have been so slow to avail themselves of this valuable means of combatting some of the most dangerous and insidious of the foes of human life."[66]

His curious turnarounds of opinion about milk most likely were noted by an eager clique rather than everyday consumers. But at the very least he lent visibility to the idea of health-promoting fermentation. In the process of acclaiming "friendly bacteria" as fighters of colonic menaces, he offered some temporary life support to the raw milk cause, which was rapidly becoming anathema to public health authorities. His contributions to the 1920s and 1930s acidophilus milk vogue and the exploitation of soy-based foods proved short-lived. In the final analysis, his most lasting (if unwitting) effect on American milk-consumption habits came from a completely different chapter in San history: the invention of precooked and toasted cereal flakes, to be dipped or poured out of a package and served cold.

John, Ella, and Will Kellogg's respective roles in this watershed episode would later touch off many family disputes. Regardless of who applied the crucial touches to the inspiration, it is plain that in 1896 John received a patent for a method of manufacturing a ready-to-eat flaked cereal food.[67] At that point the phrases "breakfast cereal" and "cold cereal" didn't exist. "Cereal" was still a word applicable to all edible grains; it didn't denote a category of processed ready-to-serve products based on them.

John soon began marketing toasted wheat flakes on a small scale. Will, who thought his part in perfecting the idea hadn't been properly credited, later went his own way and speedily founded a great commercial empire involving many different kinds of cereal flakes. The Kelloggs were not alone in exploring the possibilities of ready-to-eat products based on grains, but Kellogg was and is the name most nearly synonymous with them. Almost as soon as they had been invented, the meal most indelibly associated with them came to be breakfast, and their most inseparable accompaniment immediately came to be milk—fresh (or putatively fresh) cold milk. John Kellogg may or may not have understood what a boost he had given to the drinking-milk industry. But he surely rejoiced to see cold cereals receiving the imprimatur of nutrition experts, especially in combination with milk. It was an added spur to nationwide milk consumption by both children and adults, more durable than any of his plugs for pathogen-fighting yogurt or his other autointoxication remedies.

The unfortunate fact is that though the turn-of-the-twentieth-century restoration of soured milk to scientific respectability produced some health claims and marketing opportunities, it had not the slightest effect on the breakneck expansion of the drinking-milk industry. Neither the koumiss and matzoon fads, Henry Piffard's pleas for a reconsideration of sour milk, the Metchnikoff-inspired yogurt startups, Leo Rettger's evangelism on behalf of acidophilus milk, nor John Kellogg's various efforts toward colon reformation ever caused the great majority of pediatricians and public health authorities to view fermented milk as a pleasurable and perfectly rational alternative to the full-lactose drinking-milk that they wanted to see on all family tables. Neither did the hidden-in-plain-sight fact that milk acted on by LAB presented a strong (though not foolproof) resistance to pathogens that wasn't shared by drinking-milk. Somehow both leading health authorities and the consuming public continued to take for granted that fluid cow's milk untainted by the least suspicion of sourness was the only *real* milk. Even champions of raw milk saw no reason to question this assumption.

During the Straus-era pasteurization wars, the very real advantages of LAB fermentation had never entered debates of the "milk question." They remained invisible to the medical and public health communities at large. The only traditional soured dairy products that retained a little commercial importance after about 1920 were buttermilk and sour cream, both made by inoculating milk or a milk-cream mixture with pure cultures of LAB. The first, more properly called "cultured buttermilk," had lost all connection with actual buttermaking. The second was almost exclusively sold to Ashkenazic Jewish and some German American clienteles. Yogurt fell off the map, forgotten for the time being by all but a smattering of hard-core health food devotees. The American dairy industry entered a period of industrial-scale growth intensely focused on wringing as much full-lactose milk as possible from the creature whom dairy-industry boosters had christened the "foster mother of the human race."

No scientific basis for questioning the primacy of unsoured milk could have existed in the absence of research about the post-weaning cutoff of lactase production in most humans. In 1906 the British researcher R. H. Aders Plimmer had made a rough-and-ready attempt to account for earlier findings that lactase seemed to be produced in the intestines of younger and not older test animals, but interest in following up this lead was apparently lacking.[68] In the United States, fresh full-lactose milk was more than ever the culturally normative superfood, the object of perpetual campaigns to make it one of the cheapest items that an American family could purchase. Any contradiction between this goal and the fact that drinking-milk kept getting more expensive for an American farmer to *produce* managed to be ignored in polite conversation.

7

MILK FOR THE MASSES

The Price to Be Paid

I n 1934 the Federal Trade Commission decided to investigate how the Great Depression had managed to generate booming profits for milk dealers along with a catastrophic slump in returns for dairy farmers. The agency was unfortunately forced by lack of funds to replace a hoped-for nationwide inquiry with hearings in only two locations, Connecticut and the Philadelphia area. One well-informed, college-educated Connecticut farmer testified that the tortuous statements furnished by his local dealer to justify penalties inexplicably levied against his account were as baffling to him and his wife as "Chinese puzzles."

"It is like reading Einstein's theory of relativity and Chancellor Haldane's explanation of it?" a sympathetic FTC examiner suggested, referring to a somewhat opaque popularization by a scientifically minded British peer.

"Or Gertrude Stein," the witness replied.[1]

This chapter will examine some events roughly bookended by the run-up to World War I and the aftermath of World War II that inflated the drinking-milk industry to mind-boggling size while swathing it in abstruse pricing complexities. Among them were a sharp growth in milk production helped by the nation's first organized food policy program during World War I; ensuing efforts by the U.S. Public Health Service to promote a state-by-state strategy for commercial production of clean, safe milk; and the transformation of middlemen into dairy companies capable of implementing this agenda with the aid of new farm-to-consumer infrastructures. When the Great Depression shook the U.S. agricultural economy to its foundations and provoked rebel economists to question the revered tenets of free-market capitalism, the largest dairy companies had already swallowed up many smaller ones and acquired a hold on dairy farmers' livelihood coercive enough to stimulate talk of government-mandated supports for wholesale milk prices.

But these events could never have been set in motion without another stimulus: a marriage between dietary advice and public health policy that had been firmly cemented by the 1910s. It began with experts invoking science to declare that large amounts of drinking-milk were absolutely mandatory for every American household. It soon helped transform the drinking-milk business into a labyrinth of transactions differing from the early milk trade not in mere size but in structure.

When Nathan Straus and Henry Leber Coit began disputing the merits of raw and pasteurized milk, the bottled milk that each wanted children to have was collected, handled, and dispensed to families in a fairly straightforward fashion, with only incidental need for middlemen. But by the time of the FTC hearings, middlemen were more or less calling the tune.

The turn-of-the-century model was not radically dissimilar from x hundred bushels of apples being shipped to a city warehouse from Farmer Jones's orchard and going on to destined retail outlets. Another analogy might have been a flashlight with an on-off switch that enabled batteries of y capacity to intermittently send power to a light bulb until they ran down, at which time they would be replaced. In both cases, finite processes involving discrete quantities of some "product" were begun and completed.

Throughout the 1920s and 1930s, however, the most advanced segments of the milk industry became reconfigured on a different structural model in which large pooled aggregates of the "product" were constantly in motion. For analogies we have to look not to apples or flashlight batteries but to a city water system fed from a regional watershed. Or perhaps more adequately, an electric power grid with an uninterrupted flow of current that could be rapidly shunted here or there to adjust supply to demand in different divisions of a complex network. Payments to farmers could be easily finagled within such systems, where any individual farm's milk was almost literally a drop in the bucket—or the "milkshed," a term that had been adopted before 1920. The finagling mechanism was a set of classified price differentials governing milk meant to be drunk in unfermented fluid form and milk used for all other purposes.

At every stage, the growth of the system was fueled by a near-religious national certainty—unshaken by repeated and disastrous market gluts— that there could be no such thing as too much drinking-milk.

"NUTRITION IDEOLOGY"

The difference between nineteenth-century and twentieth-century glorifications of drinking-milk lies in what the sociologist E. Melanie DuPuis has called "the rise of nutrition ideology."[2] When Wilbur Atwater was teaching at Yale, prestigious theories about how foods nourished the body were only gradually progressing from the concept of calories to the new refinements of proteins, fats, and carbohydrates. There was no precedent for the avalanche of discoveries that began to appear between about 1900 and 1930, spurred by food chemists like Henry C. Sherman at Columbia University.

Before 1910 Sherman had established the critical importance of some mineral elements in human diets. Among these, calcium and phosphorus were found to play a decisive role in the formation of skeletal bones and to be plentiful in milk—which indeed was the biggest dietary source of calcium in the industrialized West. No sooner had the medical profession started to celebrate the importance of minerals than the great vitamin discoveries launched by (among others) Casimir Funk and Elmer V. McCollum were raising milk's reputation to still more awesome heights. By 1917 its fame as the cheapest and most digestible source of protein and calcium had begun competing for attention with the news that its butterfat was rich in a fat-soluble substance about to be dubbed vitamin A. Not long afterward, other factors eventually classified as the B vitamins thiamin and riboflavin were added to the list of milk's blessings.

Those who most immediately benefited from nutrition experts' new explorations of common foods were the experts themselves, whose pulpits for preaching to government policy-makers and mothers of families were now imposing. Drinking-milk was the object of their first concerted campaign for *minimum consumption quotas necessary to avoid dangerous nutritional deficits*. A century later, the mentality behind this edict still has great staying power despite all it has done to contribute to dairy farmers' perennial surplus problems.

When the target quota doctrine was first conceived, American consumers' faith in public institutions was far greater than it is today, with public health agencies enjoying special esteem. Medical theorists were quick to weigh in on political debates involving milk prices. An early opportunity occurred in New York City in the autumn of 1917, about six months after America's entry into World War I. Since the outbreak of war in Europe, President Woodrow Wilson had authorized massive food shipments to the Allies that had helped throw the national food chain into a frantic price spiral. Meanwhile, a farmers' cooperative called the Dairymen's League, chiefly centered in Orange County, had recently managed to boost wholesale farm prices for milk in the Greater New York area through a series of strikes that also had the effect of increasing retail prices for metropolitan consumers. By now, talk of a sinister "milk trust" could be counted on whenever such farmers' organizations sought to exercise some clout.

Health Commissioner Haven Emerson asked Mayor John Purroy Mitchel to address the perceived emergency by appointing an investigative committee. The Mayor's Committee on Milk report was issued in December. It showed that average retail prices for bottled milk delivered to homes had indeed risen sharply between 1914 and 1917, from 9 cents to 14 cents a quart. Many other common foods, however, were found to have undergone even steeper increases, the result of the Wilson administration's attempts to juggle difficult prewar and then wartime food policy choices.[3]

Some prestigious voices were wanted to prove that price hikes for milk were more outrageous than still greater price hikes for eggs or pork. The Mayor's Committee had accordingly called in the cavalry: big names from the diet-and-nutrition field, now in the first flush of its prestige as a wing of public health. The report cited Henry Sherman, Milton J. Rosenau (author of the important 1912 survey *The Milk Question*), Elmer McCollum, the renowned pediatrician L. Emmett Holt, and Graham Lusk (author of the highly regarded textbook *The Elements of Food and Nutrition*) to confirm that milk was the most valuable article of diet anyone could possibly consume. It wonderfully encouraged "a proper balance in the mineral constituents in a diet" (Sherman); promoted growth in infants and children (McCollum); and should be given to babies in the amounts of a quart a day up to the age of one year, a pint and a half up to two years (Holt). Sherman also called it "the most important single food for adults."[4] Lusk, probably voicing the thoughts of others concerned about war preparedness, commented:

No family of five should buy meat until they have bought at least three quarts of milk. Milk contains not only protein of animal origin but also a very valuable fat which has specific properties for growth . . . Milk is the cheapest form of protein you can get. It is the most complete and sufficient food that can be had. Around the dairy farms centres the proper nutrition of a nation.[5]

Some of these advisers may not have understood that ever-expanding nutritional claims for milk helped to energize attacks on dairy farmers as heartless price-gougers getting rich from poor families' suffering. But Rosenau, an eminent bacteriologist and public health officer, had shown much feeling for the producers' plight five years earlier. "[The farmer] is made the butt of the cartoonists and is hammered at from all sides," he had commented. "He is inspected and re-inspected, preached to, lectured at, scolded, and the object of legal action. He is pestered with the enthusiast, the reformer, the sanitarian, the lawyer, the baby's mother, and the baby's doctor. He is showered with advice, some of it contradictory. In this predicament he does not know which way to turn."[6]

A stubborn factor in the predicament was that the small family farms from which most milk came at the time of Rosenau's writing were mixed-use operations where farmers could divert only limited attention or cash from plant crops and other livestock to the special demands of milking. Thus he could point out that "the dairy business has been largely built up on a cheap basis," while other handicaps to a sound development of the industry lurked at the retail purchaser's end. "One great stumbling block is the disinclination of the consumer to pay a fair price for a fair article. There is much opposition on the part of the consumer to pay a higher price for milk. There is a curious psychology in this. While begrudging one cent more a quart for milk, he supinely submits to an increase in the price of everything else."[7]

As new evidence of milk's extraordinary nutritional value arrived, it helped city politicians warming to the role of consumer champions to illogically argue that retail prices must remain as low as possible. Rosenau was not the only observer to worry about the trend. In May 1918, his qualms about popular attitudes were echoed by Herbert Hoover, the head of the World War I Food Administration. Addressing the National Milk and Dairy Exposition, Hoover remarked of the dairy business: "It is an industry to certain products of which attach a peculiarly large amount of sentimental value; fluid milk is the absolute foodstuff of our babies and is equally a necessity to the very poor and to the rich. The consequence is that a rise in the price of milk may provoke more blind and fanatical opposition than any other of the food industries, not even excepting bread." He was inclined to blame high prices not on farmers but on "the enormous duplication and waste in present chaotic distribution methods."[8]

No matter where the fault lay, Hoover thought that price hikes caused "heartbreaking" reductions in the amounts of milk reaching children in "the poorer sections of the community," an evil to be "overcome by propaganda in these sections as to the necessity for milk for children." But at the same time, "Food must be seen from the new viewpoint of ammunition to win the war"—meaning both military rations for American, French, and British fighting forces and food relief for civilians in the shell-torn European theaters of war. For this reason, he argued for treating farm surpluses not as market gluts but as the foundation of invaluable national stockpiles.[9]

Of course, surpluses of fresh fluid milk could not be stockpiled. But Hoover had developed a deep respect for canned milk during his years organizing food relief in ravaged parts of northwestern Europe before the United States entered the war. "There has been scarcely a child born in the north of France, and many in Belgium, whose continued life has not been dependent upon American condensed milk," he declared, hinting at the prospect that the nation's dairy industry might soon have "the child life of the world" in its hands.[10]

The Food Administration had made itself unpopular by abandoning (for the duration) laissez-faire principles and claiming the right to arbitrate price disputes in certain venues. Trying to appease the dairy exposition attendees for unavoidable bumps in the road, Hoover acknowledged that "there is no other agricultural industry of such economic complexity" as theirs. But he insisted that the Food Administration's only mission was "to soften the shocks of war so that the food supplies of our own people and the allies may be maintained" through travails like bad weather and transportation bottlenecks. It was not meant to solve long-term problems that would have to be sorted out later by "local initiatives." The immediate goal had to be maintaining the American dairy cow population at a high enough level to satisfy ramped-up wartime domestic and overseas demands for milk. Should war "so dislocate the industry as to cause temporary periods when loss faces you," every dairyman should bravely remind himself of his role as a member of "the world's reserve army that may, at any moment, be called into battle for our existence and the existence of the next generation."[11]

Hoover repeatedly reassured the public that government intervention in agricultural markets was a one-time emergency measure and that victory in Europe would mean a return to reliable supply-and-demand norms. His hopes were misplaced. For a short honeymoon period after the end of the war, domestic food surpluses could be absorbed into European famine relief shipments while bestowing a certain humanitarian halo on the American farmer. But by the start of Warren G. Harding's administration in 1921, intractable surpluses and slumping prices were ushering in a severe and prolonged agricultural depression. As growers of major crops began complaining about the shrinking returns they now realized to offset production costs, in contrast to their (relative) earlier prosperity, economists coined a term to serve as a benchmark for prices sufficient to give farmers purchasing power equal to a prewar standard: "parity." It was a chimerical goal.

Drinking-milk was partly spared at the outset. There was a sharp decline between 1920 and 1922[12] before dairy farmers' cooperatives began to make some headway against the dealers, guaranteeing member farmers higher returns for milk and in some cases creating their own cooperative processing and distribution facilities so as to control all cow-to-consumer stages. But their success was greater in less populated rural areas such as the northern Midwest than on the East Coast, where urban consumers' lobbies commanded strong political support.[13] And at no point did co-ops manage to abolish the stubborn challenges responsible for the unique "economic complexity" recognized by Hoover: the perishability, unwieldy bulk, and seasonally fluctuating supplies of fresh milk. To distribute it to the masses, neatly dovetailed pickup, processing, and delivery schedules must be kept up, through expensive applications of technology. Long before anyone had dreamt up the slogan "Too Big to Fail," the drinking-milk industry had reached that treacherous state. Fiscal observers had begun discussing its built-in economic instability even as health and nutrition advisers sought to greatly enlarge the scale of production. How could the enterprise be sustained in permanent overall equilibrium?

PLUGGING THE PRODUCT

One weapon was what Hoover called "propaganda." The more diplomatic name was "education." Here the dairy industry and its allies in diet-and-nutrition circles poured great hopes into cutting-edge panaceas that were already being applied to other troubled endeavors: advertising and public relations.

In 1913 participants in an annual exposition called the National Dairy Show began planning a promotional effort that every segment of the overall industry—farmers as well as dealers; drinking-milk processors as well as buttermakers, cheesemakers, and ice cream manufacturers—supposedly could get behind. The next step was the formation in 1915 of the Chicago-based National Dairy Council, intended as an alliance of all dairy interests. At the 1916 show the NDC unveiled its master plan for a nonstop national publicity barrage over the next three years.

Describing themselves as "willing servitors at the cradle of humanity," the NDC organizers led off with the ringing declaration, "TO INSURE ITS EXISTENCE AND PROGRESS, THE FIRST AND MOST IMPORTANT DUTY OF THE DAIRY INDUSTRY IS TO STABILIZE AND INCREASE THE CONSUMPTION OF DAIRY PRODUCTS."[14] They identified "underconsumption" as a threat to the nation's health: "one hundred million American men, women and children consume less than one-fourth of the Milk and Milk Products which they can, and for their own good should, consume." (As shown in the New York Mayor's Committee report, this kind of target-setting was about to become entrenched nutrition ideology.) Every segment of the industry must now attack the problem through "emphatic, sledge hammer advertising" carried out nonstop on billboards, magazine pages, store window displays, a speakers' bureau, "moving picture shows," and other fronts. The goal was to increase per capita U.S. consumption from the pitiful average of one glass a day by at least 10 percent over the next three years, if not to double it. Even 10 percent would allegedly add 2 million dairy cows to the current 22-million national herdstock and increase the present total of $1.5 billion in combined profits from all dairy products by another $1.5 million. The NDC cheerleaders trusted the power of "good advertising" to raise prices by showing the public how economical and healthful drinking-milk was in comparison with other foods, while also boosting the reputation of American butter, cheese (now "practically unknown and wholly misunderstood"), buttermilk (the one form of soured milk that seemed to be gaining some permanent market share during the early vicissitudes of yogurt), and ice cream.[15] They saw prosperous, efficient farms guided by the most systematic modern business principles as the bedrock on which all other aspects of the industrial dairy enterprise would rest in future.

These goals were only imperfectly realized. Though the 1917 declaration of war strongly bolstered the campaign, wartime triggers to expanded production could not erase the self-evident biological differences between drinking-milk production and all other segments of agriculture. The demands of lactating animals also hampered farmers' efforts to act as a unified political lobby. But from the great vitamin discovery days on, the dairy industry and its allies in government have never stopped bombarding the public with exhortations to buy more milk while obstinately glossing over permanent discrepancies between supply and demand.

A prominent example in the first postwar years was the "Campaign for the Dairy Cow" launched in Illinois by the state department of agriculture's Dairy Extension Division. It called for breeding programs to eliminate the "scrubs" (descendants of Spanish and French cattle brought to the New World colonies several centuries earlier and left to fend for themselves; the term now vaguely denoted nameless bovine mongrels) that greatly outnumbered purebred dairy cows on small multipurpose farms. During 1918 and 1919 the theme was repeated in slews of informational literature (including reprints of articles by milk's tireless scientific champion Elmer McCollum) and encapsulated in the slogan "The FOSTER MOTHER OF THE WORLD." The Illinois Dairy Extension Division was working on an educational film of that title, to be shown throughout the state in order to familiarize the public with every aspect of modern breeding, dairy farming, and milk handling. It also distributed 50,000 copies of a handsome poster by the well-known illustrator Richard Fayerweather Babcock, headed by the same catchphrase and further commanding:

PRESERVE HER
IMPROVE HER STOCK
HELP HER TO PRODUCE
MORE AND BETTER DAIRY PRODUCTS

"Foster Mother of the World" carried more definite patriotic overtones than W. D. Hoard's earlier "foster mother of the human race." Babcock's image left no doubt of its meaning: a noble black and white Holstein cow draped in a laurel wreath, being acclaimed on the one side by a grateful European mother with a brood of little ones and on the other by milk-chugging soldiers preparing to crown her with another wreath. No one could have read the message as anything but congratulations to the American dairy industry for its part in defeating the Central Powers and bringing food relief to famine-stricken postwar Europe.[16]

By 1921, New York City was demonstrating its loyalty to NDC goals. "Mayor Will Drink Milk for a Week," announced a headline in the June 5 Sunday New York Times. In response to urging by the Board of Education and a "committee of citizens" (probably seeded with dairy lobbyists), Health Commissioner Royal S. Copeland had designated the next seven days "Milk Week." Mayor John F. Hylan and the commissioner had both pledged to consume a quart of milk with lunch every day of the observance as an example to growing youngsters and health-minded New Yorkers. City restaurants and hotels chimed in to offer "special milk dishes." Liggett's drugstore chain set up "milk bars." The Board of Education also provided schoolchildren with a week's worth of activities, including special assembly programs "featuring the use of milk," a competition for "a slogan to be adopted for the Milk Campaign," another for designing a milk-celebrating poster, and a day trip to two dairy farms and a "milk factory" by a club at Washington Irving High School.[17]

All states and large cities mounted similar efforts in the postwar decades, diligently working to plant healthful principles in young minds through suggested lesson plans and educational pamphlets. Agricultural and public health bureaucracies at all levels of government continued to pitch propaganda (to use Hoover's word) to mothers and children throughout the twentieth century. Their efforts irreversibly solidified an earlier century of teachings about drinking-milk that had enjoyed great prestige even before the modern mineral and vitamin discoveries.

The new ideology also made generous room for butter as a source of fat-soluble vitamins. It encouraged ice cream sales and dutifully pointed out the nutritional virtues of cheese. But the unquestioned star of the show, and the real hub of the American dairy industry, was fresh drinking-milk. An unforeseen consequence of its enthronement above all other forms of milk was to keep more and more producing farmers perpetually at the mercy of forces beyond their control. Convincing people that cow's milk was foster mother's milk never miraculously translated into bulletproof profits for producers. Propaganda could do little to keep milk produced on the farm from annually repeating its own seasonal mini-version of boom-and-bust cycles.

The NDC's vision of harmonious cooperation between producing farmers and the dairy companies that dealt with transportation, processing, and distribution soon evaporated. To the dealers, seasonal surpluses were a wonderful excuse for trimming payments to producers. "Classes" or "grades" of milk (both terms were used) were the crux of the struggle for advantage.

Rough distinctions reflecting practical reality had emerged during the early pasteurization and certification campaigns. It was clear that certified raw milk was more expensive to produce, supervise, and handle than pasteurized milk. But at the outset of the clean-milk movement many or most physicians and diet experts strongly preferred it for its supposed purity and freedom from unnatural interference. The earliest class or grade distinctions were between certified (A or 1) and pasteurized (B or 2), though the cheap "loose" milk that was neither didn't immediately vanish from grocery stores.

During a period of muddled terminology in which pasteurization gained ground over certification and loose milk was either marginalized or driven out, public health authorities began erratic attempts to classify milk by more carefully gradated sanitary standards. At the same time, the expanding dairy companies, or dealer-processors, began applying price differentials to the milk they bought raw from farmers.

The only aspect of new terminology and farmer/dealer price schedules that need concern us here is the dairy companies' policy, or theoretical policy, of placing a higher value on "fluid milk" than "manufacturing milk." The former was that intended to fill milk glasses on family tables. The latter was milk used for any other purpose. The raw material for butter, cheese, cultured buttermilk, ice cream, canned evaporated or condensed milk, and the increasingly popular powdered dried milk was lumped together as manufacturing milk, or occasionally "surplus milk."

The price classification policy remained theoretical because the dealer was the only party who got to decide whether any farm shipment of milk qualified for the more lucrative rank. All sorts of reasons could be found for disqualifying an entire lot or some portion of it from fluid-milk status. Dealers also claimed the right to allocate milk to any preferred purpose at any time when they found themselves with a temporary surplus of milk supposedly destined for processing as fluid milk; hence the term "surplus milk."

As for the public health schedules, for decades they were an inconsistent mélange of local regulations. Every city asserted the right to set its own sanitary requirements for milk sold within its limits and to use farm inspections as a means of holding suppliers to account—a constant source of urban-rural friction. The dairy companies, however, quickly saw that standardized pigeonholes and requirements encouraged their own consolidation and growth. Meanwhile, federal public health authorities deplored the national patchwork of regulations but had no jurisdiction of their own in the matter. They thought that state legislatures should begin replacing random, inconsistent city-by-city imperatives with rational statewide requirements. That, however, would have been political suicide in major dairying states where discontented farmers looked likely to form hostile blocs.

The largest dairy farmers were the most willing to go along with health-promoting standards for milk. Of course, they were also the most in tune with a general message being sounded by professors of dairy science and advisory groups like the New York Mayor's Committee. These experts were eager to promote a modern dairy industry capable of pouring target amounts of milk (determined by nutritionists' fiats) into every American.

At the turn of the twentieth century, dairy farmers had scarcely begun to emerge as a special bloc. Most of the milk that reached cities from any regional milkshed originated on hundreds of insignificant multipurpose "dirt farms" that were the despair of agricultural school missionaries.

Enlightened opinion held that they should be either reformed into efficient business operations concentrating on a strategic handful of cash crops or got rid of as a drag on the agricultural economy. In the case of milk as a crop, reformation meant war on scrub cows that grazed unimproved pasturage in spring and summer, survived (or didn't survive) the winter on meager allowances of hay instead of being fed silage foresightedly put up during the hot months, and produced very little milk per head.

The New York Mayor's Committee report cited statistics from USDA bulletins and experts at the Massachusetts and Connecticut Agricultural Colleges to demonstrate that low-yielding dairy cows were a financial burden to their owners—not to mention that "they add an item to the cost of milk which is an improper tax on the consumer." The remedy was to have owners pay for memberships in cow-testing services capable of identifying inferior specimens. They should then sell off the rejects for beef and buy properly bred replacements that gave higher yields on the same amounts of feed. From the agricultural college witnesses' estimates, the committee concluded that in ten-cow herds the cost to the farmer of producing one quart of milk from a cow capable of only 4,500 pounds a year was 7.02 cents. That figure fell to 4.74 cents for a cow who could yield at least 7,500 pounds.[18] Unfortunately, most New York State farm producers still ignored cow testing. They also disregarded the experts' arguments that small herds of seven or ten cows were far less efficient than large ones of fifty or sixty. The committee calculated the difference at almost 2 cents a quart.[19]

Rosenau, a more thoughtful observer than some of the other Mayor's Committee authorities, grasped that dirt farmers far outnumbered profit-minded dairy farmers and that non-modernized farming was a strongly rooted way of family life resistant to new marching orders. At present, he commented, "the great bulk of the milk comes from the small farm, and is there regarded only as a by-product. The small farmer keeps a few cows for his personal use. The yield is more than he needs, and he sells the excess. The farmer gives the subject small attention and finds it unprofitable to comply with the exactions of modern sanitary requirements."[20] Champions of modern diets could scarcely wait to get rid of milk produced by such antediluvians.

The pundits at agricultural schools as well as federal and state departments of agriculture were gradually winning over a younger generation, but millions of farmers ignored their calculations. The USDA Yearbook of Agriculture for 1922 estimated that in 1920 there were close to 24.5 million dairy cattle on American farms.[21] The statisticians did not explain how dairy cattle differed from other cattle, a point that probably seemed obvious to them. But many of Rosenau's "small farms" might have had only scrub cattle that indifferently furnished milk, veal (from bull calves not worth raising), and once in a while home-butchered beef (when a cow was worn out for milking). The 1922 yearbook gave the average number of putative dairy cows per farm at four for the entire United States. Twenty-seven states were listed as having five or fewer; averages in the other twenty-one ranged between over five and over ten.[22] These figures show how far farms with fifty to sixty cows were from any norm.

Rosenau had misgivings about the changes being urged upon the rural old guard: "The crowding-out of the small farmer is not to be lightly regarded, for he has human rights and society must grant him economic justice."[23] But his own suggestions for reeducating farm personnel were demanding even by the standards of public health reformers. Acutely conscious that industrial-scale expansion of dairying also meant more opportunities for pathogenic invasion of milk, he wanted milking to be done with sanitary precautions as rigorous as those in an operating theater. "As in antiseptic surgery, success can only be achieved through cleanliness and scrupulous attention to minute details and an intelligent understanding of the problem . . . I could imagine no better training for a milkman than an apprenticeship of a few months in a surgical clinic where aseptic methods may be learned. It is no exaggeration to compare the operation of milking the cow to a surgical operation."[24]

This advice may have been unrealistic, but it was far from senseless considering that virtually all milking was still done by hand, an at least twice-daily task. In addition to being the biggest single labor cost of dairy farming, it was an enormous sanitary liability. A century earlier, women had usually done a family's milking, but in most households this seldom meant more than one or two cows at a time. Milking a herd of even five to ten chafed a worker's bare hands and painfully taxed arm-wrist muscles. Reports of milkers spitting on their hands before grabbing a teat or moistening their hands with the first spurts of milk were undoubtedly the reason that older boutique dairy operations like F. Ratchford Starr's Echo Farm had insisted on rigorous handwashing with soap and water. Such requirements were currently in place at all farms certified by Coit's Medical Milk Commissions as well as those supplying Straus's "pasteurization laboratories."

When Rosenau urged adopting a surgical clinic's methods, milking machines were woefully inadequate. An expert as progress-minded as Henry E. Alvord of the USDA's Bureau of Animal Industry had had to regretfully conclude in 1899, "Cows still have to be milked by hand. Although numerous attempts have been made, and patent after patent has been issued, no mechanical contrivance has yet been a practical success as a substitute for the human hand in milking."[25] Patent followed patent for more than two decades, inflicting a good deal of trauma on cows' udders and never managing to imitate the rhythm of a suckling calf's mouth as deftly as a skilled human milker. The 1920s saw improved manual or (increasingly) electric models in which a vacuum pump drew milk from the cow's teats into a sealed collecting vessel through pulses of alternately applied and released suction, efficient but gentle enough to spare the animal pain. Still, the apparatus was difficult to keep cleaned and sterilized, and using it did not eliminate contact between human hands and the udder.

The only breakthroughs came for very large dairies that were able to invest heavily in assembly-line-scale equipment. In December of 1930, the U.S. Patent Office granted a patent to an engineer named Cyrus Howard Hapgood who was affiliated with the American branch of De Laval, a prolific Swedish manufacturer of dairy machinery. His creation was already being rolled out in Plainsboro, New Jersey, home to an operation that had recently been acquired by the now omnivorous Borden Company. The new Borden subsidiary was Walker-Gordon Laboratories, a certified raw milk dairy like no other. Defying the commonsense assumption that raw milk could be safely handled only on a small scale, it had fashioned itself into a huge mechanized endeavor that sent milk, via a fleet of refrigerated trucks, constantly en route to destinations up and down most of the Northeastern and Mid-Atlantic seaboard.

Walker-Gordon had to have been stupendously capitalized to operate as it did in the teeth of the Great Depression. The Plainsboro farm milked 1,500 cows when fifty was considered a large herd. Hapgood's patent was for a breathtakingly new assembly-line concept, the "Rotolactor," that employed advanced milking machines (probably a model from De Laval, the assignee of patents for a galaxy of inventions in many corners of the globe) fixed in fifty stanchions on a revolving platform that completed one rotation in twelve and a half minutes. Fifty cows in a group walked in file to their individual stanchions. Members of the milking staff rapidly hosed down their hindquarters with clean water, wiped their udders clean with a few efficient strokes, affixed four rubber-lined cups to each animal's teats, and disconnected the cups when she was milked out. Each cow's milk first went to a transparent Pyrex glass vessel that allowed the crew to measure individual yields and detect any visible dirt; from there all milk was piped to a weighing tank and thence to a large bulk tank for immediate chilling. As one group of cows filed away from the platform, the crew flushed out the entire apparatus in preparation for the next lot.[26]

The Rotolactor's requirements were prodigious, including a state-of-the-art—not to say futuristic—custom-built installation with electric power, huge amounts of water, efficient drainage, ultra-precise timing, and thoroughly trained personnel. Few dairy operations can have been conceived on such a scale. But in the interwar years all forward-looking dairy companies focused on a goal that Walker-Gordon's Plainsboro nerve center epitomized: to get as much milk as possible into bottles as fast as possible under strict sanitary precautions.

MILK ORDINANCES: ALABAMA AND BEYOND

Public health authorities not only shared this aim but wanted to translate it into mandatory programs that would address the joint challenges of pumping more milk into more people and curbing milk-borne illness, which was still far from being stamped out. Their proposed solutions, unlike Walker-Gordon's, strongly relied on pasteurization.

The U.S. Public Health Service fretted at the lack of statewide efforts to address milk safety and implement modern production methods. Every city, every county, every large or small jurisdiction was a different kettle of fish in which sanitary requirements might be rigorous, haphazard, or absent. In 1924 the USPHS prepared to roll out a draft of a model state-wide milk ordinance that might be proposed to legislatures or at least adopted by enough local jurisdictions to serve as a template that others might accept under political pressure. The state chosen for the experiment was Alabama. Early in 1923 the USPHS had dispatched an official named Leslie C. Frank—his job description was "sanitary engineer"—to Montgomery to work on a draft ordinance with local personnel.

Why Alabama? For one thing, Frank had had previously spent time in the Gulf coastal region trying to coordinate USPHS and local efforts toward malaria eradication. And since the dairy industry was less developed in the Deep South than anywhere else in the nation, less entrenched political opposition to policing existed there than in big northern Atlantic and Midwestern states.

The reasons for the relative backwardness of dairying in states like Alabama begin with geography, climate, and demographics. The land did not furnish enough suitable ground for pasturage or hayfields to support many commercial-scale herds. Scrub cows were more the rule than the exception. Some could give good milk if well cared for, but they rarely gave much of it. The large Holstein or Holstein-Friesian cattle, which were making great strides in Northern states, suffered serious health problems in Southern summers. The only pedigreed cows that thrived in hot weather were the Channel Islands breeds, especially the small, delicate-looking Jerseys. They were proverbial for giving creamier milk than any other breed—but in much lesser amounts than Holsteins. Besides, the Gulf Coast states were still far less urbanized than the major milk-producing regions. City-country political dissensions did not run as deep, and rural jurisdictions were more accustomed to being left to their own devices—for instance, on the subject of unpasteurized milk.

The climate ensured that fresh raw milk rapidly became "clabbered milk" or "curds" during the months that in the North had historically been synonymous with summer complaint and rising infant mortality. In the Deep South, however, attitudes were different. Clabber had once been doled out to field slaves—or, on some plantations, pigs. In luckier circles it could be considered a seasonal delicacy. The food writer Sheila Hibben, born in Montgomery in 1888, included a recipe for "Curds and Cream" in her 1932 survey of American cooking, *The National Cookbook*. It began with ladling clabbered sour milk into a heart- or diamond-shaped press to drain the curd before turning it out onto a plate to be served with "very rich cream," grated nutmeg, and sugar. "During the curds season—which lasts all summer, beginning with the first hot weather—Alabamians rarely have a breakfast or a cold supper without curds and cream," Hibben affirmed.[27] At around the turn of the century, people had happily bought a similar delicacy from Black vendors on the streets of New Orleans as *fromage à la crème*.[28] It was a summer pleasure clearly born in societies little (if at all) touched by the modernizations that reformers like Leslie Frank wanted to bring to underdeveloped states. Naturally enough, no Southern fan of clabber cared about the obscure fact that using it furnished a means—an ancient one in hot climates—of inhibiting if not wholly eliminating milk-borne pathogens by letting lactic acid fermentation take its course.

The bacteriological advantages of fermented milk were equally invisible to Frank and his USPHS colleagues, who certainly had no reason to consider its culinary merits or prize it above drinking-milk. They were interested only in how to put a stop to stubborn milk-borne disease outbreaks and get what Frank called "enough milk"[29] into the consuming public. They and the Alabama health authorities didn't expect any measure to be immediately enforceable at the state level; their hope was to encourage individual municipalities and towns to adopt an ordinance that Frank had helped draft and persuade local suppliers to go along with. For the time being, the carrot was to be preferred to the stick.

Like Straus and other earlier pasteurization adherents, Frank firmly believed that the double insurance of serious sanitary protocols and pasteurizing equipment would lastingly ensure public safety. But warned

by the example of battles in the major dairying states, he fully understood the degree of political opposition that pasteurization requirements would have to overcome little by little even in a state like Alabama
where farmers were not formidably organized. Thus the draft ordinance
embraced both a long-term goal, an interim expedient, and an accom-
modation for milk that failed to measure up to either of these. The ultimate holy grail was universal pasteurization. For the nonce, raw milk
meeting strict requirements was also given preferential status, though in
language leaving no doubt that the authorities thought it dubiously safe.
Lower-quality milk was allowed to be used—when pasteurized—for
various other food purposes. The ordinance reflected a pragmatic decision to give maximum protection to raw or pasteurized drinking-milk
at once while allowing farmers time to decide that in the final analysis
pasteurization would work in their favor.

Coit and the Medical Milk Commissions had successfully gotten raw-
milk producers to rethink the logistics and physical layout of farm buildings and equipment while accepting periodic inspections to ensure that
they were not cutting corners. Taking a leaf from their book, Frank's draft
ordinance laid heavy stress on eliminating visible and invisible dirt in
locations where milk was drawn from cows and collected for transportation.
Compliance with these precautions dictated rank in a hierarchy of four
grades verified by inspectors, reflecting different permitted bacterial counts.

There were in fact five grades, with Grade A being subdivided into
Grade A raw (exactly what it sounded like) and the more highly valued
Grade A pasteurized (meeting all qualifications for Grade A raw, but
with the extra step of pasteurization). These, the drinking-milk grades,
were to have a bacterial count no higher than 50,000 per cubic centimeter. Frank's case for the double Grade A approach was, "We should
pasteurize milk not because it is poor milk, but because pasteurization
renders any milk, however safe, still safer. We should regard pasteurization not as a means of converting poor milk into safe milk, but as a necessary addition to all other safeguards." The lesser grades (B, C, and D)
were not held to bacterial counts as low as the A grades and had leeway
for somewhat laxer procedures (for instance, the milk did not need to be
chilled to as low a temperature).[30]

The logistics-and-layout demands must have been a shock to farmers unprepared to learn that among many other regulations, every cow must be stabled with at least 500 cubic feet of air space, the floors of milking barns must have a slight grade (for drainage) and be made of cement or some other impermeable substance, and milk must be removed from the barn as soon as drawn and transferred to a religiously clean milk room for prompt chilling. Toilets or outdoor privies must be at a certain remove from milking and milk-handling premises. Water wells must be carefully sited to avoid pollution from manure heaps, which also must be prevented from attracting flies. The udders and flanks of cows must be suitably cleaned before milking; milkers must wash and disinfect their hands and be wearing "clean outer garments" for the procedure. Steam cleaning of all equipment between uses was required for Grade A milk. And the processing plants where milk was bottled for distribution were subject to similar rules.[31].

In the North, standards approaching Rosenau's "surgical clinic" analogy were already being met by farmers supplying the biggest dealer-processors, who in turn generally welcomed antibacterial measures. They were less familiar in the Deep South. But in all regions, small mixed-use farmers undoubtedly foresaw money spilling from a pocket every time they turned around. A poured cement floor was no negligible expense. A steam sterilizer was an enormous investment in itself, but the coal to keep it going every day was at least an equal challenge.

These and many other requirements were to be enforced, on behalf of all Alabama jurisdictions that adopted the ordinance, through a corps of inspectors and testing laboratories funded by the state. A farmer who undertook to comply with them was committing himself and his livelihood to a nearly inconceivable break with the past. But public health professionals were determined to persevere. When Frank's description of the ordinance appeared in the USPHS journal *Public Health Reports* in November 1924, he noted that seven Alabama cities had adopted it in the past twelve months.[32] By 1926 it had won the endorsement of the National Dairy Council, and ten states had adopted some version as a template for citywide regulations.[33] Frank argued that given the increasing importance of interstate milk shipments, letting states pick and

choose which provisions of the ordinance to enforce, and in what manner, was an invitation to dangerous inconsistencies across state lines.
He had already drawn up a new version revised in a number of details
(for instance, chocolate milk had now joined the list of milk products
subject to the ordinance's safety provisions).[34] This he proposed to submit to all states as the USPHS "Standard Milk Ordinance," with most of
the cumbersome definitions and technicalities bundled into a separate
"Standard Milk Control Code" where local enforcers could study them
in detail. The USPHS circulated a mimeographed draft of his "Standard
Ordinance and Code" in 1927, and states continued to ratify the concept
while leaving enforcement up to cities and villages.

Only after World War II did a state go further. The nation's first state-
wide pasteurization ordinance was enacted in Michigan in 1947 and
went into effect the following year. It mandated pasteurization (by either
the batch method or the now-rehabilitated flash method) for milk and
cream as well as half a dozen other drinkable milk products. Butter and
most cheeses were to be manufactured only from pasteurized milk or
cream, with exceptions for cheeses that had been cured or ripened for at
least sixty days.

Two provisos, however, indicate some temporizing in Michigan's
commitment to pasteurization. One stated that the requirement didn't
apply in the case of sales outside the state's licensing system or sales
made "by persons primarily engaged in agricultural production to
employees working on farms operated or controlled by such persons."
(This sounds as if farm workers customarily were allowed to buy milk
or cream to take home to their families.) The other suggests that the
state still had a long way to go in overcoming pockets of political resistance to pasteurization. It allowed 10 percent of the electors in any city,
village, or township to file a petition for a referendum on the question
of exempting that jurisdiction from the provisions of the act. As loop-
holes go, this was more than generous. Certainly it tells us that less
than two years after the war's end, American consumers were far from
united in firm allegiance to pasteurized milk.[35]

In 1965, however, the latest iteration of the 1927 U.S. Standard Ordinance
became the "Grade A Pasteurized Milk Ordinance," in recognition of

the fact that virtually all drinking-milk was now pasteurized. Leslie Frank would have rejoiced to see that day. It fulfilled the true but unspoken mission of the first Milk Ordinance advocates: to sweep away an entire farm-based mentality and replace it with one geared to future needs for "enough milk." Progress dictated that the unambitious small farmers described by Rosenau, with their casually tended cow or handful of cows, must give way to profit-focused farmers who marched to more pragmatic drummers and were ready to accept pasteurization as a norm.

But this model of progress had suffered many setbacks before the war. Not long after the 1929 stock market crash, drinking-milk joined the ranks of other farm commodities that had been mired in disastrous surpluses for the past seven or eight years. The intrinsic peaks-and-valleys nature of dairy cows' lactation cycles, coupled with sharp reductions in consumers' purchasing power, overwhelmed the supposed defenses of "sledge hammer advertising."

The Depression could not permanently stymie modernized production approaches and expanded sanitary regulation. But it starkly exposed splits in the ranks of rural interests and agricultural policy-setters.

The plight of farmers was a major target in Franklin Delano Roosevelt's administration's attempts to address the national shipwreck. Henry Agard Wallace, the secretary of agriculture, presided over a department bitterly divided between two factions. Status-quo champions thought that maintaining prices at the highest practical level while finding new markets to absorb surpluses should guarantee rural prosperity; a cadre of Young Turks was convinced that rapidly attacking surpluses—by desperate means, if necessary—and eradicating rural poverty should be the immediate priorities. The first clique was amply peopled with successful large-scale Midwestern farmers, the second with Eastern social scientists and high-powered lawyers. Their mutual antipathy was unsurprising.

The dairy industry was a particularly messy target for federal intervention. Wallace and his bickering subordinates did manage to get milk shoehorned into the cluster of national food commodities addressed in the New Deal's first attempt at solving the farm crisis, the Agricultural

Adjustment Act of 1933. But the new agency appointed to implement its provisions, the Agricultural Adjustment Administration (AAA), had made only fitful progress in relieving milk producers' distress by 1936, when the Supreme Court struck down the act in an opinion declaring that it usurped the right of states to regulate agriculture.

A SCATHING ASSESSMENT

While Wallace's legal team scrambled to produce amended versions of the act, some of the uneven recovery encouraged by the first initiative began to fail. The last years of the decade saw renewed economic downturns, along with disenchanted opinions from the New Deal's more contrarian theorists. Some of these had gravitated to a wing of thinking known as "institutional economics," which broke with orthodox counterparts by insisting that any exchange of money should be viewed through the prism of complex interactions among many different social forces. Members of this faction believed that supply and demand reliably regulated themselves only in the minds of pundits blind to the underreported human dimensions of both.

In 1938 the well-known institutional economist Walton H. Hamilton, who headed one of the New Deal bureaucratic workshops assigned to thresh out many issues bearing on consumer prices, published *Price and Price Policies*, a collection of studies drafted by members of the group a few years earlier. He and the other contributors had examined manifold factors governing the prices of seven commodities or articles of trade, from automobile tires to women's dresses. The young and sharp-witted Irene Till, Hamilton's ex-student and now wife, had chosen to examine the gasoline and milk industries.

Till, who had some serious legal training and a strong background in economics, had been given access to confidential AAA files. She had also combed through the abovementioned 1934 FTC hearings on milk prices, and amassed much evidence from unpublished accounts as well as conversations with farmers. Tearing into all ramifications of the milk business with uninhibited iconoclasm, she achieved trenchant insights unmatched by any other twentieth-century investigator.

Like many liberal Easterners in Wallace's USDA, she believed that the chief victims of the general agricultural debacle were farmers and consumers, the chief villains the entities that conveyed the product from the first to the second group as dealer-processor-distributors. Like Rosenau a generation earlier, she was troubled by the plight of the many small independent farmers—still the foundation of the industry—who conducted humble mixed-use family-scale operations with a few cows. "The ordinary milk producer is not engaged in the dairy business. His farm is his way of life," she wrote.[36] Indeed, "The small farmer is really not a part of our money economy."[37] In terms of power balance, the farmer-dealer situation was not unlike relations between laborers and employers—except that smallholding farmers were in no position to form trade unions and force collective bargaining on their exploiters. They were sellers in what was intrinsically a buyer's market.

As a committed institutional economist, Till had no use for talk about protecting competition among processor-distributors or the public's freedom of choice. She saw these as brazenly misleading shibboleths in an enterprise where "the machine-like precision of the processing plant" creates "an identity of ware among competitors which few industries can equal." Nonetheless, "the fiction of a buyer's choice is maintained by the industry."[38] Over the last generation or so, the largest processor-distributors had managed to acquire control over the official narrative through strategic alliances:

> Organizations educating the public to the food values of milk were established on a national scale; the public schools were stumped in glorious campaigns; the healthy infant complacently sipping his daily quart of milk was a commonplace in every newspaper. Everywhere the promotion of milk was the promotion of business. Lobby fortifications were run up in state and national capitals; pious denunciations of statutes inimical to distributor interests blared symphonically throughout the land. It was fitting and proper that the sanctions of public health and the ideals of free enterprise blended mercifully to make this position well-nigh impregnable.[39]

In her judgment, dietary experts' hymns to milk, in league with massive publicity campaigns, had played an unfortunate role in turning a biological reality into an industrialized artifact subject to bizarre price convolutions. She actually dared to question "notions of the indispensability of milk in the human diet," skeptically remark that "some dietetical experts have endowed milk with mystical properties," and treat recommended daily allowances as less than sacrosanct, since "a rigid rule for milk consumption has no more validity than any other principle which is besieged with exceptions."[40] She could even imagine that in time to come, shifts in the diet might cause milk to "become an added gratuity to human health or unnecessary. Human ingenuity may, at some time in the future, create a synthetic milk superior in taste and nutrition to the natural product; and a commodity, now regarded as a necessity, might by virtue of technology be rendered obsolete."[41]

Till would have liked to see federal policy setters conduct a serious, thoroughgoing review of the industry's bizarre ideology and structure. This did not happen. No fundamental re-examination of crucial issues ever occurred during the New Deal, or later. Nutrition advisers and public health administrators formed a solid front with the NDC in insisting on the supreme virtues of drinking-milk. Irene Till got as close to heresy on that point as anybody, but even she was more concerned with mitigating the industry's problems than taking a wrecking ball to it.

By the time her study appeared, the Depression had devastated huge segments of the agricultural economy. The first New Deal attempts to reduce farm surpluses and stabilize prices had offered financial incentives to farmers to cut production, usually by plowing under some portion of a crop or leaving some of their acreage fallow. These measures were absolutely useless to dairy farmers. Come hell or high water, they had to milk every lactating cow in the herd every day. The only surplus-control tactic open to them was culling—selling off a certain number of cows for cheap beef while hoping against hope that it wouldn't take too long to rebuild the herd if prices ever rebounded. The biggest expenses were labor (especially milking) and fodder for the cows. Agricultural school teachings about getting more milk out of every animal through scientifically planned diets will be more fully discussed in chapter 8; by the start of the Depression, they had already persuaded many hopeful farmers to adopt high-priced additions to the daily ration. Cutting back to the bare essentials of grass and hay (sometimes damaged by droughts or other unavoidable setbacks) took a toll on outputs. Average annual production per cow was 4,579 pounds in 1929, 4,033 pounds in 1934. Workforces also had to be cut to the bone.[42]

U.S. buying habits underwent drastic changes. Among dairy products, cheese was one of the first nonessentials to be discarded by hard-up families. Margarine gained ground as a thrifty alternative to butter. Fluid milk showed some resilience at first, but had entered a slump in a few years as urban consumers' incomes shrank. A 1935 Brookings Institution survey, though somewhat hampered by the difficulty of collecting nationwide data, reported that prices for milk sold by farmers to distributors had declined by 39 percent from 1929 to 1932. Overall, per capita drinking-milk consumption fell by between 7 and 12 percent from 1930 to 1933, with far greater losses in some cities.[43] The national decline would have been still steeper if rural families living on the mixed-use "dirt farms" scorned by apostles of agricultural progress hadn't begun consuming more of their own animals' milk, sometimes even adding another cow or two for the purpose.

The farmers' predicament meant even stronger leverage for the dairy companies to dictate terms. Unlike the farmers who merely harvested the product every day, they had the technological means to convert it into less perishable or even indefinitely storable forms such as canned or powdered dried milk—after agreeing to take the producers' bulky, fragile output off their hands at some price far below that mandated for drinking-milk. The general structure of the operations that sold milk to processors varied so greatly that it was nearly impossible to organize individual farmers into alliances acting to any common purpose. In fighting back against the dealer-processors, it was mainly every man for himself.

All observers could see that the milk production landscape was hopelessly chaotic. The USDA under Henry Wallace and his successor, Claude Wickard, sought to impose some order on the situation, but attempts to intervene in milk pricing were hampered by the Supreme Court's position on infringement of states' rights. Some individual states with large dairy industries also cast about for reforms. The main solution that occurred to would-be regulators was to draw geographical boundaries around urban centers of consumer demand for drinking-milk, requiring individual producers within the delineated region to pool their milk and abide by a set of pricing formulas equally applicable to all of them. This was indeed the approach that would ultimately be adopted, but it was not put into effect during the Depression era. Rescue for dairy farmers came not from reform initiatives but from another world war.

In the spring of 1941, the Roosevelt administration and Congress recognized the desperate straits of Great Britain by approving large relief shipments of war matériel and food through the Lend-Lease Act. It was a timely boost for manufacturers of nonperishable dairy products such as dried or canned milk and cheese. It also presaged further war preparation measures such as the Steagall Amendment, which authorized the secretary of agriculture to employ price supports in order to maintain adequate supplies of several crucial commodities, including milk.[44] After Pearl Harbor, all sectors of the dairy industry could count on government backing for tremendously expanded production, with the added reassurance that the Steagall price supports would be continued at least two years beyond the end of hostilities. At the same time, regulatory ceilings on retail prices restricted processors' ability to jack up their own profits.

Part of the war's immediate aftermath was a series of attempts to create something closer to a national milk price policy than Wallace and Wickard's USDA had been able to achieve. Everyone was determined to avoid a repeat of the post-World War I agricultural depression. Food production had emerged from the war in a strong position, at least partly through the Steagall Amendment price supports, which were about to expire. The 1948 and 1949 Agricultural Acts continued these protections indefinitely.[45]

But federal regulators also wanted to bring milk production into some kind of coherent price support structure accommodating both local and national interests. They ended by creating the Federal Milk Marketing Order system, an expanded version of some tentative Depression-era models. It carved up the map of the United States into a number of delineated regions—"marketing orders"—in which "handlers"—the new name for the dealer-processor-distributors—would be required to pay producing farmers certain minimum prices determined by complex, regionally tailored formulas, with a general differentiation between higher prices for fluid milk and lower prices for milk allocated to other manufacturing purposes that roughly mirrored the previous scheme of milk "classes" or "grades" described earlier in this chapter.[46] These formulas gradually became as abstruse, and as unintelligible to anyone outside a small charmed circle, as anything in the bad old days before the federal government stepped in. Far from abolishing the buyer's market, they trapped farmers selling fluid milk within the marketing order system in endless struggles to wring enough out of handlers to recoup production costs.

In 2016 the newsletter of an industry group, the American Dairy Products Institute, offered a version of a well-worn trade quip, "There is an old joke about a senior-level USDA person testifying to Congress on dairy policy and milk pricing. He said there are only three people that understood it and two of them are lying."[47] I would like to dissociate myself from either category. What I do understand is that as the postwar era advanced, the sheer incomprehensibility of producer-handler milk price schemes again became an endless frustration to dairy farmers, above all those trying to make a living within the marketing order system for drinking-milk.

At D-Day and V-J Day there seemed to be every reason for optimism, not all of which was misplaced. The demand for milk in both fluid and nonperishable forms had surged throughout the war. For a few years, dairy farmers not only came close to the elusive goal of parity with pre-World War I earning power but sometimes surpassed it. During gasoline rationing, farmers received preferential treatment as being engaged in an essential industry—thus swelling the ranks of those who had swapped horses or mules for tractors. The war also allowed them to rely more heavily on milk-stimulating grain-based concentrates in feed, an investment that many had had to forgo at the nadir of the Depression. (Grain was now plentiful because submarine warfare had curbed exports to Europe.) By creating a shortage of farm labor as young men went off to the front, it expedited the shift to milking machines and other electrified farm equipment.

At the time, no observer could have grasped the real meaning of the turnaround in milk production that the war had brought about. In hindsight, statistics on the national output of milk allow us to pinpoint crucial moments. The total was 109,510,000,000 pounds in 1940, 115,498,000,000 in 1941, 119,240,000,000 in 1942. In 1945 it was 122,219,000,000 pounds.[48] The significance of these figures is made clear by other information: the numbers of American dairy farms and dairy cows.

In 1940 some 4,662,413 farms were reported as contributing milk to the commercial supply. In 1945 the number had fallen to 4,481,384. 1945 thus marks the first year in which *fewer farms delivered more milk*. By 1950 the total would be 3,681,627.[49]

The 1940 USDA census of agriculture reported the average of milk production per cow as 525 gallons, or roughly 4,515 pounds.[50] A 1946 USDA survey gives the 1945 average as 4,789 pounds. That had grown to 5,314 by 1950.[51] The U.S. dairy cow population, meanwhile, was 21,936,556 in 1940.[52] It increased to 22,803,000 in 1945 as a result of steady wartime encouragement to dairy farmers to expand their herds. But by 1950, it had shrunk to 21,367,000. Though total U.S. milk production had fallen off somewhat in the aftermath of the main wartime push and now stood at 116,602,000,000 pounds, the dairy industry had now taken a small but irreversible step toward getting more milk out of fewer cows.[53]

Thirty-some years earlier, patriotic experts had seen World War I as a wakeup call to breed more dairy cows. Herbert Hoover had warned against letting cow numbers lapse. Less than a month after the end of the war in 1918, the dairy scientist Charles E. North had given a speech to the American Public Health Association, "The Milk Industry and the War," declaring that the only way of getting nutritionally adequate amounts of milk into the entire citizenry was to add another 20,920,000 cows to the extant population of about 23,284,000.[54] No other way of dramatically driving up milk supplies could have been pictured.

But once past the hurdles of the 1920s agricultural depression and the Great Depression, completely different visions were about to dawn for American dairy farming. Though the war had kept the industry focused more on immediate production targets than on following up scientific breakthroughs, even the fairly simple technological aids that it helped put into producers' hands presaged a model beyond the imagining of Hoover or North. Year after year from 1950 on, progressive dairy farming would involve less manual labor per gallon of milk produced, more milk per cow, fewer cows per farm, fewer farms per county or state, ever-expanding national milk harvests (with accompanying surpluses), and steeper investments in breathtaking feats of technology.

Advocates for these advances thought they would help to guarantee the nation's milk producers an adequate return for their efforts. For the great majority of farmers, that goal kept mysteriously receding through the end of the twentieth century, and afterward. Researchers in many aspects of dairy biology did their utmost to cancel the inconveniences of handling live mammals for the sake of a superperishable mammalian secretion. But no matter what, farmers still were left to deal with flesh-and-blood creatures who had to be conceived, brought into the world, raised, fed, impregnated so as to get their own lactation cycles operating through a Murphy's-Law gauntlet of things that could go wrong, and finally sold off for beef. Nonetheless, both advisers and farmers continued to place faith in new and newer technology for pushing bovine reproductive capacity to the last imaginable limits.

8

TECHNOLOGY IN OVERDRIVE I

The Animals

A dairy farmer during the early twentieth-century expansion of the American milk business had to constantly divert annoying amounts of money and attention to one major four-legged headache: the bull. No calving and no milk could be expected unless he mounted ovulating cows just like his undomesticated forebears—aurochsen—who had passed down their aggressive instincts in considerable force from the Ice Ages. When not actually on the job, he had to be fed, housed, and prevented from killing anybody. In short, he was not a trifling expense, and many farmers longed to be rid of him. Wrestling with the issue, some producers conceived the idea of co-ops in which each member would share the cost of a bull's upkeep, while being relieved of his farmside presence until it was needed.[1] This stratagem helped to lighten the problem, but only partly.

Many thousands of dairy farms are now bull-free. His place is supplied by a liquid nitrogen tank maintained at a temperature of $-320°F/-196°C$. It holds a handful or more of skinny plastic straws containing the frozen semen of sires belonging to an artificial insemination (AI) service, which specializes in getting the donor to ejaculate into a cleverly designed receptacle called an "artificial vagina." (A "teaser" cow, dummy cow, or steer usually provides the necessary stimulus.) A single ejaculation can be extended in the laboratory to produce enough diluted semen for several hundred inseminations; a live bull on a modest-sized farm is unlikely to sire more than sixty calves in a year.[2] Today probably more than 80 percent of the animals in question are Holsteins; the breed surged to overwhelming popularity among dairy farmers from the 1950s on because of its extremely large yields of milk per cow.[3]

To select a potential sire, the purchaser goes online and studies computerized data about the candidates owned by the business. A bull's name may be followed by the letters "ET," indicating that he was gestated by undergoing "embryo transfer" to a surrogate mother's uterus. The procedure is performed after a series of hormone injections that induce the biological mother's ovaries to release not a single egg but five or six eggs capable of being fertilized at one fell swoop and implanted in surrogates, who also have received doses of hormones to synchronize their ovulatory cycles.[4]

Whatever the means through which he arrives in this world, the entry under his name and identification number on the company website will tell you the traits for which he is "daughter-proven," meaning that he has the ability to transmit them in the female line. They range from annual amounts of milk produced, milkfat totals/percentages, and protein totals/percentages to physical details like the conformation of teats on the udder (for properly attaching the cups of milking machines without hurting the animal) or the soundness of hooves (a vulnerable point in large, heavy dairy cows who may spend countless hours standing on hard floors). Managers of herds look for sires who earn the highest aggregate scores in crucial categories, and nitrogen tanks on many or most dairy farms hold selections of straws ready for careful thawing to body heat (about 101°F/38°C) at the right moment.

The two trickiest parts of actually using a straw of thawed semen are detecting the brief interval when the cow is in estrus—live bulls under free-range conditions used to be better at this than humans—and inserting the straw as far as the opening of the uterus. Bulls have an advantage there as well, since the erect penis is usually just slightly less than a yard long. Instead of attempting the delicate process themselves, farmers often leave it up to a trained technician who snips off the end of the straw and fits it into the tip of an "inseminating gun," a long, thin stainless steel rod equipped with a plunger. He (less frequently she) dons a shoulder-length plastic sleeve, inserts an arm into the cow's rectum, and manually palpates it while inserting the gun into the vulva with the other hand. The rectal palpation allows a skilled pro's fingers to follow the rod's passage through the vulva and vagina before threading it through the most difficult stretch, the narrow cervix. A correct push of the plunger deposits the semen just beyond the threshold of the uterus. With luck, the result will be a healthy calf in nine months.[5] And if the farmer has paid a premium for sex-sorted semen with Y chromosomes eliminated, it will be a daughter—a far cry from the days when cows bore equal numbers of heifer and bull calves, with the males inconveniently remaining on the farmer's hands until they could be sold cheap for veal.

Such apparent efficiency has come at a steep cost. In 2000 buyers of Holstein semen were unaware that all Holstein sires in AI programs— as well as nearly all other Holstein bulls in the United States—were descended on the male side from exactly two founding bulls born during the 1960s. They in turn could be traced through the male line (recorded in the breed association herdbook) to two other bulls born in the 1880s. In other words, the independent Y chromosome lineages transmitted through artificial insemination over roughly forty years—after having been conserved through some eighty years of natural breeding—boiled down to just two. The posthumous career of a third superstar in 1960s AI breeding programs had somehow been cut short, possibly because of the belated discovery that he carried a recessive mutation responsible for a spike in two severe genetic defects among the thousands of calves born from his inseminations. Not long earlier, dairy farmers had also started to notice a puzzling decline in fertility among Holstein cows.[6]

The path from bull to nitrogen tank is only one among many illustrations of how radically the drinking-milk industry was transfigured in the last fifty-odd years of the twentieth century. This chapter will examine only a few of many technological advances that reshaped the milk industry between approximately 1950 and 2000. It is not my purpose to use "technology" as a convenient whipping boy for everything that separates modern dairying from some imaginary Sunnybrook Farm.

Thinking of technology as "applied science" may make it easier to recognize that any proposed innovation can be met with either a rush to reap promised bonanzas or caution about long-term consequences. The first choice sometimes leads to publicity-ridden backlashes followed by expensive course corrections several miles down the road.

DAIRY FARM MAKEOVERS

Agricultural advisers have been urging American farmers to adopt modern business models since at least the early aftermath of the Civil War. It was a rational idea, considering that even then urban clienteles were becoming a formidable part of the market that farmers had to address. After city-dwellers first surpassed country-dwellers in the 1920 population census, the extinction of small self-sufficient family farms was only a matter of time. Farmers who did not see that they must recalibrate their roles to satisfy city-based popular preferences—for example, getting as much Red Delicious apple stock as possible into the orchard while eliminating half a dozen favorites of older apple-lovers—would be gone in a few generations. (As of 2010, Americans living in urban areas were more than 80 percent of the population.[7])

But drinking-milk was the most precarious and unforgiving of all cash crops for farmers trying to keep afloat in an inexorably urbanizing America. If dairy farmers had not started out viewing cows as machines for converting units of fodder into units of milk, with due allowance for many other production costs that melted away gross income, they soon were forced to recognize their mistake. Having to operate in a hard-nosed buyer's market shaped by intense city-based downward pressure on retail prices was a fact of life.

Rhetoric like that in the 1917 New York Mayor's Committee report about low-producing dairy cows being in effect an unfair "tax" on consumers didn't pass unheeded by the industry. One of the sternest disciplines that farmers had to learn was to cull unprofitable members of a herd and raise average yields per cow to generally approved standards. Higher productivity was the single-minded purpose of the reproductive exploits just described—in fact, a holy grail of the entire dairy-farming community.

Early programs pursued the goal with rudimentary technology and shaky guiding principles. Experts at the USDA, state agriculture departments, and land-grant schools correctly preached that breeding was a major determinant of performance at the milk pail. But the art of cow-improving soon acquired a strong preference for judging the book by its cover. The principal breed associations, founded in the late nineteenth century, dwelt much on "feminine" or "refined" appearance in dairy cows.[8] To male admirers of Ayrshires, Guernseys, and the rest, "feminine" mostly meant a bright-eyed face in a smallish head attractively poised on a graceful neck. Less absurdly, arbiters of most breed standards praised spare contours with at most slight padding over the rib cage or elsewhere. That conformation indicated that secreting milk would be the animal's principal use of food energy, as opposed to replenishing her own reserves of flesh and fat.[9] Among six or seven important breeds that attracted fan clubs after the 1880s, those that best fitted these standards were the strapping Holsteins and the dainty Jerseys— otherwise, polar opposites on any scale of dairy cow values. Everyone recognized that Holsteins gave more milk per cow than any other breed, Jerseys less. Everyone who understood milk recognized that on the average, Jersey milk was the richest and Holstein milk the thinnest among the major breeds, though individual cows in both breeds might dramatically differ from general averages.

Over several decades during the twentieth century, Jerseys and Holsteins competed for the title of most important American breed. A 1942 bulletin from the University of Illinois dairy science department reported that among dairy purebreds and stock with strong admixtures from chosen breeds, Jerseys comprised 42 and Holsteins 40 percent of the national total.[10] A few lesser contenders including Brown Swiss, Ayrshires, Guernseys, and Milking Shorthorns accounted for the other 18 percent. The balance shifted after the war, and in the last half of the century Holsteins decisively eclipsed all competition. Many people today have never seen even a cartoon image of a dairy cow without the characteristic Holstein black and white markings. There are many reasons for this preeminence. But the chief one is incontrovertible: cows who give much more milk than others reward their owners with reduced labor costs per unit of harvested milk.

A USDA review of various dairy breeds in 1898 reported that yields of 40 to 60 pounds a day were average for Holsteins, while some remarkable specimens were capable of 100 or more for at least a few days in succession. By contrast, one unusually fine Jersey "averaged over 40 pounds a day over five months."[11] Today yields of 150 pounds a day for some period register as very good rather than astonishing for Holsteins, and 200-pound yields are not unheard-of.[12] Even allowing for the fact that the full amount is usually spread out over two or more daily milkings, an animal must be powerfully built to carry such loads without great physical strain, especially on the hindquarters and hind feet.

Plainly the productive capacity of Holstein cows has more than doubled since 1898. But USDA statistics of dairy production show only small or moderate gains up to 1950. The reason is that World War II forced the industry to wait nearly a decade for a full rollout of some late 1930s technological developments. One was artificial insemination, in which the Soviet Union had been the chief world pioneer. It soon became one of the crucial factors in enhanced milk production from U.S. dairy cows.

The usual postwar records are for average milk yield per year rather than per day. After 1952, averages began racing ahead by at least two percentage points nearly every year, and often three or four. Production per cow was 5,314 pounds in 1950. It reached 18,201 pounds in 2000 and has kept gaining ever since. The United States is now among the world's leading nations in average annual milk yields per cow (about 23,400 pounds in 2019).[13]

CREATING THE TURBO-COW

Just selecting dairy cows for the conformation points lauded by breed associations could never have produced such stupefying change in half a century. Neither could the more practical idea of selecting the daughters of excellent milkers, as well as sires with a reputation for producing distinguished daughters. The deciding factors were rigorously data-driven: ever-improving artificial insemination practices, more interventionist management of a cow's reproductive cycle, and new ways of tailoring the makeup of her feed to her performance as a milker. Today all require intense attention to reams of detailed metrics, impossible to navigate without investments in specialized software. All together they have created a uniquely twentieth-century mammalian artifact: the "high-performance" or "high-producing cow." The historian Barbara Orland, surveying signs of such developments in Swiss and German dairying earlier in the century, called the first products of improvement programs "turbo-cows"—a nickname eventually picked up by choruses of skeptics in Europe.[14]

A high-producing cow may be purebred, though by about 1910 agricultural school researchers had already begun breeding "grade" dairy cattle by repeatedly crossing purebred sires with scrub cows to establish greatly improved milking capacity in as little as two generations.[15] Some grade cows can advance from fairly good to turbo-charged records. In any case, what distinguishes a high producer is the ability to channel tremendous—indeed, freakish—amounts of energy from her feed into the sole purpose of making milk.

Genetics alone underpinned much of the early impetus toward milk yields so enormous that a nursing calf could suckle only a minor fraction of a high-performing mother's output day by day. After about 2010, farmers also began paying attention to the study of entire genomes. But such contributions have been powerfully reinforced by rearing practices. Decade after decade throughout the late twentieth century, agricultural school courses and dairy management manuals taught farmers to view any unharvested drop of milk as money down the drain—which it is, in an industry of unrelenting pressures. Letting a dairy cow nurse her calf is a prime example.

With the possible exception of the poultry industry, no other branch of animal husbandry has developed such detailed micromanagement of the product and its biological source. For generations, dairy farmers had allowed newborn calves to suckle the first colostrum, then waited at least a few days to separate the mother from the infant—who, after all, had triggered the flow of milk simply by being born. But twentieth- and twenty-first-century farmers gradually whittled away at the time this mammalian pair could spend together doing what mammals evolved to do. Not unjustly, they argued that it is more wrenching to both to separate them after some days of bonding than almost immediately after birth. The usual approach was to remove the calf from the dam as soon as possible, while trying to treat both gently. The calf might be briefly allowed to suckle colostrum, but more likely would get previously drawn colostrum from a bottle.[16]

By contrast, calves reared for the beef industry used to be routinely given free access to the mother's colostrum and then allowed to nurse for six or seven months. The calf needed, and the mother provided, an increasing flow of milk for the first ten or twelve weeks, to support growth so rapid that an 80-pound newborn might gain another 220 pounds in three months.[17] But meanwhile the calf was developing an interest in grass. Its attention was divided between milk—which went straight to the true stomach (abomasum; see chapter 1) and was promptly digested there—and plants that stimulated the first stomach chamber (rumen) to start welcoming trillions of cellulose-digesting bacteria in preparation for full weaning. The flow of milk gradually dwindled and stopped in tandem with the calf's lessening demands, until the young one was completely acclimated to a ruminant diet of grass.

Dairy farmers urgently wanted to shorten this process. They generally gave measured amounts of colostrum to a newborn before getting it started on a powdered and water-diluted formula called "calf milk replacer," a striking analogue of the elaborate baby formulas that Thomas Rotch urged on human mothers in the 1890s.[18] The goal was to speed up the transition to an adult ruminant diet. But there is a quirk here: dairy cows were not left to eat a purely ruminant diet without calculated enhancements. More than a hundred years ago, dairy scientists looked at what the animals were eating and began trying to pump more caloric energy into their feed.

The huge armies of microorganisms in a normal rumen feed on endless supplies of cellulose from grass or hay, known in the industry as "forages."

The whole microbial ecosystem has to undergo tricky rearrangements when more calorie-dense and protein-rich feeds, or "concentrates," are added to the host animal's diet. The reason for using them is simple: they stimulate a cow to give more milk, though it often is on the watery side. Their chief sources are cereal grains and soybeans, more often administered as milling by-products than in unprocessed form. The first promoters of concentrates to increase milk production soon saw that they were up against the limits of ruminal digestion. The new enrichments often made cows sick, though the animals could adapt to them somewhat when given in carefully measured increments.

The Iowa State College dairy husbandry professor Andrew C. McCandlish, writing in 1922, called on the resources of modern science to analyze feeding problems, with painstaking attention to concentrates. Since no one could yet directly observe what was going on in the rumen through fistulation (chapter 1), he was partly flying blind. The main problem that he recognized was guiding a cow through the seasons of the year. Spring grass flourished in pastures just as the amounts of milk needed by the calf were most steeply increasing and the dam was building up to peak production. Mid- and late summer, however, was a trying time. Not only did it mark the end of peak grass season, but cows needed some respite from hot, dry weather; calves were even more badly affected. A dairy herd's milk production fell off considerably after June. McCandlish advised liberal use of silage (meadow grasses or cornstalks partly fermented in silos) and soilage (leafy crops harvested green and fed directly to cows) in order to increase moisture intake. Cold weather signaled the time for strategic reliance on concentrates, which might have been used only sparingly or not at all up to that point. From late autumn to early spring, the backbone of the rations was hay, silage, and concentrates.[19]

McCandlish stressed that every cow was different and that all dairymen should do their utmost to understand her individual needs. At the same time, he clearly thought that their full-time responsibilities should include hours of strenuous numbers-crunching, aided by his charts and tables for calculating just how many pounds of various dietary components per pound of a cow's weight should go into her rations at different seasons or stages of lactation. He also recognized that some minerals and the few then-known vitamins must play a crucial role in herd health, but the idea of using them in nutritional supplements had not yet caught on.[20] The most serious decisions confronting the farmer, by his lights, were about managing seasonal transitions without subjecting the animal to too sharp a jolt between outdoor (almost completely forage-based) and indoor (concentrate-enriched) diets.

After the immediate postwar years, expert advice about feeding shifted along with a mounting emphasis on pushing the limits of high-producing cows to turbo-levels that McCandlish could not have thought possible. Breeding with an undeviating focus on higher milk yields was part of the picture, along with breakthrough insights about how feeding practices could amplify such gains.

All this progress, however, led to the less welcome realization that a high-producing cow was an alarmingly delicate mechanism, easily knocked off-kilter by an operator's mistakes. At peak lactation she could scarcely manage to eat enough to sustain her own bodily needs against the tremendous drain that secreting milk put on her system. Yet dairy farmers were—and still are—being pressed to maintain peak lactation from as many cows as possible for as long as possible. Throughout their milking careers the highest-performing members of very high-producing herds hover on the thin edge of what is known as "negative energy balance" or NEB, a condition in which they spend more energy in metabolizing their feed in order to keep up lactation than they can take in by eating more. Cows—especially high producers—may go into NEB in the critical transition period just before giving birth and during early lactation, when some rapid hormonal adjustments are taking place.[21]

Before modern dairying, cows could not have kept on depleting their own stored bodily fuel after exhausting the energy derived from their food. But a 2006 textbook of dairy cattle science firmly states that for high-producing cows in early lactation, "a negative energy balance is not only inevitable, but also desirable . . . without mobilization of body reserves, cows cannot hope to reach their genetic potential for milk production."[22]

There is another complication: feeding concentrate in large amounts tends to lower the pH of the rumen. Though acid-to-base ratios fluctuate somewhat in the normal rumen over the course of a day, the ruminal microbes that break down cellulose work most effectively at a pH between 6.5 (very slightly acidic) and 7 (neutral). When they encounter more acidic conditions for more than brief intervals, they are crowded out by competitors that prefer to act on simpler fermentable carbohydrates, creating progressively stronger acidity. If the disturbed balance of bacterial kinds is not corrected, it produces either subacute or acute ruminal acidosis. Nothing deterred, the textbook authors advise farmers, "NEB cows must be kept at the edge of acidosis if nutrient intake is to be maximized. This condition allows little room for error; acidosis is a common nutritional disorder in NEB lactation cows."[23] Translation: high-energy feeding of high-producing cows as they approach peak production is a precarious tightrope act.

Acute acidosis can be life-threatening. In the subacute form, the inner surfaces of the rumen often become inflamed and easily invaded by bacteria that migrate through the bloodstream. Their favorite targets are the hooves, where they trigger laminitis (an excruciatingly painful inflammation of the tissue layers between the horny exterior and the bone), and the liver, where they produce abscesses. Another frequent condition during the NEB period in early lactation is ketosis, which occurs when the cow starts metabolizing her own fat and by-products called ketone bodies build up to dangerous levels in the bloodstream.[24]

A separate but allied problem is that high-producing cows on high-energy diets are susceptible to mastitis, or inflammation of the udder, with the greatest danger occurring during the postpartum NEB period. There is no shortcut cure. An afflicted cow has to be put on a course of antibiotics until her milk shows no abnormalities. Meanwhile, she must be milked separately from the rest of the herd, and the milk must be discarded for several days—just how long depends on the individual drug—after the last dose.[25] (Public health authorities, who spent years waffling about antibiotic residues in meat, have been more alert about keeping them out of the milk supply.)

Throughout the late twentieth century these constant health problems became a growing threat to farmers' income. Every day that a cow had to be sequestered from the milking herd meant so many dollars deducted from total production. From 1950 on, expectations of continually increasing yields intensified; lost time—meaning almost literally every hour that a cow didn't spend in lactating—translated into lost revenue.

As soon as a heifer was born, her owner was estimating how soon she could be bred (usually between about twenty months and two years of age). Any ovulatory cycle in which she failed to conceive cost the farmer money. So did a spontaneous abortion or stillbirth. A successful "freshening"—the start of milk production after a calf's birth—set human caregivers awaiting the chance for her next breeding, probably forty-five to sixty days later. If the attempt was successful, she would conceive while still in the NEB stage after freshening. She would thus be starting her pregnancy while at or close to peak production from the last birth. About sixty days before her estimated due date, she would be permitted to dry off. Ideally, that would be the only time over a twelve-month period when she was not actually in milk.

Many cows simply could not keep up with this unforgiving pace for long without incurring acidosis-linked problems, repeated bouts of mastitis, and/or serious reproductive disorders. Holsteins, because they now provided such an enormous amount of the overall milk supply, were the worst-affected breed. The highest-producing Holsteins became known for both failure to conceive and difficult births. Part of the reason may have been a shift in the "breed standards" favored by the parent breeders' group, the Holstein-Friesian Association of America.

In the Netherlands (where they were known as Friesians), the breed's ancestors had been big, solidly built animals considered nearly as good for beef as for dairy purposes. In the United States, they were raised exclusively as milking stock from the 1880s on, but retained some meat on their bones. Images of cows in an 1898 guide to dairy breeds show a Holstein with slightly fleshy contours and a little Jersey with the almost gaunt frame and sharply jutting hip bones for which the breed has long been known.[26] But for unfathomable reasons, preferences in Holsteins' body conformation made an emphatic swerve after World War II. The Holstein-Friesian Association began lauding "dairy type"—meaning something closer to Jersey type—while also emphasizing sheer size. Angularity and spareness were rewarded by show judges, along with a remodeling of the hindquarters in which the bones corresponding to human pelvic bones formed a squarish arrangement known as a "boxcar rump."[27] Indeed, the ability to transmit boxcar rumps to daughters became a sought-after quality in Holstein sires. But some pushback emerged a few decades ago.

By 2000 experts in veterinary obstetrics recognized "dystocia," or difficult labor, as a major drawback of the breed. First-calving Holstein heifers were especially prone to prolonged, complications-ridden deliveries often followed by poor milk yields or impaired fertility. Some Holstein owners who had been around long enough to acquire a skeptical perspective on current trends eventually spoke up to wonder whether the fashionable boxcar rumps played a crucial part. Meanwhile, cows had gotten not only bonier but bigger, at an average weight of 1,500 pounds in 2000 as compared to 1,250 in 1898. Not surprisingly, calves also were bigger, further compounding the dystocia problem.[28]

DAIRY FARMS AND DAIRY COWS:
SURVIVAL OF THE BIGGEST

Breeding cows for size was intended to increase milk yields, in effect enabling a smaller number of animals to deliver a larger national supply. On paper, this goal always appeared to have sound economic arguments on its side. (It was gradually applied even to Jerseys.) In practice, it meant putting more eggs in fewer as well as physically frailer baskets. Total U.S. milk production increased from about 116.6 to 167.6 billion pounds between 1950 and 2000, while the number of dairy cows shrank from 21,367,000 to 9,210,000.[29] There are no exact figures for how many of the reduced total were Holsteins, but the breed accounted for at least 90 percent of dairy cows in 2000.

At the same time, the U.S. rural landscape lost many thousands of small multipurpose farms a year, casualties of accelerating urban sprawl. In their place appeared much-reduced numbers of large, specialized operations. Farms devoted completely to dairying had been the exception before World War II. Now they became the rule. It is difficult to cite exact figures, since the old-style mixed-use farms that had once furnished more of the national milk supply—accommodating a few cows along with assorted other livestock and some plant crops—never were "dairy farms" in the sense understood by later bean-counters. More than 4.66 million farms producing at least some milk were listed in the 1940 USDA agricultural census. Between 1945 and 1950 the number shrank from about 4.5 million to about 3.7 million; after that, mixed-use farms progressively disappeared from the picture. The survivors were wholly concentrated on producing milk at the lowest possible operating cost, which meant still more drastic winnowing-out of the smallest and consolidation of the biggest. In 2000 about 105,000 dairy farms were listed (a preface to greater losses since).[30]

The arithmetic is unmistakable: The number of U.S. dairy farms producing milk in 2000 decreased to about 1/35th of the 1950 figure, while the total amount of milk produced increased by more than 50 percent. It's another instance of more eggs in fewer baskets—enormously larger baskets, accepted by everyone as an essential vehicle for survival in a business with razor-thin profit margins.

As early as World War I the New York Mayor's Committee on milk prices had been told that big dairy herds were more profitable than small ones. At the time, "small" meant seven to ten cows, "big" fifty to sixty.[31] Many mixed-use farms had only one or two. The effort involved in hand milking meant that several men—preferably skilled—would have to be paid to milk even a thirty- or forty-cow herd twice a day. Milking machines, at first primitive, gradually improved enough to make hired milkers redundant. Eventually electrical models appeared, in time to help rouse farmers' support for state and federal rural electrification programs.

Here, too, the pace of change accelerated after World War II. Farmers found it more and more difficult to survive without risky capital investments that clearly couldn't be recouped by ten-cow milking herds.

Fifty-cow farms, considered fairly ambitious in early postwar days, soon looked as quaint as horse-drawn plows. USDA data record that in 1950 more than 98 percent of dairy operations had herds of under thirty cows, with just a few listed at anything between thirty and ninety-nine. In 2000 under-thirties shared the largest percentages together with other groups of between thirty and ninety-nine cows, totaling just over 80 percent. Herds with more than a hundred head accounted for the remaining 20 percent.[32]

But these figures by themselves convey a misleading picture. In 1987, midpoint herd size—meaning the point at which half of all cows are in smaller and half in larger herds—was eighty. The 1950 figure was not recorded but obviously was far less. The 2000 midpoint herd size was 275. Of course, it has risen exponentially in the last twenty years (probably now standing at more than 1,000).[33] 500-cow farms seem minor-league today. The percentages of milk that now reach consumers from some thousands of fifty-cow farms are minuscule, while those produced by a few dozen gigantic counterparts are enormous and rapidly growing. There is no criterion for exactly when a dairy farm becomes a "mega-dairy farm," but even proponents of Big Dairying might agree that a 5,000-cow operation qualifies. Farms with 10,000, 25,000, and more than 30,000 cows are held up by many advisers as the wave of the future.

On small prewar mixed-use farms, farmers fed cows only limited amounts (or none) of anything that was produced elsewhere. The acreage devoted to a herd's needs was divided between pasture for seasonal grazing and hayfields for winter fodder, with the possible addition of cornfields for corn silage. The labor for all this came from the farm family, perhaps with part-time or full-time hired help. As farms geared solely to dairying appeared and grew larger, other options became unavoidable. The more cows in a herd, the likelier some basic necessities were to come from off-farm. Pasturage might be leased, or hay bought, from neighbors. Farmers ran accounts with local veterinarians and with feed stores that sold the concentrated enrichments recommended by experts to boost milk production. These could be bought as separate ingredients, mixtures put up at the store, or proprietary formulas manufactured by large corporations. Vitamins and minerals eventually became necessary supplements.

The growing importance of formulated rations that could be given to cows at any chosen place under controlled conditions—often in stanchions while they were being milked—tended to make advocates of scientific nutrition impatient with the vagaries of grass growing in a pasture. Pasture management did not come cheap. It was a demanding skill in itself. The place or places had to be evaluated for good drainage, analyzed for soil mineral content, seeded with desirable species of grass, and protected from overgrazing by too many animals in too little space.[34] Even with rigorous oversight, spells of flood, drought, or other disasters were unpredictable.

Another grazing problem was that switching from a winter to a spring-summer regimen brought changes in the composition of the milk.[35] For instance, the relative amount of fat generally declined, while the balance of different fatty acids was rearranged. Urban consumers who had expected predictable uniformity twelve months a year from commercial jam in a jar or condensed soup in a can had no idea why milk in a bottle should taste different at different seasons. Reminders of seasonal factors or animal origin in a mammalian secretion that once had meant new births coinciding with new grass were not welcome to either purchasers or marketers in postwar America.

Changes of regimen by season had other disadvantages linked with farmers' never-diminishing need to streamline production costs. Official federal price supports for milk had finally materialized through the Agricultural Act of 1949, as farm-state politicians convinced Washington that permanently ensuring adequate supplies of the chief food commodities through economic ups and downs was a vital priority. The act extended previously enacted wartime supports. It established a program through which the Commodity Credit Corporation (CCC, an agency founded while the Roosevelt administration was trying to keep the bottom from dropping out of farm prices) would stabilize prices as necessary by large purchases of commodities. Milk and milk products were included. The CCC thereafter periodically bought up enough butter, cheese, and other storable forms of milk to guarantee dairy farmers some minimum wholesale price.[36]

It was a safety net of sorts, but far from adequate to protect anyone from the severe downward pressures on drinking-milk retail prices that had been a given since before World War I. Milk had been, and remained, intrinsically more expensive to produce and handle on a commercial scale than any other major agricultural commodity. Generation after generation, industry experts told farmers that ratcheting up economies of scale another notch was the road to salvation. The next notch in management strategies for the machines known as high-performing dairy cows was to reduce already pared-down production costs per unit of milk through new approaches to diet.

The broad outlines of ruminant digestion were already understood. But the experts also knew that feeding cows calculated amounts of high-calorie foods that sat somewhat uneasily with ruminant physiology stimulated higher milk production. The increased yield often meant disproportionately more water—high-producing cows on high-energy feeds required a great deal—than nutrients, so that the milk tended to be rather thin. But that scarcely would have mattered to farmers focused on pounds of output per cow if it had been easier to maintain peak yields over many months without tipping the animals over into acidosis or mastitis.

Managing even a modest-sized herd of high-producing cows on high-energy diets while staving off health problems and keeping the feed budget within limits demanded both constant attention and endless mathematical calculations that weren't going to be made any easier by putting the cows out to pasture. The advent of 100-cow and 300-cow herds, with predictions of bigger contenders still to come, meant more numbers-crunching. Many twentieth-century farmers must have wished for some way of providing each cow with a day's nutritionally balanced ration, somewhat tailored to her individual needs and fed to her at some spot close to the milking area. Livestock feeding specialists began addressing the goal during the 1960s and eventually arrived at a concept labeled "Total Mixed Rations," TMR for short.

The TMR approach as applied to dairy cows involves studying the milking records and health history of all herd members, usually separated into a few groups by factors such as stage of lactation or pregnancy. Whoever supervises the feeding program calculates desirable recipes containing all the ingredients needed to supply a day's requirements for each group. Forages, concentrates, and nutritional supplements must be assembled in correct proportions and mixed together in a particular order that enables each component to be broken down into bits of the optimum size. Computer chips embedded in tags on each cow's ears record crucial statistics about her milk every time it is drawn and also monitor her for signs of common disorders.[37]

From the start, it could be seen that the system was poorly suited to existing small and mid-sized farms. But it presented dazzling opportunities for innovators to invent much bigger operations along radically restructured lines—for example, to redesign the spaces where cows are housed, fed, and milked. On advanced dairy farms today, cows are often kept in a number of large open-sided pens with continual or frequent access to their feed. This is one version of the livestock-managing arrangements known as confined animal feeding operations (CAFOs).

All elements of the ration are precombined in large, powerful mixing machines that may be mounted on wagons, enabling operators to drive around the perimeter of a pen and pump the mixture into a bunker running along one side. The technology clearly eliminates huge amounts of human labor in mixing and distributing. And as the abovementioned textbook points out, "Every mouthful of the ration is the same, stabilizing the rumen environment."[38] At the same time, rations can easily be modified according to individual farmers' priorities with the aid of another handy tool, feed management software. In fact, farmers are free to incorporate aspects of TMR feeding into more traditional practices, perhaps even with allowance for spring pasturage. But it is often simpler to dedicate some space to plantings of grass not for pasturage but for mowing and adding to the TMR.

Those who most eagerly seized on the total-mixed-ration and open-pen ideas saw that the two factors in tandem would enable gigantic farms to operate as self-sufficient environments, freed from traditional limitations of geography and climate and filled with massive numbers of cows designed to bypass the constraints of biology. Short of putting a dairy farm on an orbiting satellite, the sky was the limit.

The trailblazing farms required stupefying investments in climate control and other infrastructure as well as an insistence on thinking outside the box. Aided by new water-management strategies, they sprang up in states that had not belonged to the chief twentieth-century dairying strongholds: Idaho, Arizona, Texas, New Mexico, Oregon. They surged to great importance in California, helping it displace Wisconsin as the top dairying state in 1993.[39] Nearly all of these states had been thought to have summers too hot and dry for large dairy cows—especially Holsteins, which are dangerously susceptible to heat stress. Open-pen installations addressed the problem with liberal provision of shade, together with cooling and ventilation systems that could lower sweltering temperatures to something approximating the animals' comfort zone. They were expensive but necessary as the consolidation of the U.S. dairy industry accelerated. While the total number of dairy farms swiftly dropped, the average number of cows per operation rose along with average milk yields per cow—the same startling eggs-and-baskets equation that I have already pointed to. Factory-scale farms dependent on TMR and advanced housing systems could not meet ideal production targets without spending whatever was necessary to keep their delicate charges pumping out maximum yields.

GLOBAL FIELDS OF DREAMS

No matter whether these installations represented brilliant triumphs over outmoded thinking about natural limits or epic-scale conjuring with square pegs and round holes, the power of the American example made improbable venues all around the globe suddenly look like aspiring dairy farmers' wishes come true.

The challenge was quickly taken up by Saudi Arabia, where the 1970s oil embargo had frightened the royal family into thinking seriously about national food self-sufficiency. One of King Faisal's sons was dispatched to the United States to tour profitable dairy farms. Finding inspiring examples in California, he returned in 1979 with suggestions for a project that eventually became Al-Safi Dairy Company, located about sixty miles southeast of Riyadh in one of the kingdom's chief oasis regions. It opened in 1981 as a mega-dairy housing some 6,500 Holstein cows brought from Canada. In 2002 a reporter for the German newspaper *Der Tagesspiegel* found about 13,000 cows living in shaded open sheds cooled from an outside temperature of 104°F/40°C to 79°F/26°C by a constant drizzle of fan-circulated water vapor. With some reluctance, a publicity spokesman disclosed that it took about 3,500 liters of water—from an aquifer some 6,000 feet deep—to produce one liter of milk. The lion's share, dwarfing that of water for the cooling system and that drunk by cows, went to irrigate the twenty-five-square-mile area that contributed fresh green fodder to Al-Safi's TMR.[40]

(To update this success story: The steady depletion of the original aquifer eventually forced the operators to drill into a still deeper one. A smaller fodder-growing area was relocated close to the replacement, which is estimated to be within twenty years of running dry. Meanwhile, the number of cows grew to somewhere between 30,000 and 50,000. And the California dairy industry belatedly began facing its own embarrassing questions about groundwater depletion, not to mention contamination from farm runoff.)[41]

Saudi Arabia is now one of the top milk-producing nations in the Middle East, part of a global scenario that recalls Christian missionaries' earlier conversions of so-called savages. Western evangelists had been trying to export their superior wisdom about farming and food to other parts of the world at least since the early twentieth century. But their proselytizing for intensive agriculture and expertly calibrated diets is now more fervent than ever. Their teaching is aimed at "developing countries," a grab-bag concept that in practice turns out to mean nearly all non-Anglophone countries outside of Europe. The doctrinal lessons usually stress the nutritional virtues of cow's milk and encourage followers to create dairy herds and milk-processing plants. Many of these actually belong to subsidiaries of Western-founded multinational companies.

Though the "developing countries" category is most often associated with the global South, it also embraces much of northern Eurasia as well as almost everything between the Zagros Mountains in Iran and the Black and Mediterranean seas. The first peoples to domesticate livestock and use milk lived in these latter regions, chiefly along the western Great Steppe as well as Anatolia, the eastern Mediterranean, and much of today's Muslim Middle East. There were good reasons that their chief milking animals were not cows but goats and sheep. The smaller animals have more tolerance for the arid climates and fierce summers that dominate the original cradles of dairying. Most cows—certainly most of the major breeds that British and American pioneers labored to perfect in modern times—are too large to dissipate their own body heat under the stress of summer temperatures that may be between 90°F/32°C and 120°F/49°C. The only important exceptions to the thermoregulation impediment are Jerseys and various land races that originated in the African and Asian tropics, especially the humped zebus of the Indian subcontinent, the somewhat similar African sangas, and some humpless cattle also prized by African pastoral or agro-pastoral peoples.[42] These heat-tolerant tropical races, however, give only scanty amounts of milk.

Western would-be educators initially felt called on to enlighten Third World governments by explaining how superior dairy cows were to goats, and Holstein (or Friesian) cows to scrubby local specimens. In theory, one good Holstein could make a farmer more self-sufficient than a dozen poor milkers.[43] It also seemed likely that the rapid urbanization overtaking all developing nations would soon recapitulate the American pattern by creating an urgent need for industrial-scale drinking-milk production to supply cities.

Attempts to separate good sense from overconfident claims in these preachings didn't develop at once. For decades the credo of intensively breeding and managing pure Holstein stock in order to keep jacking up average production per cow swept away all doubts, in both industrial West think tanks and recently converted ministries of agriculture anywhere from Thailand to Uganda. Early signs of second thoughts, in parts of the United States transfigured by the mega-dairy-farm rush as well as in developing countries, centered on two unforeseen hazards: environmental costs and herd health.

High-performing cows must have vast amounts of cool, fresh water simply to keep up production. To avoid heat stress in sweltering conditions they must be provided with still larger amounts, along with shade. In vertically integrated operations where every element from growing and harvesting fodder to maintaining nonstop cooling systems, milking and hosing down cows, hosing down floors, processing milk, and flushing out intricate pipeline systems is carried out on one huge site or complex of sites, water and energy needs are colossal. So may be the havoc wreaked on local waterways, water tables, or even aquifers. Al-Safi, the largest vertically integrated dairy farm in the world, is lucky enough to operate under the auspices of a family not responsible to voters. In countries not run by absolute monarchs, some political price must be paid for wholesale water pollution or depletion, not to mention locally severe air pollution from the largest and geographically most concentrated CAFOs. In residential areas close to mega-dairy farms—notably in Oregon, California, and Arizona but also in other parts of the world—methane emissions, an unavoidable by-product of ruminant digestion, can make the air nearly unbreathable for nearby residents.

LIVES CUT SHORT

Heat stress in conditions that Holstein cows should never be subjected to is only one among dozens of factors that over a few human generations have contributed to a horrifying decline in life expectancy among dairy cows here and abroad—above all, Holsteins. This race of large cattle originally bred in the Netherlands close to the North Sea was the worst possible choice for kickstarting modern dairying in the tropics and other regions with blazing summers. But even if Holsteins had been more adaptable to hot climates in the United States or elsewhere, the prevailing fixation on getting more milk out of cows by any available means was a recipe for driving them to the end of their biological limits. During the 1990s it also threatened to become a public relations embarrassment.

By then milk producers here and abroad could boast of staggering increases in average yields per cow, thanks to reproductive technology—with artificial insemination by elite sires as the linchpin—and energy-intensive feed-management strategies. But researchers were now ready to play another card: endocrinology.

In 1985 the *Journal of Dairy Science* published a report co-written by two members of Cornell University's Department of Animal Science and two staff members at the Monsanto Company, all of whom were involved in a projected rollout of Monsanto's genetically rearranged ("recombinant") version of the pituitary hormone somatotropin, already known to stimulate not only growth but milk production in cows.[44] Monsanto was preparing to release this product, generally known as rBST (recombinant bovine somatotropin) or rBGH (recombinant bovine growth hormone) under the brand name Posilac. Scientific controversies soon broke out over the Food and Drug Administration's review of Posilac, which was finally approved in 1993 for injection into lactating cows. Critics of what was starting to be dubbed Big Pharma promptly circulated a theory that milk from Posilac-treated cows might cause cancer in people who drank it. The claim was never clearly validated. But undeterred consumer advocates continued to denounce rBST as a menace to human health, with great success in the court of popular opinion.[45] Further squabbles ensued over whether commercial dairies that printed assertions on bottles or cartons about *not* using rBST should be required to add disclaimers explaining—accurately—that its presence or absence is chemically undetectable in the milk. Eventually many milk producers decided that whatever the facts, Posilac was more of a public relations liability than an asset. Monsanto apparently thought so too, for in 2008 it sold its Posilac division to Eli Lilly.[46]

Half buried in the furor over supposed health risks to people who *drank* the milk were the very real health risks to cows who *produced* it. Dale E. Bauman of Cornell, the principal author of the 1985 study, confidently stood by its finding that among thirty cows given either no hormones, actual bovine pituitary somatotropin, or rBST, injecting the last into the test subjects at two-week intervals over a period of 188 days had increased milk production significantly while causing no ill effects.[47] Not all dairy scientists were satisfied. Many other studies were conducted over the next few years, repeatedly leading doubters to some disturbing conclusions.

The FDA decided that any projected complications could be adequately handled by farmers through usual methods of treating high-producing cows' ailments. Its Canadian counterpart disagreed, and ended by denying approval to the drug.[48] What bothered critics were not strange new symptoms but heightened signs of exactly the problems already associated with turbo-cows. From the 188-day Cornell experiment, it seemed that Posilac had enabled high-performing cows to work up to peak production more quickly and to maintain it longer than untreated control subjects.

But what about longer lactations? (For many farmers, 305 days is a standard yardstick.) Or controlled studies of more than ten rBST-treated animals? In fairness to the Cornell and Monsanto authors of the study, no single experiment could have been realistically designed to follow thousands of cows over long lactations or throughout their milking careers. Nonetheless, only a broad years-long overview will allow observers to realistically evaluate the recombinant hormone's effects on the life spans of high-producing cows. Posilac has been one of the most visible parts of a multipronged effort to make high-performing members of any herd still higher-performing despite mounting evidence of frequent mastitis, hoof and leg damage, difficulty calving, and multiple reproduction-linked ailments.

Even before the rBST furor, questions about the ethical implications of the unrelenting quest for production efficiency in dairy cows and other farm animals had emerged in the United States and Europe. The seminal manifesto of the ethical treatment movement was *Animal Liberation* (1975) by the philosopher Peter Singer.[49] It took members of the industry several decades to start paying attention, generally more on practical than ethical grounds. In 1998, a team of researchers from Norway and the Netherlands warned that data about animal health in highly concentrated chicken, turkey, pork, and dairy cow operations signaled future crises.[50]

A more scathing polemic by Wilhelm F. Knaus, a professor of agricultural science at an Austrian university, appeared ten years later under the auspices of the Society of Chemical Industry: "Dairy Cows Trapped Between Performance Demands and Adaptability," the English translation of a short but trenchant German-language indictment. It was an unsparing assault on an entire dairy-farming model that Knaus saw as driven by shortsighted profit imperatives and pitfall-ridden technological spurs to production. His targets included intensive selective-breeding and concentrate-feeding practices that had traveled from the United States to Europe, where Holsteins were already crowding out less productive local stock as milkers. But he also spoke as an advocate for a growing international sustainable-agriculture movement that viewed employing the food energy and edible protein of grains and soybeans for livestock instead of needy humans as criminal folly.[51]

Knaus was not the first observer to draw attention to the shrinking productive lives of dairy cows, which had become too striking to be ignored by the industry. Growing numbers of colleagues in Europe and the United States were pointing out troubling declines in "parity"—not the economic benchmark that New Deal farm price policies were supposed to address, but the number of successful calvings (followed by lactations) achieved by a cow during her career in a milking herd. Eight or more parities had been unremarkable before the post-World War II campaign to increase milk yields per cow; Knaus put the 1994 average for U.S. Holsteins at 2.79, down from 3.4 in 1966.[52]

Heifers are usually first bred close to the age of two, which is taken as the beginning of the productive life span. A "heifer" officially becomes a "cow" at first calving; farmers can theoretically plan on one calving and lactation each year afterward. 2.79 parity therefore indicates a productive life span of less than three years for Holstein milking stock and a total life span of less than five. Some perspective on this figure: A dairy cow with no serious health problems can easily live to the age of twenty. A few U.S. dairy farmers were old enough to remember such cows, and more had heard about them from fathers and grandfathers. Smaller farmers especially were bothered by the notion that business as usual had to mean sending worn-out cows to the hamburger factory before their fifth birthdays. Some agricultural school pundits shared their qualms.[53] But Holstein Association USA, the successor to the Holstein-Friesian Association of America, had long had allies in animal science departments and commanding influence at cattle shows. The association stood ready to rebut any detraction of the breed as developed in postwar America—its milking records, its large size and rawboned dairy conformation, even its black and white markings. A certain minority of Dutch Friesians and their U.S. descendants had always been red and white, the result of a pesky recessive gene. For some years they were drummed out of the breed registry in order to preserve the image rigidly prescribed by the custodians of Holstein purity. (After the early 1970s red and white Holsteins began winning more respect as legitimate parts of the breed lineage.[54])

The association argued that AI programs to accentuate recognized Holstein characteristics were in the main good for the industry. Its equivalents in Switzerland and Austria angrily dismissed complaints about turbo-cows as cheap headline-chasing. But at around the turn of the century the apostles of Holsteinism found their authority being slighted by weary dairy farmers and challenged at some leading U.S. agricultural schools. An iconoclastic suggestion suddenly became respectable: outcrossing Holstein heifers and cows with sires from breeds virtually unknown in this country. Already some owners of Holstein herds had tried combating the dystocia problem by breeding heifers and cows (through AI) to Jersey sires in order to produce smaller calves. The new program was more radical.

In 1997 several California dairy farmers in the Central Valley took their dissatisfaction with recurrent Holstein health problems to a local AI service. Their discussions led to a series of crossbreeding trials carried out in cooperation with dairy cattle geneticists at the University of Minnesota. Participating farmers inseminated Holstein heifers and cows with imported semen from several different European breeds, then produced progressive crossings over a few more generations. The best results were found to come from a triple-rotation program involving Holstein dams and sires of two unrelated breeds, Montbéliarde and Swedish Red. The former, a big, sturdy red and white Alpine type, was famous in France as the standard source of milk for the prized Comté cheese. Participants in the Swedish Red part of the program eventually formed an amalgam of several popular red and white Scandinavian breeds (already noted for strong Ayrshire ancestry) under the name VikingRed.[55]

The advantage of three-way rather than two-way crossings was that they allowed the stock to sustain greater genetic diversity over successive generations. The resulting cows were an implicit repudiation of all that American Holsteins had been engineered to be by well-meaning breed-standard guardians. They were beefier, better-knit, and far less prone to medical tribulations like mastitis, laminitis, acidosis, ketosis, infertility, and dystocia. The Minnesota geneticists who had helped to develop the breeding program continued to conduct follow-up studies dwelling on evidence that in the long run Holstein-VikingRed-Montbéliarde crosses were more profitable milkers than purebred Holsteins. Their somewhat smaller average yields per cow had to be set against enormous savings to farmers in veterinary bills, lost milking days, and time spent caring for sick members of a herd. They also lived longer.[56]

The program's success inspired its American, Scandinavian, and French originators to team up in an international breeding service called ProCROSS. A few years later the Minnesota scientists unveiled another service, GrazeCross, similar to the Holstein-VikingRed-Montbéliarde model but based on triple crosses of Jersey, VikingRed, and Normande, another red and white French breed that once had been the most important supplier of milk for Camembert and Brie cheese. Montbéliardes and Normandes both had long histories as well-fleshed dual-purpose cattle equally useful for meat and milk—a stark contrast to the American dogma of specialized dairy type. The impetus for GrazeCross had come from the realization that Jerseys were becoming almost as overbred and inbred as Holsteins.

Ventures like ProCROSS and GrazeCross were not romantic exercises in banishing advanced technology from the milk business. They were practical responses to crises that American dairying had brought on itself—and disseminated abroad—through leap-before-you-look reliance on technological fixes to pursue shortsighted goals, above all the largest possible yield of milk per animal. Both farmers and dairy scientists were perfectly aware that Holstein cows can be bred and fed to give milk with impressive percentages of milkfat and protein. But the breed's highest-performing stars are better at yielding large amounts of milk than at pumping nutrients into it in any reasonable proportion to the extra volume—that is, the extra water. Had it not been for milk processors' obligation to comply with federal and state minimum requirements for the non-water components of milk, nothing would have stopped thousands of farmers from sending the local processing plant deluges of the nearest approach to plain H_2O that anyone can get a dairy cow to yield. Required minimums of other components were often met by balancing acts. Some farmers brought the overall composition of their herds' milk into the proper range by combining high producers' ample but substandard yields with much richer milk from a few cows better fitted to supply milkfat and protein. They might even keep a few Jerseys or Guernseys for the purpose.

Milk processors supplied by many farms had their own balancing act, called "standardization." It involved measuring the composition of a volume of milk received at the plant and adjusting it to tally with standard minimums spelled out in the state public health code or (for interstate shipments) the latest U.S. Public Health Service milk ordinance. The most critical figures were usually 3.25 percent milkfat and 8.25 percent SNF—defined as "solids nonfat" or "solids not fat"—by weight.[57] SNF included casein, whey proteins, lactose, minerals, and some vitamins—that is, the entire nutritional package of skim milk. Large dairies using the milk of many different farms would either boost deficient percentages by adding milk from herds known for rich milkfat and SNF content or dilute excess percentages by adding thinner milk from especially high-performing herds. Holstein herds might fall into either category—for there never was a time when some Holstein owners didn't concern themselves with superior milk rather than superior amounts. In fact, admirers of the breed were among the sincerest critics of what had been done to it.

Some of the dairy-cattle geneticists with acute apprehensions about the U.S. and global future of Holsteins were Leslie B. Hansen, an architect of the Minnesota-led triple-rotation crossbreeding programs; his

Minnesota colleague Brad Heins; and Chad Dechow of Penn State University, a supporter of the programs' aims. Their concerns about the disturbing Y-chromosome Holstein bottleneck mentioned earlier in this chapter gradually attracted attention in (and beyond) the dairy-farming community.

A 2008 article in the *New York Times Magazine* acutely portrayed the dilemmas of farmers in East Africa torn between loyalty to the beloved local Ankole cattle race and expert advice (aided by semen-supplying companies) to lift themselves from poverty by raising Holsteins or progressively crossbreeding them into the Ankole line. The author, Andrew Rice, saw that Holsteins as well as Holstein crosses were a dubious or actively destructive fit with the Ugandan grassland ecosystems that had supported Ankole cows for many centuries. Local farmers, he wrote, were "creating herds that consume unsustainable amounts of dwindling resources. And something else is being obliterated: genes. Each time a farmer crossbreeds his Ankoles, a little of the country's stockpile of adaptive traits disappears." Citing Hansen's findings about the diminishing Holstein gene pool, Rice pointed to "a serious problem with inbreeding, which has adverse effects on fertility and mortality. But overseas markets like Africa are, so to speak, virgin territory . . . In Uganda, a company called World-Wide Sires, the international marketing arm of two American breeding cooperatives, is working with aid agencies to increase dairy production."[58]

The news that a mere two sires had been responsible for virtually the entire male Holstein lineage since the 1960s eventually made it into the pages of *Hoard's Dairyman* and other publications addressed to the dairy-farm trade. In 2019 *Scientific American* took note, in a report that was picked up by National Public Radio and created a certain stir. The *Atlantic* published an article on the repercussions of a genetic defect that had finally surfaced in descendants of Pawnee Farm Arlinda Chief, one of the two founding bulls.[59] The issue, however, never approached the visibility of the rBST wars in print or online news media. It passed unnoticed by most of the general public.

The Minnesota and Penn State dairy scientists, allies in the effort to confront an approaching crisis, continued the campaign. The Penn

State team managed to locate samples of older Holstein semen in germplasm banks and began using them to produce calves who with luck might start independent Holstein lineages. (One of the Penn State calves was named "Les" in Hansen's honor.) Hansen, Heins, and their colleagues had their own living germplasm experiment in a special Holstein herd that had been maintained at the Morris Minnesota campus since 1964.[60] Some farmers came around to thinking that it might be a good idea to breed *smaller* Holstein cows instead of trying to crank up their dimensions any further. VikingGenetics, the Scandinavian company that had developed VikingRed, began advertising semen from VikingHolsteins, explicitly billed as designed to produce "resilient, medium-sized cows."[61]

Sadly, the effect of such attempts to redress the industry's past mistakes in breeding pure Holsteins—and, as is now recognized, Jerseys—has been far from transformative. After the turn of the century, segments of the dairy-farming community did indeed try to stem the toll on cows' health and longevity, and a promising commercial future did dawn for serious crossbreeding programs. But in many ways, the overall picture became darker rather than brighter after about 2008, when the artificial insemination business acquired the means of genomic sequencing. The effects reached critical momentum seven or eight years later. They confirmed, in spades, that most dairy farmers maintained faith in choosing semen from a small handful of elite bulls to father a herd's next crop of heifers. The new technology also allowed AI companies to directly evaluate a bull's transmissible qualities before he reached his full growth, simply by studying his genome—thus allowing him to become a hot property in the blink of an eye after puberty. At the same time, it encouraged the already tremendous global scope of the American AI industry. (A 2002 *Washington Post* article on Round Oak Rag Apple Elevation, the other 1960s founding bull, had quoted a delighted Holstein Association USA research director who kept running into the superstar's daughters during a trip to Chile and Venezuela: "His descendants are absolutely everywhere."[62])

World-Wide Sires had helped to convince livestock husbandry technocrats around the globe of a vast need for American genetic knowhow.

After Elevation's owner, the Ohio firm Select Sires, acquired a share in World-Wide Sires in 2001, his genes and those of stellar sons and grandsons wafted like confetti from continent to continent. The genomics revolution accelerated the process to warp speed. In a 2016 online brochure, a sire analyst for Select Sires called attention to how rapidly one generation of elite bulls as well as heifers—who were also being readied for breeding very young—could now succeed another: "With the combination of more, better and faster information, we have reduced the generation interval [see next paragraph] to about 21 months. This adds an extra generation every five years. The ability to have that type of aggression, along with a group of extremely influential sires and young heifers, has put genetic progress in overdrive."[63]

Hansen already distrusted genetic progress in overdrive. In an article titled "The Impact of Genomics on Rapid Increase of Inbreeding in Holsteins," he detailed some changes that he had seen kicking in between 2015 and 2020, the first half-decade in which trends could have been clearly documented. The worst of these was "a dramatic reduction in generation interval," meaning "the average age of parents when their offspring are born. The allure of genomic selection is choosing parents of the next generation at a very young age." The "major pitfall" here was "a corresponding increase of genetic relationships within a population . . . As individuals in a breed become more related, the average inbreeding of a breed increases at an accelerated rate." The mantra of the movement was "breeding the best to the best as fast as we can." As a result: "Genomic selection has been applied blindly" by dairy breeding companies. To be competitive, they must satisfy an "unrelenting desire and expectation" for "bulls [i.e., semen] with highest-ranking genomic evaluations." Rational though this might appear at the moment, "intense selection to maximize short-term genetic improvement may have major negative consequences in regard to the potential for long-term genetic improvement and viability of the Holstein breed."[64]

Such warnings had little effect on the mega-dairy movement and its emphasis on rapidly "breeding the best to the best" for increased productivity. Enormous confined dairy operations, invariably of high-producing

Holsteins, kept on confirming their dominant role in the U.S. dairy industry. After securing new strongholds in Southwestern and Western states, they began expanding into traditional dairy states like Minnesota, Wisconsin, Pennsylvania, and New York. There they became a direct threat to older mid-sized and smaller farms after 2015 by glutting the market and knocking the bottom out of farm milk prices.[65]

The U.S. model of mega-operations based on hyper-productive animals found a home in other industrialized nations. The whole system of belief also took root in the developing world. One reason was that Western agricultural authorities sincerely expected a steady supply of fresh milk to alleviate hunger in the world's poorest regions. Consequently, food aid organizations and their allies in many ministries of agriculture have repeatedly tried to introduce Western-bred cows to tropical countries. In some cases, purebred Holsteins are plunked down in Torrid Zone conditions where they rapidly become sick. In others, experts look to the promise of crossbreeding Holsteins with a landrace of the region—a less rash solution but one that risks depleting unique genetic reservoirs built up through centuries of adaptation to particular environments. Or in extreme cases, local interests are talked into adopting some version of the high-tech dairying operations that have seized the initiative in the United States, with massive numbers of very large, fragile cows installed in a custom-designed environmental bubble— though a bubble capable of releasing concentrated manure and methane pollution into the outside world. Advisers who conscientiously reckon with issues like Third World climatic challenges, local farmers' existing management practices, or parasites and pathogens specific to a region (e.g., the sleeping-sickness organism and its vector, the tsetse fly, in most of central Africa) may not get as favorable a hearing from local governments as ones who offer brilliant promises.

Western champions of milk-enriched diets for all the world's peoples aren't necessarily trying to sell anyone a bill of goods. In fact, they usually are actuated by the best motives. Faith in drinking-milk as the key to dietary improvement for impoverished nations is almost a birthright legacy in much of the industrialized West. Unfortunately, it has become an object lesson in skewed priorities.

From its prehistoric beginnings, dairying was entirely dependent on animal-human relationships. These were forged between peoples and herbivores living along the Great Steppe and in the Fertile Crescent. The animals made the nutritional potential of local grasses available to humans by digesting cellulose and allowing people to harvest a source of food renewable on a day-to-day basis from the start to the end of the milking season.

Thousands of years later, people living in very different environments set in motion a train of events that would eventually turn turbo-cows into cogs in a huge, dysfunctional machine. Starting by concocting pseudo-scientific theories that exalted drinking-milk to permanent and unquestioned superfood status, they wound up enmeshed in endless maneuvers meant to get around the limitations of bovine digestion, reproduction, and lactation. Today the chief rationale for putting animals' basic biological functions through the wringer is to get ever-more milk flowing ever-faster from ever-fewer cows with ever-greater economies of scale.

Will the model of animal-human relationships represented by 35,000-cow dairy operations be thoughtlessly exported to the rest of the world? One can only hope not. At least some farmers and animal science researchers have begun to recognize the toll that the blinkered goal of higher milk production and the ensuing technological juggernaut have taken on cows. With luck, they will be joined by food-lovers pointing out the toll that the same process has taken on milk itself.

9

TECHNOLOGY IN OVERDRIVE II

The Milk

Modern city-dwellers' mental maps of what they eat, and its real cost, are at best incomplete. For instance, they have trouble telling when food as nature's virgin bounty turns into food as drastically processed artifact. This is particularly true of the chilled white liquid called "milk" that reigned as the twentieth century's great nutritional nonpareil. As early as 1916, a New York State legislative committee inquiring into major food industries had commented on the outsized role that city consumers' fixed notions played in pushing down wholesale prices for milk at the farm. The consumer, the report noted, "had become accustomed to pay a certain price for a bottle of milk in the same way that he became accustomed to the payment of the street car fares."[1] Even at that date an entire supporting technology had disappeared from view for people who had grown up assuming that it was natural for inexpensive milk to materialize on their doorsteps every morning out of thin air.

A century later, the vast infrastructure that continued to be built up around drinking-milk in order to bring it from farms to stores at retail prices alarmingly disproportioned to farm prices remains just as invisible to consumers. Virgin-bounty suppositions about what reaches our tables only through stupendous feats of engineering stand in the way of understanding milk. For instance, the widespread assumption that milk is a fine natural source of vitamin D is mistaken. As it comes from the cow, it is a poor source at best. But in the 1930s nutritionists began encouraging U.S. dairy processors to fortify drinking-milk with synthetic forms of vitamin D as a handy way of slipping a valuable nutrient into most consumers' diets.[2] Because it is always there, few people wonder how it *gets* there—a case of information hidden in plain sight.

Many other realities in the story of modern milk have disappeared or are disappearing from sight through ubiquitous feats of technology. This chapter will discuss just three examples: homogenization, refrigeration, and genetic rearrangement of milk before it leaves the cow. The first is essentially a marketing ploy for stretching profits through artificial sales gimmicks—incidentally ensuring that cow's milk in American kitchens only remotely resembles the original chemical composition and structure of cow's milk. The second is a genuine necessity. Deep chilling is imperative for controlling bacterial growth in drinking-milk from the moment of production to the moment of consumption. Its importance keeps increasing as production and processing operations—farms and milk plants—become bigger, more consolidated, and more complex. In their different ways, these two interventions say a lot about the haywire priorities of the industry. But my third example deserves to be recognized and debated before it, too, becomes so usual as to pass unnoticed.

"INTIMATELY MINGLED" MILK

As explained in chapter 1, cow's milk left standing for some hours naturally begins separating by gravity into two layers: cream (containing the milkfat) on top and skim milk at the bottom. People didn't historically see separation as a defect—far from it, since dietary experts considered the butterfat the most and skim milk the least nutritious portions of the milk. That a deep, conspicuous creamline in a bottle of milk indicated superior quality had been assumed from the start of the nineteenth-century drinking-milk industry and would be a given for many years. But in 1900 the French inventor Auguste Gaulin unveiled what he hoped would be a revolutionary innovation at the Paris World's Fair, a way of "treating milk."

His idea was to "intimately mingle" (*mélanger intimement*) the milkfat component with the rest of the natural substance to produce "stabilized milk" (*lait fixé*) that would not divide into two components.[3] His machine for forcing milk through very fine apertures under pressure performed as advertised, by breaking up the comparatively large glob-ules of milkfat into globules that were too small to be affected by gravity in the water-based medium of skim milk and remained permanently emulsified throughout it.

Gaulin's treated milk attracted some notice without setting the world on fire. Critics complained about bad flavors in the milk, and some medical authorities claimed to discover that children who drank it developed scurvy. Other inventors tried their hand at homogenization under one name or other, with indifferent success. The biggest problem was milk turning rancid as soon as it left the homogenizer. The reason wasn't understood until the 1930s.

As previously explained, emulsified fat globules share space in raw whole milk not only with the suspended casein micelles responsible for forming curd but with a huge array of dissolved substances, including enzymes. A newborn calf doesn't encounter the enzymes until the milk actually travels the closed route between mouth and nipple. Only then are they able to be activated in the digestive system. Milk enzymes that become operational in the outside world are another story, particularly those in the milkfat.

Milkfat globules in milk as it emerges from the cow are encased in an extremely complex membrane that shields them from the action of lipase, the fat-cleaving enzyme. If the membrane is breached, lipase promptly attacks the contents, discharging free fatty acids into the milk. Among these, free butyric acid creates the unmistakable smell and fla-vor of rancid milk. Eventually dairy chemists recognized that it was released into raw homogenized milk when the fat globule membranes were perforated. Once the problem had been nailed down, a rough solution suggested itself: heating the milk to a high enough temperature to denature the lipase enzyme before subjecting it to homogenization. A temperature of 113°F/45°C proved to be sufficient. (It is not clear whether Gaulin himself had run into the rancidity problem; his U.S. patent application in 1902 stated that he had found milk easiest to process at 185°F/85°C.[4]) But rancidity can result from other temperature changes in handling milk.

With the main cause of rancidity identified, some dairy companies hoped to start selling homogenized milk right away. Not all technical details, however, could be ideally ironed out at once. The product attracted some enthusiastic customers between about 1932 and 1940, but the scale of expansion was restricted until after the end of the war. At that point another useful factor entered the picture: mandatory pasteurization.

The U.S. Public Health Service's efforts to get statewide pasteurization requirements enacted finally led to the first state law in Michigan in 1947, followed by a cascade of others. By the early 1950s milk processors who resisted pasteurization had mostly disappeared. The rest saw great promise in a piggybacking strategy for carrying out the two procedures together: homogenizing milk virtually at the instant it was pasteurized.[5] The fact that raw milk wasn't amenable to the much-admired homogenizing procedure helped to hasten its demise as a commercial product.

The industry was ready for rapid growth bolstered by promising technologies and marketing pitches. Small local processing plants started to either expand or vanish, while large ones widened their delivery routes. Dovetailing the pasteurization and homogenization processes, while also following one of the vitamin D enrichment methods, committed any company to processing and selling an energy-intensive product with less relationship to plain cow's milk than anything previously offered to U.S. consumers.

But what was the *reason* for adopting homogenization? It is the most radical technical change ever visited on the chemical structure of commercial fluid milk, a much more drastic reconfiguring than most forms of pasteurization. No public health agency ever pleaded for routinely employing it; no body of medical evidence ever proved that it made milk safer or more healthful. Gaulin and assorted advocates had convinced a

number of medical authorities that it was more digestible than unhomogenized milk.[6] But criteria for actually *measuring* digestibility were
shaky and sometimes contradictory, and there was no consensus on
homogenized milk's general nutritional merits. Cheesemakers, meanwhile,
almost unanimously refused to work with it. The problem was that when
the original milkfat globules were shattered into mini-globules, some of
the casein micelles suspended in the milk became incorporated into the
re-formed globule membranes and interfered with curd development.[7]
Only a few highly processed varieties such as commercial cream cheese
were unaffected.

There was just one clinching argument for homogenization: It eliminated any way of guessing the amount of cream in the milk by sight. For
housewives as well as industry experts, judging the milk's richness by the
visibility of the creamline was second nature. On average, Jersey milk
had the deepest creamline, while that in Guernsey milk was the most
striking at first glance. Indeed, Guernsey breeders had managed to avoid
being totally eclipsed by vogues for Holsteins or Jerseys by exploiting a
genetic oddity in Guernsey cows' ability to synthesize vitamin A from
grass: more of it appears in the milkfat as the orange-yellow precursor
beta-carotene than as the colorless preformed vitamin A. The cream
thus acquires a delicately inviting yellow tinge, a color that in the 1920s
spurred a group of entrepreneurs to incorporate as "Golden Guernsey,
Inc."[8] The licensed Golden Guernsey logo soon became familiar on milk
bottles. The demarcation between the lovely cream on top and the skim
milk below was the signal advantage of the product. Homogenization
advocates meant to efface such visual clues.

The food historian Mark Kurlansky was a child when homogenization conquered all during the 1950s. As he mournfully records, his
siblings and he had been perfectly happy with their beloved creamline
milk. "But one day we didn't like the milk anymore. There was something
wrong with it. It was all one color."[9] My childhood memories of the
same period are different: Either the Pennsylvania dairy that delivered our milk had switched to all-homogenized by the time I was old
enough to notice, or my parents had decided that homogenized milk
was more modern. That certainly was the idea that the industry in

general sought to convey. Boosters claimed that it had been scientifically proved to taste *creamier* than creamline milk, a triumph of promotional doublespeak.

Homogenization helped to restore continuous-flow "flash" pasteurization to respectability after it had acquired a sleazy reputation earlier
in the century. Continuous-flow technology became greatly improved
in the 1920s and 1930s, allowing a better version of the procedure—now
rechristened "high-temperature-short-time" (HTST) pasteurization—to
be done more cheaply and on a bigger scale than pasteurization carried
out one batch at a time. However, there was some dissatisfaction because
the heat of HTST pasteurization (usually 161°F/72°C for 15 seconds)
tended to shrink the creamline.[10] Homogenization solved the problem
by making the creamline obsolete. It also allowed the standardization
of milkfat and "solids nonfat" (SNF) content mentioned in chapter 8 to
continue imposing the effect of industrial uniformity, obliterating most
evidence of the subtle or dramatic distinctions that can exist between the
milk of different breeds, different cows of the same breed, or even one
cow under different conditions.

The industry's march toward undifferentiated gigantism was speeded
up by the growth of supermarkets, together with the adoption of disposable packaging, from the late 1940s into the present century. For
many consumers, buying milk as part of a weekly shopping expedition
instead of having it delivered was a joyous liberation from cumbersome
routines with heavy, breakable glass bottles that had to be washed and
returned to the dairy after every use. Disposable paper or cardboard
cartons were not absolutely new; packagers had started experimenting
with them before 1910. But the technology improved swiftly from the
first postwar years on. In addition to the new packaging's lightness and
perceived convenience, it removed a difficulty that had plagued dairy
companies while homogenization was gaining acceptance: protecting
the milk from sunlight.

Promoters of homogenized milk had already recognized that through
some chemical reaction, it often developed a musty off-flavor when
exposed even briefly to direct sunlight. Milk processors scratched their
heads over complaints from customers along delivery routes where

full bottles were left to sit in the morning sun until somebody brought them in. It also appeared that sunlight partly inactivated the B vitamin riboflavin.[11] These discoveries were a shot in the arm for manufacturers of opaque milk cartons. They were equally welcome to milk processors who saw retail delivery routes and the retrieval of glass bottles for cleaning and reuse as a costly, inefficient horse-and-buggy relic.

Homogenized had almost completely forced out unhomogenized milk by the end of the 1950s. Cheap disposable packaging replaced glass bottles a little later with help from an unforeseen development: health authorities' new war on dietary fat.

THE KEYSIAN DIETARY CREDO

Milkfat, or butterfat, had been exactly what made whole drinking-milk taste good to many North Europeans with the right genes, and what made cream creamy. When separated by churning or centrifuging, it had been the foundation of the butter industry. Nobody could have guessed how soon butter, cream, and whole milk would be demonized after the mid-1950s.

The charge was led by the nutrition researcher Ancel Keys at the University of Minnesota, who had published some highly influential studies about the relationships among dietary fats, blood serum cholesterol, and coronary artery disease. His conclusions soon rocketed to the status of accepted scientific tenets. The main thesis was that heavy use of animal-based foods—especially fats—was responsible for a huge increase in heart attacks in much of the industrialized world, in contrast to far better cardiac health and greater longevity in the Mediterranean regions. Keys reasoned that foods like beefsteaks and full-fat dairy products contained harmful amounts of saturated fat, which raised serum cholesterol levels and caused a disastrous buildup of plaque in the coronary arteries.[12] The logical preventive was to adopt a diet in which these dangerous elements were replaced as far as possible by greens, whole grains, fruits, nuts, and some favorite Mediterranean fresh vegetables, with modest amounts of olive oil or other plant-derived fats and perhaps a little fish as an occasional animal protein source. In certain ways, Keys's vision of the ideal diet curiously resembled that of John Harvey Kellogg in his righteous Seventh Day Adventist days, but with the addition of colorful, appetizing Mediterranean elements little known to American eaters during Kellogg's career.

No suggestions about dietary changes have ever swept more rapidly to a critical mass in public opinion. It took only a few years for Keys to become the voice of mainstream authority about what people should and shouldn't eat. He had the good luck to catch the attention of the news media just as an early postwar vogue of female slenderness was giving way to an obsessive cult of ultra-thinness—aiding the later spread of anorexia nervosa, a previously rare disorder—that reigned during and long after the 1960s. Fat as cosmetic nemesis and cardiovascular threat blended effortlessly into one muddled crusade.

By the late 1970s, Keys's followers had convinced influential health spokespeople and most of the news media that his theories were not only scientifically established facts but commands. The new Keysian mindset differed from all prior nutritional consensuses in aggressively proclaiming what amounted to a national state of emergency. Many prominent politicians riding the bandwagon readily deferred to the insistence of the movement's leaders that in order for their dietary recommendations to have any effect, they should be universally followed not by members of particular age or health-risk groups but by everybody—for a central doctrine of the new creed was that *the population at large must be considered a health-risk group*. Among their pressing reforms was banishing whole drinking-milk from the American diet as a contributor to heart disease and replacing it with skim (now rechristened "nonfat") milk.

These ambitions were spelled out in a watershed document, the 1977 *Dietary Goals for the United States* prepared for the Senate Select Committee on Nutrition and Human Needs under the chairmanship of George McGovern.[13] They sat better with the popular media than with scientific investigators. The first published draft of the McGovern Committee report aroused such an outpouring of opinions among researchers that later that year the committee was obliged to issue a thick volume of "supplemental views." At the time, it received little news coverage.[14]

The supplemental views were a huge mishmash of predictable complaints from industries that stood to be affected by loss of customers, admiring comments from scientists who supported the report's recommendations, and many dismayed demurrals from others who didn't. Today these last reactions seem remarkably prescient. They repeatedly questioned the wisdom of plunging an entire nation into a dietary experiment based on extremely inconclusive data—for even in 1977 Keys's ideas were far from universally shared by students of the relationship between diet and disease. The cardiologist Eliot Corday summed up some widely held reservations: "We therefore must question whether application of an unproven diet blanketed to the population as a whole would be advisable. This seems to me like asking the whole nation to wear a size twelve patent leather shoe."[15]

The committee drew in its horns. Probably its responses reflected industry pressure more than criticism from dissenters like Corday. But at the end of 1977 it issued a revised edition of the report with considerable softening of some recommendations. Among these, "Substitute non-fat milk for whole milk" was changed to "Except for young children, substitute low-fat and non-fat milk for whole milk and low-fat dairy products for high-fat dairy products."[16] Converts to the cause continued to denounce whole milk. Recipe writers who sought to obey the committee's instructions about limiting the fat content of daily diets to a certain percentage of total calories gratefully recognized that nonfat milk made their arithmetic a lot easier.

In hindsight, some kind of backlash was inevitable. When it arrived several decades later, the hardline fat-phobic campaign could be seen to have squandered much of the prestige that the public health apparatus had acquired during the careers of officials like Milton Rosenau and to have helped encourage the spread of "alternative" medical ideologies that flourished with or without verifiable scientific evidence. Chapter 10 will focus on one example, the resurgent raw milk movement of the early twenty-first century. But in the meanwhile, anti-fat promises looked like heaven-sent opportunities to every branch of the food industry.

Milk-processing companies quickly responded to the proposed dietary overhaul by promoting nonfat milk and creating homogenized versions of reduced-fat milk in several possible gradations from .5 percent to 1 percent, 1.5 percent, and 2 percent milkfat by weight. The extreme wing of fat-fighters scorned these as fit only for wimps, but each soon acquired its fans. They now enabled milk processors to knock the last nails in the coffin of genuine whole milk—meaning milk with the same chemical structure and proportions that it had on leaving the cow. The percentage-slotted categories were another triumph for disposable cardboard cartons in which each pigeonholed category of milk was offered to the public with no direct view of the contents. They also represented a new technological refinement in the processing of homogenized milk—or rather, a new exploitation of an older refinement: centrifuging.

DISASSEMBLING AND REASSEMBLING MILK

Centrifugal separation of milkfat from skim milk had been hailed as the technological godsend of the era during the 1880s. Large or small centrifuges could remove the cream from unhomogenized whole milk faster and more completely than human hands working butter churns. On farms or at fluid-milk plants, they allowed richer or thinner cream to be processed for retail sale at stipulated minimum milkfat percentages that varied from state to state, with designations like "heavy cream," "whipping cream," table cream," and so forth. They also caused butter-making facilities called "creameries" to appear in all dairying regions.[17]

The gradations of lowfat milk that appeared in the late 1970s represented milk marketers' extension of the same technology to drinking-milk. But their effect was more profound. For maximum profit, dairy processors realized that the best procedure was to separate *all* milk as it arrived at the plant and recombine it to each state's minimum standards for any given category, including "whole" milk. In most states and in interstate commerce, this was supposed to contain 3.25 percent milkfat and 8.25 percent solids nonfat (SNF) by weight (see chapter 8).

Some perspective on these figures: A manual of dairy chemistry published in 1975—just too early to take lowfat dairy products into account—gives the average milkfat content of milk from six major dairy cow breeds as varying from 3.52 to 5.05 percent, SNF from 8.69 to 9.35 percent.[18] In other words, homogenized commercial "whole" milk was already far from whole when compared with undoctored milk harvested from cows. Well-managed Holsteins at the time were easily capable of 3.52 percent fat and 8.69 percent SNF. The 3.25 and 8.25 requirements already allowed dairy processors to retool "whole" milk to arbitrary standards. No commercial processor would have dreamed of simply pasteurizing and bottling genuinely whole milk. Consumers had not so much lost a taste for milk as forgotten that milk itself had any taste—that it could be anything other than an anonymous chilled white fluid, toted at intervals from refrigerated supermarket dairy case to home refrigerator and increasingly lectured about by nutritional censors.

The technological ability to "crack" petroleum into different hydrocarbon fractions has many different practical applications. By comparison, the ability to take milk apart and ingeniously reassemble it into simulacrums of its former self like some kind of child's puzzle serves little if any useful purpose. But from the first salvos in the antifat campaign, the industry saw dissecting-and-reconfiguring games as a profitable response to successful recent attacks on whole milk—so successful that not long after the McGovern Committee issued its findings, local politicians began getting up campaigns to supply *only* nonfat or lowfat milk to children in public school systems across the country. A few decades later, some cities extended the effort to an absolute ban on whole milk for schoolchildren, and in 2010 the Obama administration followed suit for schools participating in the National School Lunch Program.[19]

Somehow commercial "whole" milk—which is really anything but whole—never benefited from a general rethinking of the cardiac health ideology that began in the early 1990s and will be discussed in chapter 10. Parts of the ideology have been adjusted or frankly discredited. Government spokespersons have changed their tune on many questions—but they never have reversed themselves on an abhorrence of whole milk that defies rational explanation.

Perhaps one should not marvel at this attitude. After all, the thinking that made genuinely whole cow's milk a scientific mainstay of modern Western children's diets a few centuries ago was remarkably evidence-free. The conversion of milk-processing into a lesser analogue of petroleum-cracking, for the sake of unproved health benefits, is only too typical of the strange marriages between technology and quasi-science that keep on allowing the industry to find new sales opportunities. But we should recognize that no one has ever conclusively proved sustained improvement in cardiac health or life expectancy for children who drink lowfat or nonfat milk, or for adults who swear allegiance to one of the zero-to-2-percent choices.

Such uses of homogenization technology may not fall afoul of laws against adulteration. But they are a form of denaturing. They illustrate how thoroughly everyday consumption has been transformed into an illusory caricature of free choice and self-expression. Faced with as many alternatives in the dairy case as the toothpaste aisle, shoppers cannot be blamed for failing to reflect on anything preposterous, not to say pointless, in the maneuvers necessary to customize one substance into all these possibilities. After all, the original non-customized substance has been almost completely banished from commerce, with the aid of medical dogmas that took a long time to be questioned.

Pasteurized unhomogenized milk has made a small-scale comeback in recent years—but unfortunately, only as a *recherché* item for sophisticates who frequent expensive specialty shops, not anything tailored to ordinary consumers and ordinary budgets. Most people raised on homogenized milk find the unhomogenized version strange or frankly off-putting at first taste, a situation not improved by the fact that milk today almost always takes at least a few days to get from the farm to a consumer's refrigerator. Strangely enough, milk deliveries were faster in horse-and-buggy days than they are in the age of space flights. The interval today is usually long enough to allow the cream of unhomogenized bottled milk to collect in the neck as a semi-solid plug that resists being smoothly stirred back into the skim part and tends to form unwanted little clots or oil slicks in the user's morning coffee. This is the sort of snag that could be addressed if anybody saw a wider market—but realistically speaking, isn't likely to be. Almost the only consumers who now consider fresh unhomogenized milk more "natural" than homogenized are raw milk enthusiasts.

COLD AS SAFETY NET

My second example of profoundly game-changing dairy technology is refrigeration. Homogenization may be a piece of profit-minded technological fiddling made to fit in with now-disputed medical directives. Refrigeration, however, is one of the great necessities without which commercial drinking-milk could not reach some 333 million Americans. It is also virtually invisible to those who live with it as an everyday convenience. For a simple example, think of the numberless Americans who love nothing so much as downing a glass of ice-cold milk or swigging it straight from the carton. What might they say if asked why people in this country want to drink milk so thoroughly chilled as to lose anything like milk flavor?

In fact, freshly drawn milk at cow temperature (101°F/38°C) would be a serious shock to dyed-in-the-wool milk-chuggers. For them, deep chill and neutral flavor—along with perfect homogeneity—signal milk's true natural character. It is never more satisfying to devotees than when drunk at refrigerator temperature, at or a little under 40°F/4°C. Its best-loved qualities are pure artifacts of recent refrigeration technology.

Perhaps the claim should be qualified a bit. If we take "technology" in a sense broader than the latest bells and whistles in kitchen infrastructure, then the use of chilling technology is far from new. The knowledge that freshly drawn milk stays "sweet" longer when cooled than when exposed to warm ambient temperatures was common three or four centuries ago, and must be much older than that (though most humans

took less interest in "sweet" than soured milk until relatively recently).
We have ample evidence of the use of cold spring water—probably at
temperatures a little lower or higher than 55°F/13°C—in colonial-era
American farm dairies and springhouses. The first households to adopt
this means of chilling had no way to know that cold temperatures discouraged the growth of food-borne bacteria across a broad spectrum.
But by World War II the principle would be drummed into schoolchildren everywhere.

Commercial harvesting of ice from frozen winter ponds or streams
began in the United States during the early nineteenth century, and it
soon began to be used as a thermal preservative for perishable foods
such as milk. In Nathan Straus's time, many middle-class New York
households depended on "iceboxes"—insulated wooden boxes chilled
with blocks of ice periodically supplied by the iceman. (Confusingly,
the word "refrigerator" was often used for iceboxes during this period.)
It would be forty or more years before mechanically cooled electric or
gas refrigerators mostly supplanted literal iceboxes as everyday kitchen
appliances, to the joy of public health authorities who foresaw more families drinking safer milk. In hindsight, however, the new refrigerators
decisively reinforced consumers' amnesia about the natural qualities of
milk from cows. If you have never lived without a refrigerator, it is
hard to think of chilling as intervention or interference in the destiny
of a biological secretion, and milk that has *not* been profoundly chilled
seems to have something wrong with it. Today American consumers
have yet to fully embrace forms of milk processing and packaging that
dispatch it to supermarkets at room temperature.

REFRIGERATION RELAY: THE COLD CHAIN

What makes it possible for devotees of cold, cold drinking milk to belt
it down as casually as water is an unbroken relay system known as a
"cold chain." The system is older than the name, which was invented
to describe a way of handling temperature-sensitive medical materials

such as vaccines.[20] For today's milk, it could be said to begin in the liquid nitrogen tanks at onsite semen-storage facilities of artificial insemination services. After a nine-month interruption for bovine pregnancies, the chain resumes (though with less drastic chilling) precisely when milk leaves a lactating cow's udder and is piped into a refrigerated tank on the farm. From then on, its temperature is closely monitored through all stages of processing and packaging, with the goal of keeping any detours into ranges above 40°F/4°C as brief as possible. U.S. retail purchasers have been educated since infancy to keep the chain intact until the very instant of swallowing the milk.

The proposed temperature guidelines in Leslie Frank's draft of the 1924 Alabama model milk ordinance had in effect attempted to establish a cold chain—though nobody had yet coined the term—with then-available technology. They had called for cooling milk from the cow to 50°F/10°C or less within one hour after milking, or two hours if it was going straight to a processing plant. The same upper limit was to be observed once milk was pasteurized.[21] Bacteriologists then recommended it as the best—or the most realistic—temperature for keeping bacterial counts within the range permitted by the ordinance. Improvements in refrigeration eventually permitted the top limit to be reduced to the lower figure now considered the ideal refrigerated-storage temperature.

The gradual refinement of the cold chain for drinking-milk was bound up with enormous changes in dairy farms and processing plants. As always, milk was a buyer's market in which the processors regularly got to set the terms. During the early 1950s they decided on some factory retoolings that made it more convenient to pick up raw milk from farms on an every-other-day schedule. The switch from once-a-day pickups posed serious difficulties for farmers, who already had incurred forbidding expenses in keeping milk cold when versions of the 1924 ordinance began reaching more jurisdictions. The usual practice was to place the standard ten-gallon milk cans in large containers of ice water after milking. Getting enough ice for the purpose was a substantial expense. From the farm the milk generally was shipped to the city in railroad cars, for which requirements of cooling with blocks of ice eventually were imposed. As truck haulage gradually supplanted railway shipping, a schedule of daily pickups from the farm became usual, until one day it wasn't.

Standing twice as many cans in ice water at once to accommodate the new schedule was a logistical challenge. In what was by now a sadly familiar pattern, many dairy farmers simply gave up and sold their cows while the others invested in an expensive new necessity: a bulk milk tank.[22] This was a covered stainless steel vat, usually (in the early 1950s) of between 100-gallon and 300-gallon capacity. It was double-walled, with an insulating space between the inner and outer walls, and equipped with a refrigeration system for rapidly chilling the milk. Since unhomogenized milk couldn't sit for two days without the inevitable cream separation, bulk tanks also had motorized agitators to keep the contents evenly distributed.[23] Milk was piped from the room that housed the milking machines and pumped into the vessel. Milk trucks cooled with ice, meanwhile, had undergone their own metamorphosis into refrigerated tank trucks into which two days' worth of milk could be directly pumped from the bulk tank. At the plant, it was pumped into other chilled systems, making the cold chain more seamless. Milk cans became collectors' items.

The remaining dairy farms, of course, were larger and more heavily capitalized than ever before. So were the milk-processing plants that had dictated the switch in pickup schedules. In both cases, public health authorities were happy to see slovenly little farms and substandard little processing plants disappear. (Well-maintained small farms and plants often suffered the same fate.) The larger facilities that replaced them amid the advance of exurban sprawl undoubtedly got more drinking-milk to more people in safer condition. But as in the case of new, improved dairy cows, there was a sizable downside.

The efficient functioning of the cold chain demanded that at nearly every moment between bulk tank and supermarket dairy case, drinking-milk should be in motion with only short interruptions. As processing plants inexorably got bigger, they also got faster. Volume was of the essence, but so was speed—especially in temperature control. Milk arriving at the plant had to be pumped at once into gigantic refrigerated silos before being shunted into centrifuges for separation of cream and skim milk. Once separated, these had to be almost instantaneously heated to the necessary temperatures for homogenization and pasteurization and promptly rechilled, keeping the unavoidable break in the cold chain as brief as possible. Batch pasteurization methods as outlined in chapter 5 were a poor fit with the speeded-up tempos of the new production lines and soon gave way to the continuous-flow-high-temperature-short-time pasteurizing process.[24]

But even HTST pasteurization couldn't satisfy the industry's search for time-saving advances, including ones that might make the last links in the cold chain unnecessary. In the United States at least, cream was the first object of these efforts. Demand for it had shrunk as the war on fat expanded, so that longer shelf life became a priority for cream earlier than for milk.

The new methods that became and still are popular for processing cream are generally lumped together as "UHT" (ultra-high-temperature) pasteurization or "ultrapasteurization." They shave 13 or 14 seconds off the HTST process by exposing the cream to heat far above the boiling point of water (usually 280°F/138°C for 2 seconds), a radical departure from the older pasteurization principle that a liquid being pasteurized should always remain well under boiling point. The taste of cream suffers less than that of drinking-milk because the fat-free portions of milk undergo more chemical disruption—including lactose caramelization and the release of some sulfur compounds—in the heating process than the milkfat. But from the start, ultrapasteurized heavy cream aroused consumer complaints because it lost some viscosity in heating and became thinner than simply pasteurized cream. Stabilizers and emulsifiers were routinely added to vaguely simulate creaminess, but failed to overcome the allied problem that the product took much longer to whip than cream pasteurized at conventional temperatures. Nevertheless, non-ultrapasteurized cream quickly disappeared from supermarket shelves. Shoppers today must hunt far and wide for it.

In addition to trimming more than a dozen seconds from one stage in processing, ultrapasteurization came close to actually sterilizing the product rather than just eliminating some pathogens. Processors in this country didn't focus on exacting criteria of sterility for packaging cream. But the idea caught on faster in Europe than in the United States as a treatment for milk, which had more rigorous technological requirements than cream. The aseptic method trademarked as Tetra Pak in Sweden quickly became familiar for packaging milk and fruit juices. It relied on maintaining near-perfect sterility while the liquid was pumped into complexly laminated containers in a process that telescoped the creation and sealing of the package and the pouring of the milk into a few seconds.

The cold chain ended there; the resulting product could be stored at room temperature for months—and here the convenience of ultrapasteurized milk couldn't stop it from encountering decades of consumer resistance in the United States, where people associated drinking-milk with deep chill. To Americans, milk that wasn't drunk at refrigerator temperature was somehow unnatural. That reaction testifies to nearly a century of cultural conditioning as arbitrary but immovable as dressing newborn babies in the "right" color for their sex. Only in the past twenty or so years has milk *not* sold in the chilled dairy case made headway in the United States.

CONSEQUENCES OF REFRIGERATION: CHILLING THOUGHTS

The most important purpose of chilling milk has always been maintaining a barrier to bacterial growth. Cold and heat, meaning refrigeration and pasteurization, are the twin pillars of dairy sanitation. But as processing technologies for drinking-milk got bigger and faster, the necessary engineering infrastructures—including refrigeration apparatus—grew more complex, with more potential lurking spots for bacteria throughout the system. Manufacturers worked tirelessly to eliminate such liabilities as corners and seams, install cleaning technologies capable of reaching every inch of the system, and monitor conditions at every crucial point. It is fair to say that the products emerging from today's giga-plants are bacteriologically safer than commercial dairy products ever have been. But though slipups may be rare, those that do occur have vastly greater scope for harm than similar failures in the past. A dairy plant that processes several million pounds of milk per day can spread infections to many more people than a small 1950s plant of 200,000-pound capacity. One valve mistakenly left open for a few seconds in a vast labyrinth of pipes can allow raw milk to mingle with properly pasteurized and chilled milk, contaminating huge volumes at a time.[25] Many milk-borne illnesses have been traced to post-pasteurization contamination of drinking-milk or other dairy products. But there is another connection between bacteria and the refrigeration story.

As explained in chapter 6, the lactic acid bacteria (LAB) responsible for most natural souring of milk—an important if not infallible defense against some milk-borne pathogens in preindustrial epochs—are either thermophilic or mesophilic. That is, they multiply most speedily at temperatures roughly falling within a range of respectively 104°F/39°C to 120°F/50°C or 70°F/21°C to 90°F/32°C. But a large group of organisms form a third category. They are psychrophilic or psychrotrophic, meaning that they either actively prefer or can well tolerate the standard temperatures of modern refrigerators. They can slowly but inexorably multiply in refrigerated milk, making their presence very nastily known after prolonged sojourns at 40°F/4°C. And some are tough and versatile, able to live at quite high temperatures and to survive in out-of-the-way niches.

Whereas LAB feed chiefly or exclusively on lactose, the principal carbohydrate of milk, psychrophiles and psychrotrophs mostly attack milkfat and milk proteins.[26] Their existence in milk naturally escaped scientific notice until refrigeration had given people a chance to observe that milk stored for a long time at cold temperatures usually developed horribly rank, bitter flavors. Rather than harboring dangerous toxins concealed under a harmless semblance, it became too frankly inedible to fool anyone—the result of bacterial action releasing evil-tasting byproducts of fat and protein breakdown. Conditions hospitable to these spoilage organisms hadn't been usual in the early days of milk pasteurization. Milton Rosenau and colleagues had specifically sought to find time-temperature combinations that would leave some of the original LAB intact and able to start working again if milk refrigerated at 50°F/10°C were allowed to sit at room temperature for a while. Besides, consumers bought and used up milk daily or almost daily in pint or quart amounts. The switch to HTST pasteurization altered the playing field, especially after processors started selling milk in larger containers.

In August 1964, a *New York Times* headline proclaimed, "Plastic Is New Entry in Battle of the Milk Bottles." The reporter, Robert A. Wright, revealed that the newest "combatants" meant to see to it "that most American families, who have no problem buying a quart, increase their purchases to a few gallons of milk a day. This objective promises a revolution in the packaging of milk—in gallon-size plastic bottles."[27] Hopes of getting people to buy a few gallons a day fell through. Rather, the habit of buying milk by the gallon (or half-gallon) plastic jug caught on quickly because it allowed people to shop less often for milk. The result was that larger amounts of milk, pasteurized through a process that eliminated LAB, could sit around far longer in home refrigerators. Cold-tolerant bacteria usually didn't multiply to the point of spoilage within less than two weeks—but thrifty purchasers who thought they could make a gallon last that long might be unpleasantly surprised.

But spoiled milk in home refrigerators was only the tip of the iceberg. Dairy microbiologists gradually learned that many bacteria with different temperature preferences have the ability to collect in organized communities called "biofilms"—highly adhesive single-species or multi-species matrices that show up in processing factories. They plaster themselves to surfaces such as the walls of pipes and holding vessels, or find likely sticking-places on gaskets or conveyor belts. They seem to be particularly fond of stainless steel, rubber, and various plastics. And as their presence was proved beyond doubt, concern mounted about their apparent ability to checkmate—or at least partly thwart—vaunted advances in plant-cleaning systems.

Until the mid-twentieth century the tanks, pipelines, and pumping equipment in milk-processing plants had to be opened or disassembled after each day's use and rigorously cleaned by hand—a serious limitation on the volume of milk a plant could handle on a daily basis. But during and after the 1950s, advances in the manufacture of stainless steel, heat-proof glass, and durable plastics enabled milk processors to build astronomically larger facilities that could operate continuously for days on end, with scheduled pauses for "cleaning-in-place," or high-pressure pumping-out of the system with improved sanitizing solutions.[28]

Clean-in-place technology was considered nearly foolproof for decades. Biofilms shattered the illusion soon after 2000. They proved to be a stubborn bacterial safety hazard on any surface in a processing system that was repeatedly brought into contact with milk, cold chain or no cold chain. They can be astonishingly resistant to removal by cleansing and disinfecting agents, abrasion, or heat. (Dental patients who have had plaque cleaned off their teeth know how unpleasant it can be to remove biofilms, and how predictably they grow back.) Because they are so persistent and talented in adhering to inaccessible spots, they can contribute tremendously to post-pasteurization contamination problems in dairy-processing plants dealing in products from cheese to drinking-milk to ice cream.[29]

The biofilm problem is now well-enough recognized in the industry to make unforeseen mass-scale catastrophes unlikely though far from impossible. But one particularly insidious frequenter of biofilm communities merits special attention. It is *Listeria monocytogenes*, a member of a genus of bacteria ubiquitously distributed in natural environmental reservoirs—for instance, soil and water.[30] *L. monocytogenes* is amazingly tenacious and versatile. It is a psychrotroph capable of flourishing even in ice cream. But it also likes warm temperatures and does well up to about 113°F/45°C. It is hardy in both moist and dry conditions, as well as highly tolerant of some natural antibacterial preservatives including salt and acid (it can survive in extremely salty brined cheeses and many pickled foods). And unlike many less dangerous psychrotrophs, it doesn't affect the smell or taste of the foods it colonizes—meaning that it can be transmitted through milk and many other products without arousing suspicion. The symptoms of listeriosis can include gastrointestinal upsets, fever, joint pain, headache, and in severe cases meningitis or other central nervous system effects. It is particularly dangerous to the elderly, pregnant women, and newborns. The Centers for Disease Control and Prevention has estimated that some 1,600 cases occur in the United States every year, including about 260 fatalities.[31]

L. monocytogenes didn't attract serious attention as a health hazard until late in the twentieth century. It began turning up in the news after 1983, when the first extensively researched study was published in the *New England Journal of Medicine*. Milk was found to be only one of its favorite substrates; it also invades various kinds of delicatessen cold cuts, certain cheeses, and dry fermented sausages. It has been implicated in outbreaks traced to raw fruits and vegetables. Its first positive identification as a source of food-borne illness came from a batch of coleslaw.[32] It can form biofilms by itself in manufacturing plants, or join multi-species communities. Though it can be eliminated from milk by correct pasteurization, it is one of the most frequent culprits in contamination through post-pasteurization lapses.

The identification of L. monocytogenes in food was one of several early wakeup calls suggesting to epidemiologists that their mental picture of pathogenic threats needed serious redrawing. As recently as the late 1970s, it had not been mentioned in textbooks of epidemiology or food microbiology. Many public health officials, and many doctors in private practice, thought that medical science had gone far toward eliminating the causes of most major food-borne illnesses. But by the end of the 1980s, they would find themselves confronting a number of "emerging" infectious diseases, meaning ones that had never been previously identified among patients or that had suddenly appeared far outside usual geographical limits. Reports of strange illnesses traceable to a large range of foods catapulted the names of the new—that is, newly recognized—organisms to headlines throughout the country. Several will be discussed in the next chapter in connection with the history of the current raw milk movement. L. monocytogenes, however, deserves to be examined in relation to the cold-chain story.

In nearly all cases of L. monocytogenes spread through milk and dairy products, the infection has been ultimately traced to raw milk. But "nearly" is not "always," especially in industries dependent on fantastically elaborate technologies.

Public health experts like Leslie Frank could assume that chilling plus pasteurization plus rechilling took bacterial enemies out of action in milk. Then came the discovery that chilling could make it fair game for psychrophiles and psychrotrophs. The fact that they multiplied in milk more vigorously the longer it was refrigerated introduced some caveats about a trusted technological resource. And when one of the bacterial cold-lovers turned out to be a dangerous pathogen, health authorities had to recognize that at times refrigeration could be a liability in food safety strategies.

As "new" pathogens emerged, microbiologists had to devise testing procedures to detect their presence in farm buildings, bulk tanks, factories, supermarket shelving, home pantries and refrigerators (or even freezers), and the systems of patients. For *L. monocytogenes*, the issue was confused by the difficulty of distinguishing it from harmless members of the *Listeria* genus until genomic sampling and amplification methods allowed more precise observations during the 1990s. It also took time to add the new offender to existing lists of mandatory tests for raw and pasteurized milk.

The ubiquity of the organism as a soil microbe made it especially hard for farmers to strategize against. There were endless opportunities for *L. monocytogenes* to enter the milk, starting with what the cows were eating. Even pasture grass might (though rarely) be suspect. Badly cured, moldy hay could be a reservoir, as could corn (or other) silage not fermented to a low enough pH to inhibit the growth of *L. monocytogenes*. Some cows might be asymptomatic carriers that shed the pathogen in their manure, contaminating bedding or stalls and infecting the rest of the herd.[33]

The U.S. dairy industry has not managed to take listeriosis in its stride, but it has usually managed to contain it through extra vigilance and more strenuous technological monitoring while exploring new cleansing and disinfecting agents. At that, dairy farmers and processors probably have done better than people in many other segments of food production because they have a history of being *legally required* to think about minute details of sanitation—unlike, say, cantaloupe or spinach growers, who were nearly blindsided by listeriosis cases traced to their farms or transportation systems. But *L. monocytogenes* has plainly shown up the limitations of an uninterrupted cold chain—a technological bastion that has been relied on for generations—in preventing the spread of milk-borne pathogens.

From a bacteriological point of view, the description "moving target" is just as applicable to refrigerated as unrefrigerated milk. Refrigerating milk once it has left the cow interrupts natural fermenting processes—once of great importance to dairying peoples—that never can be resumed without impairment. But refrigeration doesn't make the moving target stand still. Cold temperatures slow down the course of events but also deflect it in different directions and toward different outcomes, often either unpleasant or dangerous. Refrigerating milk—and in relatively sterile containers—remains an urgent necessity in any region where people expect to keep it without souring or other changes for more than a few hours. But it can give aid and comfort to some bacterial enemies.

There is no going back to any supposed good old days in either countries with long-established dairy industries or developing countries where entrepreneurs are trying to turn drinking-milk into a nutritional grail. Still, it is realistic to assume that the *L. monocytogenes* situation is just the beginning. The question is not *whether* some future milk-borne pathogen will show up apparently out of nowhere, but *when*. Perhaps no single piece of technology will be directly to blame; it may be more a matter of many simultaneously intensifying strains on threatened resources such as soil, water, and air, or bovine biological capacities. The first hint may occur in this country, or in one of the many Western-inspired attempts to kickstart large-scale industrial dairy farming and processing elsewhere in the world. Certainly not all dairy farms or processors should be considered equal contributors to a potentially approaching crisis. But those who embrace real, stupefying gigantism—especially in climates and ecosystems that are a bad fit with dairy cow metabolisms—already bear heavy responsibility for environmental depletion and deserve calling to account before they can inflict more. Emerging pathogens are all but guaranteed to be part of the cost, and they may be as challenging to trusted food safety technologies as *L. monocytogenes.*

As future threats arise, a huge industry already swathed in stupendous, energy-intensive technological complexities will be forced, at great expense, to add still more layers of complexity to address unfamiliar predicaments. The super-labyrinthine workings of the dairy business will become even more unintelligible to the general public than they are already. The number of points at which something can go wrong in the system undoubtedly will increase, giving the back-to-nature dissidents to be introduced in the next chapter more opportunities to portray the mainstream industry as public enemy number one. Sadly, a piece of industrial engineering can look like the solution to a food safety problem for the better part of a century and then turn out to be inextricably entangled with other problems.

THE NEXT FRONTIER: DESIGNER MILK?

As ideas about cow improvement advanced over the last decades along with both refinements and frustrations in milk processing, some dairy scientists began to glimpse another horizon: To what extent, and for what purposes, might it be possible to *reconfigure milk before it leaves the cow?*

One of the most highly publicized initiatives began in New Zealand after researchers found a strange feature in the casein makeup of different cows' milk. It was discovered to be genetic in origin, and might never have come to light had not Holstein cows (usually called Friesian in New Zealand) gone a long way toward eclipsing all other commercially important dairy breeds in every part of the globe by the 1990s. An Auckland pediatrician named Robert Elliott began expounding a theory that the distribution of childhood diabetes in developed- and developing-world countries uncannily matched the use of milk that contained or lacked a particular variant form of casein or more correctly, caseins.[34]

The micelles described in chapter 1 that contain most of the calcium and protein in cow's milk are actually composed of several different casein fractions designated by the Greek letters α, β, and κ. These can occur in variant forms through tiny alterations in the sequence of individual amino acids making up the protein. Elliott's interest focused on two variants of β-casein that he had concluded had widely dissimilar metabolic effects: β-A1 and β-A2. Both were very widely found in milk from up-to-date dairy herds, in which Holsteins now figured heavily. The breed appeared to be the main source of β-A1, which had the strange property of being easily broken down in the small intestine to release β-casomorphin-7, a substance with a range of unusual bioactive effects. This did not occur in β-A2.

It was soon clear that the only mammals whose milk contained β-A1 were domestic cows—more precisely, cows of North European and British origin. They included Holsteins, Ayrshires, and Shorthorns. Wherever Holstein sires had been employed to "improve" another breed, some admixture of A1 occurred in the milk. Pursuing the genetic thread of the mystery, researchers hypothesized that cow's milk had originally contained only A2, the form found in all other ruminants' milk; the A1 deviation appeared at some point when ancestors of the northern cattle breeds evolved as separate landraces. In any case, inheritance doesn't follow strict Mendelian dominant-recessive logic. Cows with two exclusively A1 or A2 parents (A1A1/A2A2) will give exclusively A1 or A2 milk, while those of mixed parentage (A1A2) will give milk containing both β-casein variants and pass on some degree of the mixed condition to their offspring— meaning that the milk will have at least some β-casomorphin-7 activity.

In 2000 a pair of converts to Elliott's thesis launched the "A2 Corporation," hoping to market a genetic test they had devised to measure the admixture of A1 and A2 in a cow's (or bull's) ancestry, and also planning to sell milk guaranteed free of the undesirable protein.[35] The allegations against A1 milk came to center on harmful immunological effects, and the number of medical conditions that β-casomorphin-7 was theoretically linked to soon included not only diabetes but cardiovascular disease, autism, and schizophrenia. The A2 Corporation and the arguments behind the anti-A1-milk campaign eventually garnered a great deal of publicity in New Zealand and Australia. By 2010, A2 fever had begun spreading to the United States.

Proponents set to work to eliminate the problem at the source by selecting genetically tested animals and breeding A2 to A2 parent so as to create pure A2 stock. Guernsey cows proved to have already won some kind of genetic lottery: Their milk showed almost no trace of A1 ancestry. The breed began recovering an éclat that it hadn't possessed since the "Golden Guernsey" days many decades earlier. The dairy industry at large, however, put up some serious resistance to the A2 vogue, claiming that several studies warning against the threat of A1 milk actually came from people connected with the A2 business enterprise.

Over time, investigators with no dog in the fight failed to find convincing evidence that β-casomorphin-7 played a significant role in any of the illnesses that the company and its sympathizers had cited. They did, however, consistently find that milk-drinkers who switched from A1 to A2 milk reported some reduction in digestive problems such as stomach cramps or loose stools. Sales pitches for A2 milk gradually shifted to this more defensible ground.[36]

Many milk producers and processors ignored or pooh-poohed the whole A2 affair. Others rapidly appreciated that almost any "functional" food with both a slightly obscure scientific aura and an easy-to-pronounce name could attract a lucrative market. Publicity for the new marvel paid off: consumers who kept up with health news began asking for A2 milk even, or perhaps *especially*, when they knew that it cost more than ordinary milk.

Artificial insemination services took notice. No breed was categorically excluded from sharing in the genetic blessings of A2, so Holsteins (or Friesians) were not doomed to carry an overwhelming A1 inheritance. Guernseys might come close to unblemished A2A2 status, but Holsteins usually had a fair amount of A2 ancestry from somewhere in the mix. With genetic testing and purposeful breeding programs, interested farmers could gradually eliminate β-casomorphin-7 from Holstein milk and join the movement with clean A2A2 credentials.

A2 milk brightened the hopes of product-development gurus who had already foreseen a promising future for designer milk—milk genetically targeted to some highly specialized purpose before the cow who gave it was born. In the case of A2, the goal of getting the milk into production still had to be addressed through usual dam-and-sire insemination programs, one generation at a time. The only new factor was computer-assisted precision in obtaining information—first, analyzing the amino acid profile of a particular milk protein to detect a single genetically determined anomaly and on observing a resulting effect, devising a test for identifying animals with and without the anomaly in question. Direct intervention in the bovine genome for the purpose of changing milk's composition wasn't at issue.   .

INSIDE THE GENOME

But direct intervention was already being contemplated in many branches of the livestock industry. Sudden advances in genome mapping and sequencing during the 1990s produced a flood of searches for practical applications—not least in the food industry, where the possibilities of gene editing promised to telescope lengthy improvement projects in both the vegetable and animal kingdoms into a few years. The public relations backlash against GMOs, or genetically modified organisms, was swift and daunting. All news media soon reverberated with attacks on "Frankenfoods." That catchword unfortunately lumped together many efforts involving the new technology of gene transfers.

In the case of milk, transgenic experiments have been too diverse to merit one knee-jerk reaction. It also should be noted that they tend to proceed more slowly and uncertainly than early cheerleaders hoped, with plenty of stumbles along the way including considerable mortality in embryos and newborns. The length of cow pregnancies also has encouraged researchers to substitute goats (who give birth in five rather than nine months) as test subjects in transgenic milk experiments.

One class of projects aims to address endemic problems with dairy animals' own health by nipping them in the bud—that is, the udder. An early example in 2005 sought to make cows more mastitis-proof by introducing a trans gene into cloned Jersey heifers that contained a cocktail of properties including the ability to manufacture lysostaphin, an antimicrobial agent powerfully effective against *Staphylococcus aureus* that is produced by a rival member of the *Staphylococcus* group.[37] The animals' udders did indeed secrete enough lysostaphin to destroy *S. aureus*, the commonest bacterial source of mastitis in high-producing dairy herds. Unfortunately, the researchers had left the job of evaluating lysostaphin's safety in milk destined for human consumption to future public health colleagues. The experiment was a success, but the project died. Other interventions intended to get some natural antimicrobial substance into cows' udders may well incur the same difficulty. And from an animal welfare viewpoint, protecting lactating cows from mastitis by reducing the stresses to which they are subjected seems like a saner priority than trying to make them more resistant to infections triggered by just those stresses (i.e., aggressive breeding and feeding for maximum milk yield under crowded conditions in mega-dairies).

There is also much interest in reconfiguring the major chemical components of milk through gene editing. Fat, especially saturated fat, is a favorite target. Milk from cows engineered for overall fat reduction or higher unsaturated fatty acid percentages may present some sales advantage, though perhaps not as decisively as at the height of Ancel Keys's influence. Dairy scientists had previously tried to achieve the goal by adding sources of unsaturated fatty acids to the animals' feed. This was an awkward balancing act, since the bacteria that digest the food arriving in a cow's rumen generally compensate for variations in the makeup of food rations by working overtime to maintain the usual equilibrium. One of the world's premier centers of dairy science research, the University of Guelph in Ontario, developed a method of augmenting the amounts of several desirable fatty acids in cow's milk by supplementing the feed with herring meal; the milk was successfully marketed as "Dairy Oh!" by the Canadian dairy firm of Neilson. Transgenics pioneers aimed to bypass such laborious strategies by adding or deleting "letters" in a cow's genome.

Enthusiasm ran high in China, where the government had started promoting milk consumption as a key contributor to national growth—in the physical as well as the economic sense, since nutrition advisers claimed that getting enough cow's milk into children could make them as tall as Americans. In 2006 Premier Wen Jiabao had publicized a program for distributing free milk to schoolchildren in Chongqing by declaring, "I have a dream, and my dream is that each Chinese person, especially the children, can afford to buy one *jin* [about half a kilogram, or half a liter] of milk to drink every day."[38] The mentality eerily recalls a quip made by U.S. Vice President Henry A. Wallace during the first months of World War II: "The object of this war is to make sure that everybody in the world has the privilege of drinking a quart of milk a day."[39] Wallace had spoken half in jest; Wen was dead serious. But his dream was ill-matched with certain human genomes: those of the Han Chinese and most other peoples in eastern Asia. Normal loss of lactase function somewhere between weaning and puberty means that the lactose in a *jin* of milk would cause mild or severe abdominal distress to nearly all adults, though not necessarily to children of school age.

Western medical authorities had not yet stumbled across the lactase nonpersistence issue when they began proclaiming an association of milk-drinking with increased size and strength. In Meiji-era Japan (1868–1912), the state was sufficiently influenced by propaganda about Western-style diets as a driver of national progress to begin importing cattle for meat and milk. Much later, the association of drinking-milk with vigorous health was reinforced under the postwar American occupation, when children began receiving milk (usually reconstituted from imported dried milk) as part of a school lunch program.[40] But China's race to catch up with the West in milk power didn't seriously take off until the late 1980s, more than a decade into the post–Mao Zedong development initiatives urged by Deng Xiaoping.

China is now the world's largest importer of milk, chiefly in dried form, with New Zealand as the most important supplier. But planners who see milk as a strategic food-security bulwark have long been thinking about how to increase domestic production while also acquiring stakes in overseas enterprises. The population has eagerly complied with calls to drink milk as a patriotic duty. But people were scared off the domestic product in 2008 when whistleblowers revealed that major Chinese processors had falsified quality-control tests for protein content by adulterating powdered milk and infant formula with melamine, a widely available plastic that improved the nitrogen score of milk. Thousands of children were sickened, sometimes with permanent kidney damage. For years afterward, most people prudently bought imported brands. Still, the Chinese appetite for milk was unabated.

The Beijing authorities continued to pump money and knowhow into expanding the domestic industry and forming international business partnerships, with an almost slavish eagerness to adopt the technological stratagems recommended by Western advisers. Mega-dairy farms and processing facilities have notably flourished in Inner Mongolia, notwithstanding semidesert conditions throughout much of the region. Ambitious research projects are ongoing at the Agricultural University of Inner Mongolia.[41] Some seek to "improve" the lipid profile of milk to reduce the proportion of saturated fatty acids and include more omega-3s, a purpose ardently embraced at research institutions everywhere in the world. Others concern the elephant-in-the-room issue of adult lactase nonpersistence in almost the entire population of China.

A team of dairy geneticists at the university's college of life sciences garnered international headlines in 2012 by introducing into fourteen bovine fetuses a gene meant to curb secretion of lactose. Only one of the transgenic subjects survived the experiment, but she had the researchers eagerly foreseeing herds of clones yielding low-lactose milk.[42] Since nothing further was heard of that plan, one may surmise that the heifer didn't perform as hoped. But six years later another of the school's research groups unveiled a more advanced approach based on precise gene-editing techniques. This time the same gene—which presumably is able to secrete lactase in the udder, preventing the full complement of preformed lactose from appearing in the milk—was directly inserted into a predetermined site on the genome.[43]

It is difficult to think of these exercises in manipulating cow's milk into a form that could not meet the dietary needs of a nursing calf as anything but an example of cultural brainwashing. Various gene-editing efforts are going on in other countries where national food-policy setters are trying to kickstart a dairy industry. The desirability of creating cows genetically programmed to give milk that humans of all ancestries can drink by the pint or quart seems self-evident to leaders of Western dairy science and their non-Western acolytes. (In the developed world, other efforts to enzymatically remove the lactose from milk have met with some commercial success, as noted in chapter 11.)

To suggest that people who can't digest lactose should simply avoid drinking-milk violates every principle of marketing. And so, in defiance of all reason, lactase nonpersistence continues to be talked and thought about as a medical problem in need of a solution, anywhere from North America to East Asia.

Other gene-editing or transgenic experiments concentrate on altering the casein configuration of milk. Publicity over A2 milk has stimulated hopes of directly deleting the A1 gene from the genome and replacing it with A2. Another line of investigation aims to create cows that will secrete milk with more β- and especially κ-casein, which play the largest role in curd formation. The idea is to obtain larger and more rapid cheese yields from a given amount of milk. The New Zealand team that worked on the project pointed out some novel features of the reconfigured milk without troubling to ask whether real cheesemakers (who generally have had no trouble accepting the less drastic technology of producing the milk-coagulating enzyme chymosin from recombinant bacteria) would find the quality of the curd acceptable.[44]

But it seems unwise to automatically dismiss all experiments with milk from transgenic cows. Lactase nonpersistence may be the subject of widespread medical delusions, and it is less than certain that fiddling with milk lipid content will improve anyone's cardiovascular health. True allergies to cow's (or other animals') milk are another question.

Lactase-nonpersistent people who for some reason think they must consume milk will encounter difficult and unpleasant symptoms. But lactase nonpersistence is neither an allergy nor a life-threatening condition. Much rarer, but also much more dangerous, are genuine milk allergies—immunologic reactions to several cow's milk proteins. They present special risks in infants and small children, whose immature immune systems may respond to foreign proteins with symptoms ranging from rashes or hives to anaphylactic shock. The chief triggers are β-lactoglobulin, a whey protein that doesn't occur in human milk, and casein. Cow's milk has about ten times more casein than human milk, and there are marked differences in the composition of the casein micelles. Hence babies who aren't breastfed may not be able to tolerate formulas based on cow's milk; formulas using soy milk or other plant-based substitutes often have their own problems. There are more rational arguments for creating transgenic cows to meet bona fide needs in an admittedly small number of newborns and toddlers than for catering to larger market segments that take their cues from headlines about lactose or saturated fat.

This isn't to say that the technology of editing bovine genomes in order to eliminate β-lactoglobulin or allergenic casein fractions is at present anywhere close to foolproof. Some attempts to produce cows without the β-lactoglobulin gene seem to have met with modest success. Cows that manufacture casein with allergens deleted probably will be more difficult to bring into being because of the extremely intricate structure of casein micelles.

Another class of transgenic experiments raises ethical questions for which there are no easy answers. They involve reformulating cow's or goat's milk in the udder for human medicinal purposes—for instance, to produce antithrombin for people who lack this crucial factor for controlling the blood-clotting process, or myelin basic protein to counter the destruction of the nerve-protecting myelin sheath in multiple sclerosis patients.[45] The logistical obstacles to getting carefully judged amounts of the desired substances into actual milk are formidable enough that debates about turning dairy animals into "pharming" instruments may remain more hypothetical than concrete for some years. But bitter showdowns can be predicted in future as the technology develops.

How should consumers respond when they are unsure whether food is a pure gift of nature or a tainted artifact of human contrivance? One way of signaling that you reject the Faustian bargain of the latter is to insist on eating everything raw, or at least some venerated article of diet. The most familiar example today is organized support for legalizing the sale of unpasteurized milk, a contentious issue that demands careful scrutiny.

10

REVIVING THE RAW MILK CAUSE

NATUROPATHY AND HEALTH

The beliefs of today's leading raw milk advocates are rooted in a German-derived movement dedicated to physical culture and diet reform that was transplanted to the United States shortly after 1900 and christened "naturopathy." The original tenets—which have been put through various later contortions by people calling themselves naturopaths—were straightforward. First: anyone could acquire a truly sound body through invigorating exercise, sunbathing, fresh air, and food in its pristine state. Second: no such thing as disease could conquer the vital force in a body so fortified. "Disease" in the usual sense was a myth invented by the orthodox medical profession to foist toxic remedies on unsuspecting patients. But properly understood, it was "a process of purification of the system," a telling description by the California practitioner Otto Carqué.[1] The one reliable preventive of disease was to stop unnatural outside agents from invading the system—and heat processing, including cooking and milk pasteurization, transformed raw food into an unnatural outside agent.

Other threats included alcohol, tobacco, tea, and coffee. Above all, no drugs or vaccines must breach the body's defenses, a conviction in which naturopaths found common cause with homeopaths against "allopathic" (i.e., mainstream) medicine. "Allopathy" was originally a derogatory word for medical methods that forced foreign substances into the system. When Pasteur's germ theory of infectious disease was adopted by most of the medical community after the 1880s, anti-allopaths stuck to their guns in opposing the use of vaccine injections—the most alien of all alien intrusions into a living bloodstream—to prevent smallpox, measles, typhoid fever, and all other pathogenic foes.[2]

Bernarr Macfadden (the name was his own improvement on the insufficiently manly-sounding "Bernard McFadden") was the most prominent early twentieth-century exponent of naturopathy. His ideas of health and nutrition reached millions through an enormous, anarchic publishing empire in which magazines and books dedicated to physical fitness, sex education, and nutrition advice shared the boss's eclectic attention with pioneering efforts in the true-confession genre. Gifted at reading the pulse of the American public, he didn't mind occasionally bending naturopathic principles for the sake of audience appeal.

In *The Miracle of Milk* (1923) Macfadden presented a "milk diet" that, unlike the one administered to John Harvey Kellogg's patients at Battle Creek, was meant for home use and didn't include such favorite Kellogg interventions as milk enemas. The diet was framed as a lengthy rest cure for subpar systems. He strongly recommended using raw milk, but with typical expediency assured readers that the pasteurized version would do if supplemented with citrus juice.

Before beginning the diet, patients had to prepare the system with a several-days' fast. They then worked up gradually to about six or seven quarts a day, slowly sipping one glass at a time by a sucking technique that Macfadden advised as a way to half-simulate the natural rhythm of infants at the breast. No solid food was permitted.[3]

His attitude toward the difficulties that many patients reported when trying to swallow huge daily amounts of fresh milk without suffering diarrhea, abdominal discomfort, or nausea shows a talent for nonchalant rationalization that was also typical. Like George Cheyne two centuries earlier, Macfadden thought such symptoms indicated the disturbed digestion's need for corrective measures.[4] Since he knew no reason that lactose could produce unpleasant symptoms, he couldn't have reached what now would be the most obvious conclusion about the effects of "sweet" milk on many people's digestions. But he did prudently leave some leeway for patients to drink buttermilk or other kinds of soured milk. The idea that lactic acid fermentation might make milk more digestible for many people was now reaching more dietary advisers, though the supreme importance of unsoured drinking-milk was still taken for granted.

Macfadden and fellow naturopaths soon showed themselves able to mount obstinate, sustained challenges to what the mainstream medical profession considered progress. Throughout much of the century, their *bête noire* was the American Medical Association, which also earned the lasting enmity of New Deal loyalists for preventing health-care provisions from being included in the 1935 Social Security Act.[5] For many decades, New Dealers' successors in the Democratic Party railed against the association as the very model of a reactionary lobbying group. Dietary nonconformists, probably inspired by the earlier campaigns of nineteenth-century English and American anti-vaccine activists, assailed allopathic physicians as a "medical monopoly" in cahoots with public health tyrants, a charge that the AMA had invited by electing itself to personify and in effect regulate the profession—or in the view of naturopaths, to strangle competition.

A like-minded handful of heterodox thinkers attracted large followings after World War II: the German-born and naturopathically trained Gayelord Hauser promoting blackstrap molasses, wheat germ, brewers' yeast, and both fresh and powdered skim milk; Adelle Davis (strongly influenced by naturopathic theories) deploring nutrient robbery through misapplied heat while firmly endorsing raw whole milk; and Jerome Rodale (a teenage devotee of Macfadden) pointing to the dangers of large-scale mechanized farming with its heavy reliance on pesticides, herbicides, and the popular new synthetic nitrogen-based fertilizers. The anti-authoritarian zeal of these advocates would not only attract members of the 1960s protest movement but go on resonating with veterans of the movement when their death-or-glory dreams slumped into futility after the 1968 presidential campaign. A sizable post-hippie backlash against mass-produced food and factory farming proved to have lasting energy. It helped to fuel a renaissance of farmer's markets—and also to plant the seeds of a new consumer base for raw milk, which had spent many decades in obscurity.

Raw milk partly shared in a cultural sea change during which some tokens of the original hippie ethos—beards, yoga, marriage-free sex— merged into middle-class respectability. It could look like an inter- esting, mildly transgressive novelty to people whose prior image of a lactating organism had been the family refrigerator. At the same time, ex-communards who had learned to milk their own cows, long-experi- enced farmers weary of wrestling with the federal milk marketing orders, and city slickers inspired by the growing cachet of the terms "artisanal" or "farm-to-table" all began to glimpse attractive possibilities in small independent dairy operations.

In hindsight, it is clear that milk battles as fierce as those of the Straus- Coit era were not far off.

The political showdowns of the 1960s had instilled into old New Left loyalists a permanent knee-jerk mistrust of the "Establishment," an ill-defined but lethal cabal of Orwellian power-wielders. It was second nature to them not merely to suspect but to *presuppose* bad faith and bad motives on the part of people in authority. Among their more durable gifts to future generations was a fondness for conspiracy theories involving greedy, cunning manipulations by corporate and governmental interests. Not long before, naturopaths with a similar mindset had been given to vitriolic invective against orthodox medical procedures. (In 1925 Bernarr Macfadden's tabloid newspaper *The Graphic* had greeted the news that the sitting president had gotten vaccinated during a smallpox outbreak with the headline "IS REPORT OF COOLIDGE'S VACCINATION PUBLICITY STUNT OF PUS TRUST?"[6]) Equally hostile assumptions were now being assimilated into the late twentieth-century Zeitgeist. Simultaneously, governmental health authorities were now declaring flat- out war on raw milk as a public health menace. If they expected to stamp out any vestiges of opposition, they were seriously deluded.

The Food and Drug Administration had first tried to ban interstate shipments of all unpasteurized milk meant for retail consumption in a 1973 revision of the U.S. Public Health Service Pasteurized Milk Ordinance. The small remnants of the certification program had managed to stay the order by requesting an exemption for certified raw milk. The Department of Health and Human Services—the parent agency overseeing the FDA—let the question ride for more than ten years. But in 1984 Ralph Nader's consumer advocacy group Public Citizen, with FDA backing, brought an action against HHS Secretary Margaret Heckler asking that the department be required to lift the stay and reinstate the ban. The federal district judge who heard the case did not go so far as to grant Public Citizen's demand for a new ban on intrastate raw milk sales, but she did direct HHS to restore the interstate shipment ban. The department complied in 1987.[7]

The effect was more symbolic than substantive since, as Heckler argued, only a small percentage of retail milk sales involved raw milk transported across state lines. (Exact figures about this percentage don't and never did exist; raw milk sales can easily go unreported, and a great deal of raw milk consumption takes place privately among families on dairy farms.) But the new ban signaled a more aggressive attack on parties trying to elude pasteurization requirements.

Public Citizen and the FDA cannot have asked themselves whether the zero-tolerance policy they were trying to enforce might be a gift to the other side. The hippie revolution as such was over, but it had helped to legitimize political pushbacks against official medical and public health positions. Nobody foresaw that the 1990s would usher in the most shattering transformation of information technology since the invention of the printing press, or that one result would be the online dissemination of endlessly fragmented factoids, theories, dogmas, heresies, conjectures, and balderdash competing for attention with scientists' unromantic attempts to validate hypotheses before handing them over to the town crier. The big comeback of the raw milk controversy dates from this turbulent decade. Its reappearance was part of the fallout from the war on heart disease mentioned in chapter 9.

AFFAIRS OF THE HEART

In their haste to address what Ancel Keys had declared to be a public health emergency of cholesterol-clogged arteries, the American Heart Association and the nation's major news media spent decades papering over widespread dissent among researchers investigating the causes of cardiovascular disease. The issue that finally exposed cracks in the official façade was the desirability or undesirability of hydrogenated shortenings, welcomed by the AHA and its allies as potent cholesterol-fighters. Only two scientists had bothered to do serious firsthand research on the physical effects of their component partially hydrogenated fatty acids. They were the biochemist Fred Kummerow at the University of Illinois and Mary S. Enig, a nutritional chemist at the University of Maryland.

To explain the importance of the partial-hydrogenation question it will be necessary to summarize a few facts about the chemistry of dietary fats. All are chiefly made up of "triglycerides," intricately constructed molecules that consist of three fatty acid molecules attached to a molecule of glycerol (one of the organic compounds called "alcohols") like three pennants on a flagpole. Each fatty acid has a chain or "backbone" of carbon atoms, and each carbon atom along the backbone is also attached to two hydrogen atoms. Fatty acids come in a fantastic range of possible lengths and configurations.

A major variable in the structure of fatty acids is their degree of "saturation." One or more of the carbon-and-hydrogen threesomes on the chain may be missing one hydrogen atom. In that case, the straight backbone makes a swerve or kink where only a single hydrogen atom is attached, and the single carbon-to-carbon bond at that point is replaced by a double bond. If the molecule has none of these junctures that leave it without its full possible complement of hydrogen atoms, it is said to be "saturated." If it has one, it is "monounsaturated"; if two or more, it is "polyunsaturated." Fats—broadly speaking, meaning triglyceride mixtures—with large percentages of fully saturated fatty acids are usually solid at ordinary room temperature and melt only when exposed to heat.

The more polyunsaturates in the mix, the lower the temperature at which the fat will melt. Any fat that remains liquid at room temperature is called an "oil."

The rapid promotion of Keys's theory that highly saturated solid animal-derived fats should be swapped as soon as possible for oils rich in monounsaturates and polyunsaturates was a boon for edible-oils manufacturers. The campaign against saturated fats also gave a huge boost to a handy technological fix already known to makers of shortenings and vegetarian margarines: "partial hydrogenation," which involved forcing oil to absorb extra hydrogen atoms under high pressure at high temperatures, in the presence of nickel as a catalyst. In effect, it artificially (though incompletely) saturated a polyunsaturated oil, allowing it to become solid at room temperature. Procter & Gamble's Crisco had been made by this process since 1911. Other players in the edible-oils industry now flocked to partial hydrogenation as a blessedly artery-sparing alternative to butter and lard.

The unforeseen pitfall was that in the hydrogenation process, polyunsaturated fatty acids acquired a peculiar structure otherwise seldom seen in nature. The preceding flat two-dimensional description of a carbon chain doesn't take into account its arrangement in three-dimensional space. In naturally unsaturated fatty acids, any hydrogen "singletons" lie along one side of the carbon backbone of the molecule. In partially hydrogenated fatty acids, their position is shifted to the other side. These two configurations are distinguished by the Latin prefixes *cis* (on the near side) and *trans* (on the far side). Enig believed that the *trans* fatty acids now becoming prominent in American diets profoundly disrupted normal cell metabolism.[8] Kummerow, who had found them in the artery walls of test subjects, had gotten a mild caveat about them included in a dietary-guidelines statement that the AHA was about to release in 1968. To his lasting anger, it was deleted under pressure from an industry group, the Institute for Shortening and Edible Oils.[9]

The first prominently published report that *trans* fatty acids might be harmful didn't appear until 1990. A small Dutch study in the *New England Journal of Medicine* found that they not only raised the dangerous LDL (low-density lipoprotein) portion of blood cholesterol but lowered the amount of desirable HDL (high-density lipoprotein).[10] In a significant break with their earlier fidelity to the Keysian position, major news organizations began calling attention to a scientific finding that contradicted it.

As further studies confirmed the bad news, media coverage of the entire cholesterol thesis became more probing and less deferential. Medical luminaries who had recently been in the driver's seat found their credibility badly damaged. Public opinion swung from ill-informed belief in the earlier teaching to not much better-informed skepticism.

There was worse to come by the turn of the century. Earlier warnings about a heart disease epidemic, whether real or suppositious, were suddenly overshadowed by masses of statistical data that revealed an all-too-real health menace. The percentage of Americans diagnosed as clinically obese had started rising in the late 1970s and continued to soar ever since, with especially worrying data on childhood obesity. The prevalence of type 2 diabetes had followed the same track.[11]

AHA allies could no longer sustain the fiction of a united medical front on all issues related to diet and heart disease. A growing chorus of observers claimed that epidemiological data suggested a direct relationship between dietary elements tailor-made to match expert recommendations several decades earlier—lowfat and low-cholesterol substitutes, new products rich in *trans* fatty acids, products re-engineered to derive fewer calories from fat and more from carbohydrates including sugar— and increases in obesity and diabetes.[12]

Fred Kummerow, who had expressed his doubts about *trans* fatty acids in the "Supplemental Views" to the 1977 McGovern Committee report *Dietary Goals for the United States*, found himself vindicated. A widespread rehabilitation of onetime voices in the wilderness eventually occurred. But it did not include Mary Enig, who had been relegated to pariah status and obliged to self-publish most of her findings on *trans* fats. She remained a marginalized figure, perhaps because of a combative personality that had propelled her into fiercely berating representatives of the majority view at scientific conferences. The journalist Nina Teicholz, who later interviewed witnesses to such scenes while working on her book *The Big Fat Surprise* (2014), recorded firsthand impressions like "paranoid" and "off-the-wall."[13]

But approximately when early rifts were appearing in the official anti-fat united front, Enig formed a friendship that would make her known at least in certain circles. Her new acquaintance was Sally Fallon, the woman who would transform the raw milk movement for the next generation.

THE KEY ADVOCATE

Fallon was born Sally Caroline Wetzel in Santa Monica, California, in 1948. She had arrived in Washington, DC, in the early 1990s when her then husband, John Baptist Fallon, decided to leave a Wetzel family aerospace engineering business and set up as an independent aerospace consultant.

Some years earlier Sally Fallon had come upon a book by Weston A. Price (1870–1948) titled *Nutrition and Physical Degeneration*. Price was a dentist who during the 1930s had visited many societies in remote parts of the world seeking evidence to support his belief that modern Western diets were a mass of nutritional mistakes responsible for endemic dental problems and many other physical disorders. So-called "primitive" diets, he had argued, had everything to teach people harmed by much-vaunted progress.[14] His theories made immediate sense to Fallon, the mother of four children whom she wanted to bring up by sound nutritional principles.

Like the naturopaths, Price had singled out refined white sugar and flour as disastrous elements of modern civilization. He also commented approvingly on the use of animal fats, liver and other organ meats, and both fish and fish roe to supply crucial nutrients in preindustrial societies. (He ignored India, Japan, China, and other countries with vegetarian traditions.)

Fascinated by Price's account of his world travels seeking to document a relationship between the superb physical condition that he reported observing in the peoples of various preindustrial societies and the foods they ate, Fallon began planning a book of her own. It was to be both a cookbook and a teaching tool, with recipes and nutritional information fused in a grand synthesis of arguments against the misguided, deceptive dietary advice being handed down by modern pseudo-authorities. The most damnable of their falsehoods, in Fallon's view, was the claim that meats and animal fats were nutritionally undesirable. She saw them as vital, irreplaceable elements—especially when eaten raw or only lightly cooked—of healthful diets modeled on those of unspoiled societies like the ones Price had visited. Raw milk wasn't originally the chief focus of her attention, though it is now the issue she is most closely identified with.

Enig became part of the enterprise after Fallon read an article that she had contributed to a small magazine and recognized a kindred spirit. Fallon, who had no scientific background, promptly hired Enig to tutor her in the fundamentals of food chemistry. They soon were filled with a sense of common mission, well reflected in a jointly signed fire-breathing letter, meant to rebut a previous reader's letter, that appeared on the editorial page of the *New York Times* in March 1994. It began, "The vegetarianism-will-save-the-world monster has raised its mendacious head in 'Help Your Heart and Your Planet' (letter, Feb. 19) . . . Analysis of studies linking heart disease to meat consumption shows serious flaws in their data bases and underlying assumptions."[15]

The letter foreshadows the preoccupations of the book that would be issued in 1995 by a small California publisher as *Nourishing Traditions: The Cookbook that Challenges Politically Correct Nutrition and the Diet Dictocrats*.[16] Fallon shortly made the work a stepping-stone to a new calling as teacher and activist in the large, amorphous motivational and self-healing field. She left her marriage and founded a publishing company of her own called "New Trends" that she used to issue a revised and enlarged edition of *Nourishing Traditions* in 1999. She also started an organization meant to be a clearinghouse for information on the dietary convictions that she was advocating: the Weston A. Price Foundation, WAPF to followers. Her new husband, Geoffrey Morell, was a founding member. He is a New Zealand-born, Washington-based naturopath whose website identifies him as a specialist "in the field commonly called magnetic, intuitive, spiritual or psychic healing."[17]

Under the WAPF aegis Sally Fallon Morell began a quarterly journal, *Wise Traditions*, as well as an enterprise called the Campaign for Real Milk—meaning raw milk. Price himself was deeply interested in the influence of seasonal pasturage on vitamin content in milk, but didn't directly address the benefits of rawness. Fallon Morell, however, was convinced that WAPF's agenda, including raw milk, was seamlessly linked with his teachings.

Like many people in the story of modern milk, she was the right advocate arriving at the perfect moment to exert some pull on future events. She was a key advocate because she was a determined, single-minded person able to combine deep anti-Establishment beliefs with natural charisma and public relations savvy. The moment was perfect because her particular brand of savvy included a gift for *using online media* almost as soon as they appeared on the horizon. The raw milk cause was already positioned to return from relative obscurity to broader public recognition, but the change almost surely would have been less dramatic without the help of cyber-resources and somebody with wonderfully quick instincts for applying them.

But another reason for Fallon Morell's success in resurrecting this particular issue is the breadth of her attack on modern American food's progression toward a state of de facto tyranny. She was able to argue forcefully against mandatory pasteurization because she succeeded in portraying it as symptomatic of a larger evil, the medical-industrial-public-health complex's power to dictate what foods consumers could get their hands on. The range of possibilities had shrunk alarmingly and kept on shrinking, leaving people with artificially constricted dietary choices that in her opinion had had terrible consequences for the health of all citizens. What she thought was at stake was the right of Americans to choose foods they considered healthful. Her perceived mission was to focus attention on a goal that supporters variously characterized as "Food Rights" or "Food Freedom"—or "Take Back Your Health." *Nourishing Traditions* became and remains the chief guidebook of the movement.

The cover blurb claimed that the author "unites the wisdom of the ancients with the latest independent and accurate scientific research in over 700 delicious recipes that will please both exacting gourmets and busy parents."[18] Because of the way in which the recipes are tailored to match Fallon Morell's dietary convictions, it is misguided to judge them by the standards of "exacting gourmets," but they certainly are a lively collection in which it isn't hard to find flavorful and attractive dishes. As for the alleged "wisdom of the ancients" and "latest independent and accurate scientific research," they are deployed with more resourcefulness than care for facts.

After Fallon Morell's eye-opening encounter with the ideas of Weston Price, she had read everything she could find to corroborate his arguments and built up a large collection of books and articles by people who shared her thinking. She worked many passages from these writings into *Nourishing Traditions* by devising an ingenious two-column format for the recipe chapters. (These followed a lengthy introduction in which Fallon Morell stated her theories about the principal elements of diet.) Recipes occupied the inner (right-hand and left-hand) columns of each two-page spread, while the narrow outer (marginal) columns were filled with sidebars in smaller type that showcased nutritional claims on a huge range of subjects, as expounded by Fallon Morell herself or dozens of her trusted authorities.

Caveat lector—let the reader beware—is a prerequisite for approaching the enormous smorgasbord of assertions in the sidebars. All were meant to support or illuminate Fallon Morell's general world view. Her starting premise was that the diets and food traditions of preindustrial societies are treasuries of "intuitive wisdom" or "unerring native wisdom" whose benefits have been confirmed by trustworthy modern scientists, though blinkered "diet dictocrats" may pretend otherwise. These societies produced healthy children who grew up to be healthy adults, free of industrial-world deformities like crooked teeth or bad eyesight. The modern prevalence of both acute and chronic illness is directly due to the nutritionally impoverished, denatured impostors that now pass for food. The crisis calls for adopting an enlightened dietary agenda rich in animal fats, red meat and organ meats (particularly liver), eggs, whole milk, bone-based stocks, fish, whole grains, vegetables, fruits, and many fermented foods. Animal-derived products supposedly deliver their vital nutrients best when consumed raw, milk being the prime example; Fallon Morell also recommended trying to frequently incorporate some raw meats into the diet. She denounced many modern dietary traps including lowfat, low-cholesterol diets, nearly all soy-based products, highly processed vegetable oils, coffee, tea, and nutrient-deprived white flour and sugar.

Some of this belief system deserves consideration, and *Nourishing Traditions* is remarkable for its attention to issues that many consumers and home cooks hadn't thought about in 1995 or 1999. Fallon Morell was deeply concerned about the loss of genetic diversity in a food system dependent on a rapidly shrinking handful of major crops as well as commercially significant cultivars. She pointed to the ubiquity of toxic contaminants in the food supply as a direct threat to human health and the disappearance of pasturage for cows as a sign of how debased milk had become.

But the significant insights of *Nourishing Traditions* are hard to disentangle from an idiosyncratic personal mashup of ideas drawn from any source that confirmed Fallon Morell's views and attacks on any that called them in question.

Food is a subject disastrously suited to the politics of mistrust, an invitation to obsessive phobias. There is a slippery slope between thinking that highly processed products like white sugar, white flour, and pasteurized milk are nutritionally inferior to less technologically altered counterparts and proclaiming that without exception they must be foul poisons being peddled to the public by greedy, cunning manipulators bent on hiding the truth. From its subtitle on, the book radiated devotion to the second attitude. So did the raw milk movement as resurrected by Fallon Morell.

THE KEY OBSESSIONS

Where the all-too-real sins of major food industries and failings of prestigious dietary advisers are concerned, fiery accusations based on preconceived notions seem to have little difficulty replacing diligent reviews of evidence. Starting with *Nourishing Traditions*, Fallon Morell appeared to have her mind made up about three issues that now conspicuously preoccupy raw milk backers: dietary enzymes, the germ theory, and immunity to disease. All had been of great concern to twentieth-century naturopaths.

Enzymes had been a major reason for the naturopaths' opposition to cooked foods. Early vitamin researchers had quickly realized that most vitamins were "coenzymes," or collaborators with a large class of proteins called "enzymes" that were capable of cleaving complex molecules into segments and smaller building-blocks and that regulated virtually every chemical reaction in the body. Their vitamin partners were nonprotein compounds without which enzymes could not carry out reactions; the enzyme side of the alliance was destroyed at cooking temperatures.

At some point before 1930 Edward Howell, then a staff member at a naturopathic sanatorium in Illinois, had an epiphany triggered by the discovery that enzymes were denatured by heat.[19] It was the start of a long career dedicated to selling "N-Zime" capsules containing putatively live enzymes while inveighing against what he believed to be the worst error in the history of diet, the practice of cooking.

Naturopathic theory already held that heating food was an unwarrantable form of interference with its natural qualities. Howell claimed to have discovered the scientific basis of this in the action of enzymes. The crux of his argument was that unless a diet rich in raw foods keeps pouring the vital energy of enzymes into the body, the system will eventually use up its own finite "enzyme potential" and be ravaged by innumerable ills at an untimely age. He singled out the pancreas as the organ worst affected by eating cooked—meaning enzyme-depleted—foods, asserting that they force it to work overtime and prematurely exhaust its supply of enzymes.

These arguments are unrelated to anything that biochemists say about the role of enzymes in digestion, cell metabolism, or other physiological processes. They observe that far from having a finite supply, the body continually manufactures hundreds or thousands of enzymes under its own steam, without more needing to be shoved in to stoke the boiler. Most of the enzymes in food cannot tolerate strong acidity. They are knocked out by hydrochloric acid in the stomach, thus invalidating claims about the need for ingesting them in either raw foods or N-Zime capsules. The digestive system itself secretes the enzymes most crucial for metabolic purposes. For instance, alkaline phosphatase, which regulates calcium uptake, is produced in the small intestine.

Medical facts notwithstanding, the Howell version of enzymology has won many converts over the years, including Fallon Morell. In *Nourishing Traditions* she devoted a number of sidebars to claims from fellow believers like "This supply [of enzymes], like the energy supply in your flashlight battery, has to last a lifetime. The faster you use up your enzyme supply, the shorter your life."[20] Whatever that reasoning lacks in dependability, it can't be faulted for catchiness. And it continues to shape the case for raw milk as seen by advocates such as the physician William Campbell Douglass II, a longtime Fallon Morell ally whom she cited in the book as contending, "Phosphatase is essential for the absorption of calcium, but *the complete destruction of phosphatase is the aim of pasteurization!*"[21]

To straighten out this scrambled complaint: The particular time-temperature conditions at which the alkaline phosphatase in raw milk is inactivated are also those at which the major milk pathogens are inactivated. For this reason, checking milk for the absence of ALP is a convenient way of confirming adequate pasteurization. "Enzyme loss" nonetheless remains one of the most popular rallying cries of the movement.

More troubling to mainstream medical observers is a prominent streak of germ-theory denial that also has regularly surfaced among raw milk proponents since the publication of *Nourishing Traditions* and the founding of WAPF.

The first naturopathic opponents of allopathic (i.e., mainstream) medicine had reasoned that what allopaths called disease germs were not the cause but the result or byproduct of infectious illness. A body purposefully maintained in a state of health by pure and nourishing food, physical exercise, sunlight and fresh air, and freedom from contamination by coffee, tea, tobacco, alcohol, and of course drugs and vaccines was supposed to have the inner vitality to repel infections. Symptoms like fever, pain, or vomiting actually represented a healthy system's purposeful counterthrust to expel toxins that were accumulating in the blood.

In this theory Fallon Morell saw correlations with Weston Price's reports about the radiant health of peoples whose diets hadn't suffered the introduction of sugar, jam, white flour, and canned foods. There is no telling what Price—who had barely glanced at causal relationships between diet and infectious disease—would have made of her conclusions, which would help to line up a sizable bloc of WAPF in the anti-Pasteurian camp.

Pasteur during his lifetime was no stranger to quarrels with colleagues, nor was he always candid about the details of his experimental procedures.[22] After his death, anti-allopaths claimed to have discovered that he had both plagiarized and discredited Antoine Béchamp, a contemporary biochemist. By their accounts, Béchamp had shown that minuscule structures that he called "microzymas" were the true building blocks of living organisms, capable of metamorphosing into multiple forms within the system throughout all life processes rather than invading it from without like Pasteur's supposed microbes. Nobody else has ever demonstrated the existence of microzymas, but they are often invoked by WAPF supporters.[23]

In another favorite accusation, Pasteur was a jealous lifelong rival of the great physiologist Claude Bernard. Bernard is known for formulating the concept of a stable internal environment, the *milieu intérieur*, maintained by complex interactions among different mechanisms that keep variable conditions (for example, body temperature) within predetermined limits. Under the name of "homeostasis" this is now a universally accepted principle of physiology. But Pasteur thought it was of no importance. Opponents of the germ theory report, with no biographical evidence, that he acknowledged the error on his deathbed, confessing that Bernard had been right all along about germs being nothing and the *milieu* everything.[24] This suggestion is accepted as fact by various leaders of today's raw milk movement, including Fallon Morell. Her most recent book, cowritten with another anti-Pasteurian, casts doubt on the existence of viruses and posits that the great 2020 COVID-19 pandemic should have been recognized not as a virus-borne disease but as radiation poisoning from exposure to 5G frequencies.[25]

The WAPF-fueled raw milk movement also places great emphasis on the issue of immunity—and here it encounters a field of knowledge in a state of rapid and bewildering expansion. The number of medical conditions now thought to be rooted in autoimmune disorders is staggering, and grows daily. Immunology is becoming steadily more leagued with microbiology through accelerating advances in molecular genetics. At the same time, however, the subject is also becoming more entangled with popular misconceptions about "boosting" one's immune system. Immune systems unfortunately cannot be boosted like team spirit or octane content. But the fact that the countless interlocking mechanisms that make it up are not to be effortlessly re-tweaked by vitamin pills or miracle foods—including raw milk—doesn't deter millions of seekers from placing faith in such quick fixes.

Once again, the raw milk movement draws on ideas first developed by the founders of naturopathy, who had contended that keeping the body superbly conditioned by exercise, avoidance of pollutants, and proper diet repels disease as surely as neglecting these protective factors invites it. Taking the broad-spectrum preventive effects of raw milk as a given, WAPF adherents assert that it has the ability to ward off ailments common among people who drink pasteurized milk. Among such conditions, members of the movement frequently single out allergies.

Allergies are inflammatory responses to substances—allergens—that for incompletely understood reasons cause the immune system to mount an antibody charge against a perceived enemy. There is nearly complete medical agreement that allergic disorders, from rashes and hay fever to severe asthma and anaphylactic shock, have become radically more frequent in the last half-century, especially among young children. There is also a growing suspicion that at least one possible reason for the alarming surge in allergies is a lack of early childhood exposure to a large range of microorganisms in the everyday environment.

Raw milk partisans are certain that raw milk is the perfect preventive-cum-remedy for allergies in both children and adults, the immunity-booster par excellence. Their argument is that it is full of (in John Harvey Kellogg's phrase) "friendly germs" capable of destroying pathogenic enemies. The most obvious problem with the claim is that anti-pathogenic effects can't possibly kick in until the milk has gone sour. Another weakness of the allergy-fighting argument is that no single food can make up for a whole skein of now-missing environmental factors that millions of children used to encounter from infancy on. Buying raw milk from a farmer (much less a health food store) is scarcely a substitute for having been born on a farm and grown up in constant none-too-sanitized contact with farm animals, while habitually drinking raw milk dipped out of a farm bulk tank (as thousands of families living on small or mid-sized dairy farms cheerfully do today, with very few cases of milk-borne illness).

Nonetheless, further investigations into the effects of either pasteurized or raw drinking-milk on allergies and other immunological conditions seem to be well worth pursuing, especially in the light of the many discoveries now being made about the human gut microbiome.

The work of Ernst Moro and Henry Tissier in isolating particular colonic bacteria (chapter 6) provided some of the first hints that the lower digestive tracts of people and other mammals housed complex communities of microbes with profound influences on the health of their hosts. Microbiologists' ability to map the diverse makeup of these populations was advanced enough by about 1990 to have had some researchers talking about the "micro-ecology" or "microbial ecology" of animal intestinal tracts. The terms that started becoming standard about ten years later were "microbiome" for an ecological system of living organisms with their supporting environment and "microbiota" (generally supplanting the earlier "microflora") for all members of the total population.

The concept caught on with dazzling speed, aided by dramatically accumulating evidence for the thesis that in many ways, microorganisms have a better claim than people to be called the real rulers of the planet. And in many ways, their success rests on the ability of different microbial kinds to live in ever-shifting balances with each other—sometimes competitive, sometimes mutually stabilizing, always interactive.

In 2000 the word "microbiome" hadn't made it into the newest edition of the *American Heritage Dictionary of the English Language*. But by 2007 the National Institutes of Health were prepared to unveil a plan for the Human Microbiome Project, an ambitious attempt to map and inventory the microbial realms of the human mouth, skin, gut, vagina, and respiratory tract. The NIH microbiome effort stood on the shoulders of the earlier Human Genome Project, which had harnessed the breathtakingly new resources of gene sequencing and molecular biology to decode the strings of "letters"—i.e., the nucleotide bases adenine, cytosine, guanine, and thymine—that spelled out the complete genetic messages of the forty-six human chromosomes. The aim of the Human Microbiome Project—still unrealized—was to sequence the genetic makeup of all the microorganisms in all five microbiomes.

It was swiftly recognized that the general balance of organisms in microbiomes furnished new insights into healthy and disordered immune systems. Not surprisingly, the gut microbiome had a special fascination for students of food and nutrition. It obviously deserved to be studied in connection with another new magnet for headlines: a class of microorganisms that had been christened "probiotics."

The modern concept of "probiotics" started with animal nutrition. In the mid-1970s, when the reputation of antibiotics was about to come under a harsh second look, some researchers studying livestock rations had a hunch that feeding chickens and pigs certain live bacteria might make them put on weight faster and help confer resistance to infections. These enrichments of feed soon outgrew the experimental stage, and by 1989 they were common enough for the British microbiologist Roy Fuller to publish a brief historical survey.[26] It took about another decade for the idea to cross the species barrier and be suggested as an adjunct to human health. Probiotics were still too new to have received more than a quick mention in the 1999 *Nourishing Traditions*. But soon the claim "Contains Probiotics" had migrated from yogurt-carton labels to advertising copy for toothpaste, pet shampoo, lip gloss, baby wipes, and laundry detergent.

The popular appeal of probiotics is surpassed only by popular confusion about just what they are. If pressed on the question, most people probably would fall back on some mention of "good bacteria" that make you healthier. The World Health Organization definition isn't much clearer: "live microorganisms which when administered in adequate amounts confer health benefits on the host." In fact, regulators trying to impose some logic on the labeling of probiotic products in this country are still floundering amid their various claims as foods, drugs, nutritional supplements, or "personal products." When it comes to requirements for demonstrating some measurable health benefit from a precise amount of any one microbial kind, today's probiotic marketing is the Wild West.

In all fairness, working out an adequate definition for probiotics will be no easy task. But where products taken by mouth are concerned, applying the label to any organisms that fail to reach the gut microbiome in a viable state should be regarded as dubious advertising. Several Lactobacilli and Bifidobacteria (especially *L. acidophilus* and *B. longum*) certainly make the cut. Most lactic acid bacteria don't, because they cannot survive a blast of hydrochloric acid in the stomach followed by further seesawings of pH in the small intestine. Raw milk proponents unfortunately spend less time thinking about such distinctions than indiscriminately hailing probiotics as further reasons for shunning pasteurized milk as "dead," while insisting that raw milk is chockablock with live bacterial benefits. In reality, few truly probiotic microbes can be gotten into milk—raw or pasteurized—without carefully managed seeding from cultures of particular lab-grown strains.

The gut microbiome is not to be brought into better order by swallowing most products touted as "probiotics." "Prebiotics" are another matter. These are not live organisms but a family of specialized carbohydrates that cannot be digested in either the stomach or the small intestine. They arrive more or less intact in the colon, where fermentation by hordes of bacteria breaks them down into components that can be absorbed into the blood or excreted via the rectum. Their effects on the gut microbiome are more clearly demonstrable than those of most purported probiotics.

Most prebiotics are plant-derived and are generally classified as "fiber," either insoluble (like bran) or soluble (like the pectin from fruits that is used to set jams). But a sizable number occur in other sources, especially human milk. Chemically, most of these substances are "oligosaccharides" composed of several simple sugar units ("monosaccharides"). The units are linked together by tough, stubborn bonds that resist digestion by any substances the body secretes on its own in the intestinal tract. A few kinds of fiber are "polysaccharides," containing more than ten monosaccharide units. The monosaccharide building blocks may be glucose, galactose (the sugar that links with glucose to form lactose), or fructose (which links with glucose to form the sucrose familiar to us in table sugar).

Impenetrable as the names may seem, it is not difficult to grasp some of these peculiar saccharides' roles by recalling what happens to most of us on eating kidney beans, navy beans, or other members of the large *Phaseolus* botanical clan. Jerusalem artichokes and a few other foods often produce the same effect, which can be explained delicately as "breaking wind" or more plainly as "farting." When these otherwise indigestible substances arrive in the colon, they finally meet microbes capable of fermenting them until they release carbon dioxide, hydrogen, and methane—which unfortunately have only one means of escape. The bright side is that saccharide breakdown by fermentation frees up a rich source of food for the rest of the neighboring microorganisms, encouraging the development of a diverse but stable colon microbiome that can modulate some immune responses. That is also the role filled by the many oligosaccharides in breast milk. Several hundred are known, and together they assist the immunological seeding of the infant gut. By contrast, there is little evidence that any reportedly probiotic bacteria in raw cow's milk can plant permanent colonies in the gut. The case for prebiotic foods being able to affect the makeup of the colon microbiome is stronger. Bovine milk, raw or pasteurized, contains few oligosaccharides in comparison with human milk. But lactose itself behaves much like oligosaccharides (though with more distressing effects) in the digestive systems of adult humans who have lost the pre-weaning ability to produce lactase.

"FREEDOM MILK"

Whatever its merits on clear-cut and less clear-cut scientific issues, the raw milk cause gathered huge political momentum as Fallon Morell built WAPF into a dynamic shaper of opinion. One of the foundation's early moves was to create a subsidiary meant to draw voters' attention, the Farm to Consumer Legal Defense Fund (FCLDF). Spearheaded by the Florida attorney Pete Kennedy, the defense fund project renewed the calls for "medical freedom" and denunciations of "medical tyranny" previously sounded by champions of naturopathy and other unconventional therapies. But it proposed two further initiatives. One coordinated dozens of efforts to introduce bills legalizing raw milk sales in every state that currently prohibited them or loosening especially onerous restrictions in other states. The second teamed up dairy farmers with potential customers through a contractual device called a "herd-share" or "cow-share" agreement. The idea was to have farmers sell shares in either herds or individual cows to people who wanted the milk—making them part owners and sidestepping any law that forbade sales of raw milk per se.

These moves were well designed to cement the movement's sense of community by inviting raw milk aficionados into fellowships of citizen-activists as well as confidential, law-skirting relationships with farmers. FCLDF also gave the issue political visibility in state legislatures, allowing activists to hone lobbying skills and cultivate useful connections. What struck a chord with thousands of voters was not just the medical rationale presented by WAPF but its strategic appeal to Americans' historic belief in individual liberty. The freedom-to-consume plea now stands as a pillar of the movement. In 2012 a recent convert confided to the *New Yorker* reporter Dana Goodyear that when he drank raw milk from clandestine suppliers, "maybe it tastes better to me because it's freedom milk. It just has a little rebellious flavor in it. To me, it's the new civil rights. It's Rosa Parks."[27]

The American history of naturopathy and other schools of alternative medical thought abundantly proves that the association between unorthodox therapies and civil liberties is not new. But somehow the latest incarnation of the raw milk movement has captured freedom fighters' imaginations more strikingly than any other food-related cause I know of. It has turned believers into a corps of Tom Paines who treat raw-milk drinking as an inherent individual human right.

The rallying cry "Food Freedom" now seems to be the single biggest mobilizer of political opinion on behalf of raw milk. It sparks frequent petitions to legislators. The 1987 FDA ban on interstate transport of raw milk meant for human consumption became a focal point for protest. Starting in 2009, Representative Ron Paul of Texas repeatedly (and unsuccessfully) introduced a bill to overturn the ban with the declaration, "My office has heard from numerous people who would like to obtain unpasteurized milk. Many of these people have done their own research and come to the conclusion that unpasteurized milk is healthier than pasteurized milk. These Americans have the right to consume these products without having the Federal Government second-guess their judgment about what products best promote health . . . I urge my colleagues to join me in promoting consumers' rights, the original intent of the Constitution, and federalism by cosponsoring my legislation to allow the interstate shipment of unpasteurized milk and milk products for human consumption."[28] Paul left office in 2013, but his son Senator Rand Paul of Kentucky also supports the effort.

Raw milk advocacy unites strange political bedfellows. Since 2014 Representatives Thomas Massie (a Tea Party Republican from Kentucky) and Chellie Pingree (a progressive Democrat from Maine) have repeatedly introduced an "Interstate Milk Freedom Act" meant to bar any federal agency from interfering in sales of raw milk and milk products between any two states where they are legal.[29] More than a dozen Republican and a handful of Democratic House colleagues cosponsored the most recent attempt in 2021. No success can realistically be expected at the federal level in even the distant future. But as of 2022 the FCLDF listed twenty-eight states in which either retail-store or direct on-farm sales were legal, as well as seven others that countenanced cow-share arrangements.[30] The cause is well supported in states like Wyoming and Montana where "Tenthers," or adherents of a movement to curtail the powers of the federal government by invoking the Tenth Amendment to nullify federal laws that infringe on states' rights, have a strong political presence.

But while the cause gained political traction in the name of liberty, epidemiologists and public health officials were finding more reasons than ever to push back against the fiction that raw milk was some sort of panacea. The Price Foundation and the legal defense fund seemed uninterested in how swiftly and frighteningly the terms of milk-borne pathogenic threats were changing.

THE BACTERIOLOGICAL SHAKEUP

By the time of the postwar campaigns for statewide pasteurization laws, federal and state public health officials confidently assumed that modern medicine had gained the upper hand over most food-borne contagions. They could not have been more mistaken.

Already in the interwar period, microbiologists had found two previously unidentified zoonoses that invaded cows' reproductive organs and udders and could be transmitted in milk: brucellosis and Q fever. The discovery that the latter, spread through a tick-borne organism named *Coxiella burnetii*, could resist usual pasteurization temperatures more successfully than any other pathogen led to hiking the recommended temperature for batch-pasteurizing from 140°F/60°C to 145°F/63°C. Signs of far more alarming developments began to appear during and after the 1970s.

A few puzzling "emergent" or "emerging" organisms, meaning ones that had never appeared before or that had suddenly found a foothold in new geographical areas, were unexpectedly being reported in the American food supply.[31] One early arrival, *Listeria monocytogenes*, has been introduced in chapter 9. Its stubborn resistance to refrigeration and other measures that would inhibit most microbes, and its knack for taking hold in inaccessible corners of food-processing lines, were dismaying to food safety experts. It rarely causes huge outbreaks in the same manner as water-borne diseases like typhoid fever or cholera, but has a frightening tendency to target pregnant women and their fetuses.

Another new—or newly emergent—organism was *Campylobacter jejuni*, which caused acute and prolonged gastroenteritis sometimes followed by other symptoms such as blood infections and arthritic pain. It had not been seriously studied until the late 1970s, when detective work by several microbiologists unexpectedly exposed it as an enormously widespread pathogen responsible for many cases of food poisoning. Like listeriosis, *C. jejuni* infections had been enabled to run rampant by factory-farm methods of raising livestock—in this case, poultry. The crowded quarters into which chickens are jammed in many operations are ideal for breeding epizootics.

By comparison, raw milk is involved in relatively few *C. jejuni* cases. But of course, the amount of raw milk consumed in the United States is minuscule compared to the amount of pasteurized milk, a fact that pasteurization opponents often fail to consider when arguing that raw milk poses little or no microbial threat. No reliable statistics exist on the total amount of unpasteurized milk that finds its way to American consumers (a situation not helped by its semi-clandestine status in many states and the maneuvers employed to skirt legal prohibitions). It must be a tiny percentage of the 226 billion pounds produced in the United States in 2021. That does not mean that raw milk should be dismissed as a *C. jejuni* transmitter.

Still more alarming pathogens were being discovered in the U.S. food supply. Many were classified among the large, prolific *Salmonella enterica* subspecies, which seemed to be generating some new serotype (immuno-logically distinct variation) every year, including one that was specifically adapted to cattle, *S. Dublin*. Others belonged to the tribe of microbes that Theodor Escherich began investigating in the 1880s. Most members of the vast *Escherichia coli* group are harmless, and some are actively useful. A few, however, have been found to secrete a bacterial toxin that the Japanese researcher Kiyoshi Shiga had identified decades earlier as the cause of acute dysentery symptoms produced by an unrelated organism. They are now named, in his honor, "Shiga toxin-producing *E. coli*" (STEC), and are among the most virulent forms of *E. coli*.

In the 1980s, one particular variant, *E. coli* O157:H7, was identified as the pathogen responsible for several outbreaks of illness, but it was not until 1993 that a huge number of cases traced to hamburgers from the Jack in the Box fast-food franchise sparked a national uproar.[32] Four children died when the pathogen spread to their bloodstreams and triggered a massive systemic collapse known as "hemolytic uremic syndrome" that virtually destroyed their kidneys and damaged other organs. Nearly 200 more people had to be hospitalized; the pathogen was specifically identified as the cause of 732 illnesses (though in such cases it is usually suspected that many more may not have been reported).

A young Seattle attorney named William Marler took on the case of a ten-year-old girl who had barely survived the long, ghastly ravages of *E. coli* O157:H7, and eventually won a settlement of more than $15 million.[33] It was the start of a notable career representing plaintiffs in cases involving food-borne illness. His reputation as a tough advocate to have in one's camp brought the Marler-Clark firm to the attention of another STEC victim's mother. This time the suspected food was raw milk.

Mary McGonigle-Martin, a Californian with a strong belief in health foods, had had good firsthand experiences with raw milk in her twenties. (California then had some of the least restrictive policies of any state on raw milk sales.) Some years later she came across glowing testimonials to its benefits for children and decided to start her seven-year-old son Chris on it. For several weeks the experiment seemed to go well. But in September 2006, Chris became appallingly ill and spent months in hospital hovering between life and death. The state health and agriculture departments quickly launched an investigation and quarantined the milk of Organic Pastures Dairy Company in Fresno, the farm that had supplied the milk.[34]

Chris Martin survived and has been able to carry on a mostly normal life, but with severe and permanent organ damage. In 2008 McGonigle-Martin and her husband, Tony Martin, brought suit against the store where she had bought the milk and Mark McAfee, the owner of Organic Pastures. The case became a stormily debated *cause célèbre* for raw milk opponents and proponents.

Clusters of symptoms in raw milk cases tended to be more scattered and the trains of evidence less clear-cut than in the Jack in the Box outbreak. Bill Marler, partnered with a California firm, again managed an out-of-court settlement. But there were complicating issues in Chris Martin's illness that left room for doubt, and not only in the minds of McAfee and pro-raw activists. For one thing, raw spinach contaminated with *E. coli* O157:H7 had just been proved to have been the source of a large California outbreak, and the little boy had indeed eaten raw spinach a few days before he got sick. For another, doctors were never able to conclusively find O157:H7 itself in his system. And the state investigation had failed to turn up positive bacterial evidence on McAfee's farm. Chris had, however, undeniably developed the hemolytic uremic syndrome that represented the most acute peril in other catastrophic O157:H7 cases.

Mary McGonigle-Martin and Bill Marler remained firmly convinced that raw milk from Organic Pastures farm had nearly cost her son's life through *E. coli* O157:H7. She became an indefatigable campaigner against legalization of raw milk in other states. In 2009 he started an online newsletter, "Food Safety News," that tracked issues related to food-borne illness. Among many other activities, the Marler-Clark firm also launched a blog named "Food Poison Journal" and the website real-rawmilkfacts.com, clearly meant as a foil to WAPF's realmilk.com. Bill Marler and other representatives of the firm often participated in legal challenges to the cow-share and herd-share stratagems that were gaining popularity among the opposition.

The battle lines were already shaping up when, almost at the same moment that Sally Fallon Morell and WAPF were pumping new life into the raw milk cause, defenders of pasteurization acquired a formidable ally. Hostilities speedily ratcheted up by several notches.

THE CZAR

John Sheehan arrived at the FDA in 2000 with the mission of overseeing food safety, including milk safety. He had come to Washington by way of Cork, Ireland (he had a degree in dairy science from University

College Cork), and Denver, where he had worked for a dozen years as a quality-control manager at Leprino Foods, a privately held company. His title, which has undergone a few tweaks over the years, is Director of the Division of Dairy, Egg, and Meat Safety in the FDA's Center for Food Safety and Applied Nutrition.

Three facts about Leprino are well known in dairy-manufacturing circles: it is the world's largest maker and supplier of mozzarella cheese, chiefly "pizza cheese"; it sells nothing under retail labels of its own; and it is obsessively secretive about its own affairs and those of the Leprino family. When in 2017 a reporter for *Forbes* managed to obtain an interview with CEO James Leprino, the event garnered notice as a once-in-a-lifetime breakthrough.[35] This background perhaps is a key to the extraordinarily guarded profile that John Sheehan maintains in dealing with the media, his preferred forms of communication being cut-and-dried official bulletins and on occasion prepared testimony.

His qualifications for running a crucial division of a major federal health agency are not clear. Reporters seeking to interview him about raw milk rarely get further than a recapitulation of the FDA's official position, which he has been presenting to state legislatures as written testimony—he is seldom known to testify in person—for at least fifteen years.[36] The gist is that raw milk, whether certified or uncertified, is unfit for human consumption. Or as he famously told a writer for the now-defunct *FDA Consumer Magazine* in 2004, drinking raw milk is "like playing Russian roulette with your health."[37] Frustratingly from that point of view, the FDA has no authority to stop anybody from buying or selling raw milk in states where the gamble is legal. But it can and does enforce the 1987 USPHS Pasteurized Milk Ordinance prohibition on transporting raw milk across state lines for purposes of human consumption. In 2008 Sheehan announced a renewed crackdown on the practice.[38] And his exhortations no doubt strengthened a number of states—Ohio, Oregon, and Illinois, among others—in mounting their own crackdowns on raw milk farmers.

The FDA now treats unpasteurized milk as a substance so dangerous as never to be tolerated in the tiniest amount under any circumstances. (In 2006 a *Washington Post* reporter was moved to think of comparisons with marijuana or heroin.[39]) The agency's policy is endorsed by the American Public Health Association, state health departments and public health associations, the American Academy of Pediatrics, the American Medical Association, the National Environmental Health Association, and many other groups of health professionals. Sheehan's allies in combating attempts to legalize intrastate raw milk sales also include the National Milk Producers Federation, Dairy Farmers of America, and the International Dairy Foods Association.

In short, mainstream health-care authorities and the dairy industry present a seamless united front against raw milk. The trouble with governmental-industrial united fronts is that in a society where rugged individualism is glorified, this kind of unanimity can inspire as much defiance as compliance. Sheehan's success in eliciting firm declarations of opposition to raw milk from a spectrum of prominent allies has not only turned him into a convenient bogeyman for members of the rebel faction but strengthened their commitment to the Food Freedom argument.

The food-rights issue had strongly appealed to David E. Gumpert, a veteran business reporter with an interest in health-and-nutrition questions. Finding common cause with Fallon Morell and WAPF, he soon became one of the most persuasive legal apologists for the movement. He commands more respect than most of his allies among outside observers for his coverage of the raw milk story on the blog "The Complete Patient" and in several books, most notably *The Raw Milk Revolution* (2009).[40] His journalistic training gives him a care in sorting out facts and a skill in evaluating points of view that set him apart from many of the raw milk zealots.

Gumpert began detailing the stories of many face-offs between raw milk farm-dairy owners and law enforcement officers. In various cases, police or sheriff's deputies had conducted lengthy sting operations reminiscent of attempts to nab drug lords, ransacked premises under cover of search warrants, confiscated or dumped milk and other dairy products, and subjected people to browbeating interrogations. These maneuvers were often conducted with a presumption of guilt that might have been expected from a Spanish auto-da-fé. Though local rather than federal, they couldn't have been better chosen to evoke the specter of medical czardom, with Sheehan as Ivan the Terrible.

Gumpert, who made a point of talking to people with both pro and con opinions and conscientiously strove to be fair-minded, could scarcely mention Sheehan's name without being roused to snarling invective. What rankled him most was that Sheehan declined to communicate in any fashion with any representative of the raw milk cause. He repeatedly turned down (through underlings) or ignored Gumpert's requests for interviews as if they had come from the Flat Earth Society.

Authoritarian crackdowns and dismissive rebuffs are precisely the right way to whip up small waves of dissent into cascades of activism. They are also a great breeder of cultish loyalties. Sheehan seems never to have doubted that simply repeating his case against raw milk and ignoring its advocates would make the problem go away. The real result has been a dangerous and rapidly widening communications gap, intensified rather than lessened by much of the accompanying media coverage.

Neither Sheehan nor Fallon Morell is willing to concede that any shred of a defensible idea could possibly attach to the other's cause. Meanwhile, each party acts as if bent on justifying the other's worst accusations. The crucial question ought to be how to prevent milk-borne illness in an era of emergent pathogens like *L. monocytogenes* and *E. coli* O157:H7. Instead, the public health disciplinarians behave as if no menace needs to be more relentlessly hounded out of existence than the pro-raws, who respond by clinging all the more fiercely to a litany of fanatical beliefs.

Journalists who report on the issue generally fall into the trap of presenting a "contest" between sides as if the possible outcomes were little different from "Yes" or "No" on a referendum vote or the Patriots' or Steelers' chances in the playoffs. It's a trap because the questions involved can't rightly be reduced to simple either-ors. What's really called for is an effort to thoughtfully evaluate the failings and strengths of the warring parties without taking anybody's claims at face value.

The worst liability of WAPF and the fiercest raw milk partisans is their contempt for scientific theses or explanations that run counter to their dogma. They have precipitated the matter so far into the realm of alternative facts as to convince most of the medical community that Sheehan's stance is the only rational one—the more so since for all practical purposes WAPF has commandeered the right to speak for anybody who wants access to raw milk. No other lobbying group independently argues for the cause. The most obvious analogy is the National Rifle Association, which by obscuring the fact that not every American gun owner has the same agenda puts many members in the position of having to explain that they are not Wayne LaPierre clones.

But if addiction to scrambled science is the pro-raws' great weakness, they should be applauded for an urgently needed contribution: they have almost single-handedly brought the bloated absurdities of the mainstream drinking-milk business to public attention. They have denounced the toll that prevailing strategies for wringing the largest possible amounts of milk from cows take on animal health and the environment. They have shown that milk can be something other than a flavorless, featureless white fluid that travels from supermarket dairy case to family refrigerator with no thought on the consumer's part about where it originated.

The signal virtue of the pro-pasteurizers is their insistence that milk-borne pathogens are real, not (as some WAPF ideologues maintain) imaginary. Sheehan and his FDA division have rightly refused to let ignorant prattle about raw milk having the ability to kill pathogens or pasteurized milk being a sinister conspiracy pass uncontested. But they aren't necessarily advancing the ultimate goal of food safety any more effectively than the raw milk apostles. Though they spend less time spinning pseudoscientific fantasies, they are remarkably obtuse about how attempts to control people's behavior can go wrong. They don't acknowledge that they are faced with a genuine grassroots protest movement that, in the usual manner of protest movements, questions aspects of the social order and springs from a sense that some institution has betrayed people's trust. Draconian crackdowns are the most foolish possible response to the reborn raw milk cause.

It should also be mentioned that though it has more substantial arguments on its side than the opposition, the pro-pasteurization public health apparatus is capable of sloppy and alarmist hype. The most egregious examples are a series of CDC reports, much cited by independent journalists, that have linked increasing consumption of unpasteurized dairy products with increasing outbreaks of illness caused by *Salmonella* and *Campylobacter* variants, STEC (e.g., *E. coli* O157:H7 and other Shiga toxin-producing organisms), and *Listeria monocytogenes*. A 2017 report estimated that if all U.S. milk and cheese were pasteurized, averages of 732 illnesses and 21 hospitalizations a year would be prevented. It predicted that illnesses and hospitalizations would increase in direct proportion to any increase in consumption of unpasteurized milk and cheese. Consumers of these products, the authors warned, "are 838.8 times more likely to experience an illness and 45.1 times more likely to be hospitalized" than consumers of pasteurized dairy products. "Unpasteurized products are consumed by a small percentage of the US dairy consumers but cause 95 percent of illnesses," they asserted. Thus, "outbreak-related illnesses will increase steadily as unpasteurized dairy consumption grows, likely driven largely by salmonellosis and campylobacteriosis."[41]

Figures like these may look like precise numerical proof of how dangerous raw milk is. But they don't necessarily prove what they claim to prove. The weakness of many cautionary pronouncements circulated by public health authorities is that they lump together all unpasteurized milk and cheese with no further investigation of circumstances. The authors of the 2017 report were statisticians, not epidemiologists or microbiologists. Details about individual cases were not relevant to their argument. But an epidemiologist trying to draw inferences would have needed to ask specific questions: Did a victim thoughtlessly drive into the countryside and find a farmer willing to illegally sell raw milk on the sly, or did the milk come from a farm with a state license program regulating raw milk sales? Did the cheese come from a trained cheesemaker or an ignoramus who had managed to get hold of some raw milk? What was the health status of the farmer's herd, and what was the bacteriological condition of the farm bulk tank? What curd-setting method had been used for the cheese? Journalists on the health-and-nutrition beat are remiss if they don't dig below the surface of claims coming from either raw milk devotees or public health authorities.

WHAT IS ADEQUATE TESTING?

Only the most fanatical Food Freedom extremists would try to maintain that raw milk production and sales don't require some degree of supervision by state (and perhaps county and municipal) public health departments. What supporters and adversaries disagree about is how to evaluate reasonable proof of safety. Those who oppose compulsory pasteurization argue that where official risk assessment is concerned, no other food has been judged by as forbiddingly absolute a standard as raw milk. By their lights, singling out raw milk for harsher restrictions than other pathogen-spreading foods shows arbitrary and systematic prejudice. They find ammunition in events like a 2006 California *E. coli* O157:H7 outbreak ultimately traced to raw spinach and responsible for 205 illnesses and three deaths, according to CDC records. This was the episode during which Mary McGonigle-Martin's young son Chris Martin and a handful of other children who had consumed raw milk contracted O157:H7. Inspectors from the California departments of health and agriculture had at once descended on the source of the milk, Mark McAfee's Organic Pastures farm, with guilty-until-proved-innocent alacrity. Organic Pastures was never conclusively proved to be the source of these cases, but from the McGonigle-Martin party's not irrational point of view, absence of proof is not proof of absence.

Since coming to the FDA, John Sheehan has stuck to the position that though very clean raw milk may contain next to no pathogens, testing can never irrefutably prove that it is 100 percent pathogen-free. He is correct. The point at issue is whether that is a reasonable benchmark.

The crux of the matter is that testing standards and methods originally devised in another age of microbiological visualizing were based on assumptions that may or may not be in need of revision. The default means of estimating bacterial populations for more than a century has been the standard plate count. It relies on culturing bacteria on plates of agar or some other growth medium and diluting a sample through progressive culturing stages until the initially astronomical numbers of colony-forming units (CFUs) are low enough to be clearly viewed on a microscope and counted with some degree of confidence. Standard plate counts were always known to be useful guides rather than

super-accurate analyses. They allow lab technicians to make rough estimates of how long milk being sampled has been held since milking,
and how favorable or unfavorable to overall bacterial growth its handling on the farm or at the processing plant has been—in other words,
how relatively clean it is. In one variation of the plate count test, counts
of coliform bacteria, meaning members of the diverse *E. coli* clan and
some similarly shaped relatives, are used as a relatively quick and simple marker for gauging the milk's prior exposure to fecal bacteria. Most
states that permit raw milk sales require standard plate counts, coliform
counts, and several other tests with stipulated maximum limits.

The principle on which earlier microbiologists relied was that whole
populations of microorganisms exist in competitive balances with each
other; when any one kind falls to extremely small numbers in proportion to its major rivals, it has for all practical purposes been crowded
out of the bacteriological picture. The object of sanitary stipulations for
handling milk was not to destroy every last remnant of all the major
pathogens but to reduce them to negligible totals confirmed through
standard tests. Maximum permissible bacterial counts were the foundation of Henry Leber Coit's certification program for raw milk.

But to Sheehan they are inadequate safeguards. Is it or is it not reasonable to set more rigorous standards in a time of newly emerging
bacterial threats? More precise methods for measuring microbial populations are at hand. Gene sequencing, for instance, eliminates uncer-
tainties about questions like whether milk contains *L. monocytogenes*
or some harmless member of the *Listeria* genus, a difficulty that sorely
taxed detection methods a couple of decades ago. Flow cytometry
allows observers to establish—not estimate—the total number of cells
in a sample; a version called BactoScan™ is already coming into commercial use.[42] Almost certainly there will be pressure in future to apply
several sensitive new tests to raw milk before approving it for sale. If so,
there will also be arguments in state legislatures about where tests are
done and who bears the expense.

It is not certain, however, that raw milk should now be held hostage
to Sheehan's distrust of usual test results. In this case, he has exposed
himself to the charge of being as ideologically driven and intolerant as
his opponents. His Russian roulette analogy is scarcely more defensible

than their hymns to raw milk as a miracle cure. Setting aside the fact that with very clean milk the chances of dangerous illness are smaller by many orders of magnitude than those you get by spinning a six-shooter, the special antipathy with which he has singled out raw milk for regulatory annihilation is conspicuous enough to do more harm than good to the pro-pasteurization cause.

COMMANDMENTS OR CONVERSATIONS?

Pro-pasteurizers who are really interested in milk safety need to do some serious rethinking of the current situation. They must recognize that Fallon Morell's swipe at "dictocrats" justifiably touched a nerve with a certain segment of the eating public. Through the Campaign for Real Milk and the realmilk.com website, she helped to fashion people of like interests into that unprecedented twenty-first-century institution, a cyber-community devoted to sharing information, or what the participants consider information. Real Milk believers and other Food Freedom advocates eagerly exchanged personal stories, tips on sources of milk or other prized foods, and galvanizing reports on medical bigotry and governmental abuses of power. Again and again, they expressed their frustration with a status quo in which the mere act of deciding what foods to take into one's body for the sake of health was not recognized as legitimate.

The targets of their resentment were not interested in listening to them, only in being listened to. Spokespeople for the public health bureaucracy and the mainstream medical profession were simply unprepared to deal with Internet-spurred citizen activism. They could scarcely understand that large numbers of laypeople might develop their own perceptions of health issues in defiance of what accredited experts were telling them. In fact, august members of the public health sector and the medical profession had trouble grasping that the enormous prestige they'd come to take for granted hadn't always been theirs by divine right. They were unequipped to confront sudden and dramatic shifts in popular views like those now being expedited by websites and blogs.

Their communication skills have been understandably slanted toward handing down wisdom from on high rather than trying to exchange ideas through person-to-person discussion. These attitudes must change— not because preventing milk-borne illness shouldn't be a top priority but precisely because it *should* be. Harsh zero-tolerance enforcement of raw milk prohibitions is an ideal recipe for encouraging connoisseurs of "freedom milk's" forbidden charms to take pride in breaking the law.

For health professionals to sit down and chat about medical issues with nonprofessionals as if scientific qualifications didn't matter surely would be an abdication of their mission. But they must start considering how to prevent channels of communication from getting hopelessly blocked. This is just what Sheehan's FDA division and most, if not all, state public health agencies have declined to do on the issue of raw milk. It's another form of abdication, considering the fact that millions of Americans now embrace medical pluralism—that is, incorporate aspects of nontraditional, non-Western medicine into their general beliefs—or go further by challenging some fundamental principles of modern medical science. Little if anything in the usual professional curricula fits future doctors or public health personnel for what now needs to be a crucial part of the job: studying ongoing pop nutrition and health vogues and trying to understand their underlying rationale at least enough to carry on civil—though if necessary, probing—conversations with people who espouse them. It's a facet of professional education that deserves the highest priority in curriculum redesign if health providers are to regain the trust of an increasingly suspicious and defiant public.

The growth of the food rights movement is a measure of how badly out of touch with the current climate the supposed guardians of health have become. Or to put it another way, how little hope many citizens entertain that accredited physicians and government functionaries can understand their concerns.

In the last few years, the most recognizable symbol of the gulf between the medical establishment and disaffected citizens has been the anti-vaccination movement, which in the last few years has formed strong links with a far-right wing of the Republican Party exploiting the confused COVID-19 scenario. The raw milk and Food Freedom movements so far are not affiliated with one political party but represent a spectrum of far-left, far-right, and middle-of-the-road protesters drawn together by the conviction that the government has no business putting anyone's health-based food choices off-limits. It would be prudent to forestall these causes from being taken over by people with more inflammatory political agendas.

The Food Freedom movement has undeniable appeal to many. Americans instinctively tend to support, or at least feel uncomfortable about legally restricting, the freedom for citizens to do whatever they say they have a right to do. An unfortunate result has been to cheapen the concept of civil rights by indiscriminately laying claim to them, while making a shambles of political discourse. A flagrant example is Ron Paul's reasoning about removing barriers to the interstate flow of raw milk for direct retail sale. It assumes that nothing should stop people who "have done their own research and come to the conclusion that unpasteurized milk is healthier than pasteurized milk" from getting all they want.

One need not be an enemy to civil liberties to be apprehensive about that approach. The factual slagheaps created by laypeople "doing their own research" in real or suppositious medical science were egregious in Bernarr Macfadden's lifetime and must now be admitted by even the most ardent civil libertarian to be an anarchist's paradise. It has proved impossible to set generally agreed-on limits to free choice even about something as clearly subject to abuse as commercially hawked nutrition supplements. (Senator William Proxmire, an impassioned fan of vitamin pills, permanently forestalled the FDA from regulating them as drugs through an amendment tacked on to a health bill in 1976.[43]) Supposing that raw milk were proved tomorrow to be as miraculous as self-appointed spokespeople like Fallon Morell say it is, many in the raw milk community would still concede that a few ballpark rules ought to be agreed on. The issue desperately calls for good-faith discussions between pro-raws and pro-pasteurizers who are not blinded by dogmatism.

11

THE FUTURE

Earning a living from milk was complex and demanding when U.S. farmers first were talked into expecting drinking-milk to become the most lucrative possible dairy product. It became still more difficult throughout the twentieth century, with many disappointments along the supposed road to riches.

The programs of dairy science that were founded for dairy farmers' guidance at agricultural colleges addressed the need for serious, detailed instruction in matters ranging from ruminant metabolism and crop management to bacteriological safety and bovine obstetrics. Decade by decade, agricultural school teaching became more exclusively focused on telling students how to operate in the commercial drinking-milk market while facing constantly mounting fiscal worries and technological demands.

Meanwhile, dairy science professors' assumptions about the average size of a farm kept being revised upward. Faith in economies of scale as a survival mechanism became a conditioned reflex, while operations that once would have been considered large—say, 300 cows—came to seem small and the very smallest farms were dismissed as negligible elements. But the picture is changing today, at least to the extent that small farmers can make their voices heard more clearly than in the recent past. Current developments in dairy farming call into question some former certainties.

With few or no exceptions, farms that produce raw milk for retail sale have built-in limitations on size. It goes almost without saying that they require more painstaking attention per cow and per unit of milk harvested than mega-dairies. Of course, raw milk dairyists operate independently of the Federal Milk Marketing Order system and the punishing encumbrances of the commodity milk market. But it is noteworthy that some people now are pursuing similar goals on small farms devoted to producing and selling *pasteurized* milk outside the market order system. In fact, one of the signal contributions of the raw milk renaissance is the example that pioneering farm-dairy operations based on raw milk have set for other hopeful new dairy farmers who want to avoid the marketing-order straitjacket without incurring the special demands of raw milk.

These two groups ought to have something to say to each other as fellow-rebels against the mentality of gigantism that has overtaken the milk business. It may be that small-scale dairy farming can help establish some common ground between pro-raws and pro-pasteurizers. Nobody understands better than these innovators what dairy farmers have suffered through long years of government policies that cheer on obliteration of the smaller by the bigger in the name of advantageous economic streamlining.

BEHIND THE GRIM STATISTICS

"Get Big or Get Out," the truculent slogan of Secretary of Agriculture Earl Butz in the early 1970s, glorifies a view that was making a mark on the U.S. agricultural economy well before Butz took office. That attitude spurred damn-the-torpedoes pursuit of short-term profits by encouraging single-minded concentration on intensive planting of soybeans and corn to the exclusion of lesser crops. It encouraged the rush toward consolidation that was already driving dairy farmers out of business. And it was echoed as recently as 2019 by another secretary of agriculture, Sonny Perdue, who told reporters covering the World Dairy Expo in Madison, Wisconsin, "In America, the big get bigger and the small go out."[1]

The big certainly have gotten bigger and the small have gone out. In 1940 the U.S. Census of Agriculture reported 4,663,413 U.S. farms with milk cows. The numbers steadily decreased every decade thereafter, with especially jolting declines between 1964 (1,133,912) and 1969 (568,237).[2] In 2003 (when the National Agricultural Statistics Service had assumed the record-keeping job) there were 70,375 dairy herds. By February 2020, there were 31,657, and the U.S. dairy cow population was approximately 9.3 million.[3]

The human toll behind the statistics of "the small go out" is incalculable. It is no exaggeration to say that farming is among the most physically and mentally grueling occupations in America, and that dairy farming places especially relentless burdens on people who are still trying to hold on to small or mid-sized operations. Almost day by day, the obstacles to making a living by selling milk in a buyer's-market framework become more forbidding. One all-too-usual escape route is simply giving up and selling off the herd, often followed by selling off the land. Another is much darker.

In 2018 the investigative journalist Debbie Weingarten wrote that on average, "it costs a farmer approximately $22 to produce a hundred-weight, or one hundred pounds, of milk. But the market price for milk is significantly less. While the price of milk constantly fluctuates, farmers are currently paid as low as $15 per hundredweight—30 percent less than the cost of production." She also reported that a little earlier Agri-Mark, a major New England dairy cooperative—for at least a century, co-ops have failed to reliably provide higher incomes for small and mid-sized dairy farmers than the big commercial processor-distributors—had sent participating farmers in the Upper Connecticut Valley region of Vermont and New Hampshire a link to suicide prevention hotlines along with its most recent checks.[4]

Farmers who haven't chosen to expand ad infinitum pride themselves on a dogged self-reliance that carries them through tough times—but not the kind of tough times that they now face. The bad news fluctuates a little from year to year, but never takes a prolonged turn for the better. Growing waves of rural despair, with dairy farmers among the worst sufferers, attracted fitful media attention in the 1990s. By degrees, agricultural authorities in once-prosperous farm states hit hard by upheavals in the U.S. farming landscape realized that they had mental health crises on their hands—worsened since 2020 by the COVID-19 pandemic. Efforts to help farmers cope with depression and fiscal panic now include Pennsylvania's AgriStress helpline, Wisconsin's Farmer Wellness program, New York's NY FarmNet website, and the Minnesota Farm and Rural Helpline. Some bills with similar aims, as well as riders to annual farm bills, have been introduced in Congress.

Some of these initiatives acknowledge that small farmers shouldn't be left to "go out" like doused matches in an American agricultural economy embodying the Sonny Perdue mentality. Small farmers have a good deal of popular sympathy—if not focused political clout—on their side. What's becoming increasingly obvious is that where dairying is concerned, they may be able to turn their lives around by declaring independence from the mainstream milk-marketing system.

The raw milk movement helped show the way by resurrecting direct farmer-to-consumer sales. A dairy farmer in business for herself or himself is likely to know every cow in the herd by name and also to know most customers by name. In contrast to economies of scale, such intimacies of scale restore something that millions of people sense they have lost: a direct producer-consumer relationship.

Retail sales of milk with no intermediaries are worth reviving for the sake of both parties. The farmer can charge prices commensurate with actual production costs. The purchaser knows who is accountable for the quality and safety of the product, whereas assigning responsibility can be hard when anything goes wrong with batches of pasteurized milk from big processors. Though the exponential growth of the twentieth-century industry certainly allowed millions of people to buy milk with some confidence in its safety and forever abolished the atrocity of the city swill-milk trade, it also projected a smaller cluster of potential risks onto an immensely larger screen.

TURNING THE TABLES?

Producing raw milk for retail sale in states where it is legal requires a different sort of focus than producing raw milk destined for quick shipment off the farm into the tortuous mazes of the commodity milk market. The independent producer necessarily bears a heavier weight of individual responsibility, most easily shouldered with a small herd yielding small volumes of milk. By awakening an interest in single-source milk from working farms, the raw milk movement already has accomplished a great deal. But it also has pointed the path to other business opportunities—not necessarily involving raw milk per se—that offer farmers an escape from the constraints of the mainstream drinking-milk industry. American-made cheese was one of the first alternatives to the commodity milk market to display bright commercial prospects after several generations of neglect. In fact, its fortunes had started to rebound before raw milk re-emerged as a cause. Shortly afterward, butter also enjoyed a certain resurgence.

Thousands of U.S. businesses had deserted cheese and butter production during the late nineteenth-century expansion of the drinking-milk industry. Cheese was especially hard-hit, with both national production and per capita consumption suffering drastic slumps. As noted in chapter 7, a 1916 release from the National Dairy Council described cheese as being "practically unknown and wholly misunderstood." It was scarcely better off in 1950, when per capita consumption was 7.7 pounds a year. The 2020 figure—40.2 pounds—demonstrates how sharply attitudes have changed, starting roughly between 1975 and 1980 and never turning back.[5] By the mid-1990s supermarkets were carrying an amazingly expanded range of both imported and domestic factory-made specialty cheeses. At the same time, domestic artisanal cheesemakers had won followings in more elite circles—and their interests dovetailed perfectly with the interests of dairy farmers wondering if raw milk might enable them to operate in a seller's rather than a buyer's market.

Farmstead cheese operations using raw rather than pasteurized milk from the farmer's own cows, goats, or sheep, as well as artisanal cheese operations using raw milk supplied by a farmer or farmers, sprang up in all states. The number of such cheesemakers probably stood at around 1,000 at the start of 2020 (it is not known how many were forced out of business by the disruptions of the pandemic).[6] Though raw milk is essential for achieving the highest quality in certain cheeses, some boutique cheesemakers achieved at least fairly good results with others using pasteurized milk from small farms. In both cases, the end product involved small volumes of milk carefully and knowledgeably handled.

Meanwhile, butter made its own more modest comeback from the doghouse to which Ancel Keys's anti-cholesterol campaign had temporarily banished it. A 1982 article on current trends put annual per capita consumption in the United States at 18.6 pounds in 1909, 4.5 pounds in 1978. A reversal—undoubtedly spurred by concerns about *trans* fatty acids in margarines—set in at around the mid-1990s, and the 2020 figure for butter was 6.3 pounds.[7] As with cheese, many small-scale startups have appeared, presenting an undervalued article in a new light and displaying artisanal American-made butter with special sales claims (e.g., Jersey cow's cream, Vermont pastures, bacterial culturing) as more than equal to imported rivals. And there have been still more beneficiaries of the discovery that the mainstream drinking-milk market doesn't have to be the only game in town. Yogurt, ice cream, crème fraîche, cultured buttermilk—the opportunities for boutique-scale entrepreneurs catering to local clienteles are steadily expanding.

Newly emboldened refugees from the mainstream drinking-milk enterprise, and novices hoping to make a living as independent dairy farmers or processors, are no longer rarities. They are a diverse lot united by knowing that *the special quality of their milk will directly register in everything they produce,* instead of being drowned in a vast flood of milk from thousands of farms. These small businesspeople have managed to turn the tables on one of the major shapers of the twentieth-century dairy industry: differential price classifications.

The idea that particular criteria should dictate a hierarchy of farm prices for milk was as old as the rivalry between raw milk certified by Henry Leber Coit's standards and milk pasteurized to Nathan Straus's specifications. The latter, initially viewed with suspicion by many medical authorities, was for some years relegated to second rank in schemes of superior and inferior milk "grades" or "classes." As medical authorities gradually decided that the pasteurized article was far safer for babies, the regulations drafted by the U.S. Public Health Service as a model that states might implement introduced a more complex set of classifications based on maximum permissible bacterial counts in milk meant for different uses. Drinking-milk was at the top of the ladder; milk meant for various manufacturing purposes was assigned to lower rungs. A little later, the big dealer-processors who were assuming control of the dairy industry adopted similar criteria to set wholesale prices for the milk they bought from farmers. Milk destined for retail sale as drinking-milk commanded the highest prices; milk meant to be turned into cheese, butter, and other non-fluid or non-full-lactose products was judged by lower bacteriological standards and priced accordingly.

The crucial inference here was that milk meant to be consumed in unfermented fluid form, primarily though not only by babies and children, should be superior in quality to all others and that the farmer should earn more from it. Likewise, prices for milk directed to other manufacturing purposes should reflect its second-best (or still lower) status.

Over the years the classes of manufacturing milk have been subjected to various shuffles in the Federal Milk Marketing Order system. Today Class I is still fluid milk and cream. Class II includes ice cream, yogurt, and cottage cheese; Class III includes most ripened cheeses as well as cream cheese. Butter now shares Class IV with powdered dried milk. If these groupings don't seem entirely logical, they aren't. The lack of logic begins with the fact that the supposedly privileged Class I drinking-milk is often if not always a terrible money-loser for small and mid-sized farms.

The comeback of the raw milk cause, with the defections from the bloated commodity milk market that it helped to inspire, has inverted the original standards of the milk classification scheme for dairy farmers who produce milk and other dairy products for retail sale independently of the system. They are now free not only to produce milk *better* than the featureless Class I stuff that reaches millions of home refrigerators but to charge what they think reasonable for it as drinking-milk, cheese, yogurt, or butter instead of settling for Class III or Class IV status. "Better" milk, in this case, means milk that contains more milkfat, protein, and solids nonfat (see chapter 9)—in other words, milk richer in everything that milk ought to have other than water.

Small-scale producers conducting their own farmstead operations can make choices that would be pointless or counterproductive within the marketing-order framework. So can those who elect to sell their output to artisanal producers.

THE NEED FOR INSTRUCTION

Unfortunately, these hopeful trailblazers may not always know exactly what they're doing. Eager converts to the raw milk cause may brush off well-founded safety warnings as unnecessary. People looking to set up small farm dairies and pasteurize their own milk may have difficulty finding anything matched to their interests in agricultural school curricula or cooperative extension programs. The problem is that for several generations, few capable instructors have had occasion to address the interests of students thinking of careers outside the commodity milk system. Those interests are assuming some urgency as well-meaning but sometimes ignorant people jump on the raw milk bandwagon.

The raw milk movement itself produced the first real attempt in more than a century to address the question, "How can raw milk be safely produced and sold?" It came from Mark McAfee, the founder of Organic Pastures in Fresno, California.

Organic Pastures (now renamed RAW FARM) is actually enormous for a raw milk operation (more than 1,200 cows), and has had occasional run-ins with state health authorities for high bacterial counts and other problems. It was at the heart of the 2006 controversy about the illness that young Chris Martin suffered after drinking raw milk from Organic Pastures (though also after consuming contaminated spinach known to have sickened other people; see chapter 10). McAfee is one of the most hard-line exponents of WAPF's teachings about the phenomenal healing powers of raw milk. But he also keenly appreciates the special responsibilities that go with producing and selling it.

In 2011 McAfee announced the founding of the Raw Milk Institute (RAWMI), an organization meant to systematically educate people in what it takes to run a clean, safe raw milk farm dairy with pasture-fed cows.[8] As he explained, nobody should confuse merely unpasteurized milk with raw milk that is clean and good-tasting. The latter depends on intelligent handling of land, animals, and an extraordinarily perishable substance. Responsible raw milk dairyists must thoroughly understand standards of rigorous sanitation, as well as the technological means to maintain them without letup from the instant the milk is drawn until it is tested for bacterial content and filled into bottles or jugs for prompt sealing.

RAWMI and its rawmilkinstitute.net website began producing literature and instructional videos meant to guide would-be farmers through the process of setting up a risk assessment and management program (RAMP) and scrupulously carrying it out, "from grass to glass." McAfee has drafted a set of common standards for raw milk producers to familiarize themselves with and observe.[9] He also envisioned being able to publish a list of certified farmers who had successfully completed the training course and brought their herds and processing facilities into compliance with RAWMI requirements. In the event, many farmers enrolled in the program but only a small number (about 250 as of early 2022) sought to join the list.

The RAWMI training course nonetheless continues to be useful. When it was devised, the dramatic growth of the raw milk movement was suggesting to both ex-mainstream farmers and a new crop of complete novices that raw milk dairying could be a promising career. RAWMI and the common standards were meant to address a glaring need for solid, methodical instruction in a demanding occupation—and to demonstrate that raw milk producers were serious about their responsibilities.

A prominent opponent took notice. The food-safety law firm Marler Clark (which had had various quarrels with McAfee, starting with the

Chris Martin case) published a substantial article on RAWMI in its online newsletter "Food Safety News." It was not the hatchet job one might have expected. The writer, Cookson Beecher, predictably left the last word to "the risk isn't worth it" warnings. But her tone toward McAfee and the new institute was thoughtful and not without respect. The RAWMI goal, she wrote, was "to use science-based food-safety principles to shore up a strong foundation for the growing raw-milk movement." For his part, McAfee candidly acknowledged his worries about torch-carriers for food freedom who scorned attempts to agree on needed safety principles. "It's usurping the cause if you're only thinking about your freedom," he told Beecher. "Freedom and food safety are connected. I'm free as long as I produce safe milk." At present, consumers visiting a farm may take "some pretty roses planted near the house" and a freshly painted barn for assurance that "things are being done right . . . We want them to be able to see their farmers from an expert's perspective." He pointed out that the jumble of different state regulations and the unlicensed and/or illegal raw milk underground subvert food safety practices. Conceding that zero-risk guarantees are unattainable, he argued that nonetheless "things can be managed in ways to significantly reduce the risk."[10]

RAWMI's proposed certification program changed the mind of no pro-pasteurization spokesperson contacted by Beecher. But to see a leader of the raw milk movement trying to cross party lines and educate people about difficult realities—while being listened to with respect—was a welcome surprise to at least a few. Here was a level-headed conversation between representatives of very different views about raw milk, taking note of variable factors and presenting an alternative to accusatory and counter-accusatory absolutes about raw milk safety.

This is exactly the sort of interchange that has been missing from the pasteurization wars. It brings raw milk out from the lawless fringes that are encouraged rather than discouraged by Sheehan-style ukases. If the raw milk cause is to do more good than harm it must operate in the open, with public demonstrations of good faith such as the RAWMI instruction program.

It is time for agricultural school curricula to address more diverse needs than they once did, including help in devising business plans for students who want to bypass the marketing-order system and conduct small, specialized operations using pasteurized milk. And in states where raw milk sales are legal, I see no reason that agricultural schools cannot take a leaf from the RAWMI book and discuss how to make raw milk operations as safe (and profitable) as possible. A future where raw milk is driven underground is at risk for more, not less, milk-borne disease. A future where well-instructed farmers can conduct raw milk dairying in the open will be far saner.

Sanity will also be served if dairy farmers who have chosen to go the raw milk route, counterparts who sell pasteurized milk, and others who sell milk to artisanal producers can work together to take advantage of their common standing as privately held small businesses. They might publicize themselves as comparable to, say, independent pharmacies that have held out against competition from giants like Walgreens and Rite Aid. An association of farm dairies could be useful in building customer base, perhaps by devising a logo certifying members' products as proudly independent of the marketing-order system and hence free to surpass its uninspiring standards.

There are many reasons to hope for a brighter future in sectors of the dairy industry where small farmers and other producers can make a mark. But it would be unrealistic to think that these encouraging developments presage a more enlightened future for the mainstream drinking-milk business.

DOMESTIC OVERSUPPLY AND LESSENING DEMAND: THE SEARCH FOR SOLUTIONS

Nothing is going to dislodge supermarket drinking-milk from its towering economic importance. It is certain to continue along the track of expansion, consolidation, and increasingly complex technological infrastructure that it has pursued for almost three quarters of a century.

Big Milk is going to become Bigger Milk. Its absurdities are also sure to become more entrenched. The greatest of these is the plain fact that Americans are drinking less milk while dairy farms are producing more of it.

The trends are far from new. Contrary to popular impressions, the decline in milk-drinking hasn't resulted from recent developments like the rise of plant-based substitutes for cow's milk. U.S. per capita annual consumption of fluid milk and cream peaked at 399 pounds in 1945 and has been declining ever since.[11] In 1975—well before a market for soy milk, almond milk, and the rest had emerged—it was 247 pounds. In 2019 it was 141 pounds.[12] The comparable figures for total U.S. milk production are approximately 122.2 billion pounds in 1945 (the result of a final war effort), 115.4 billion pounds in 1975, and 226 billion pounds in 2021.[13] In fact, most years since 1980 have seen increases in total production.

Increased production and declining consumption of anything would be cause for alarm in any enterprise less bizarrely structured than the U.S. dairy industry with its jerry-built system of prices and price supports, the latter carried out as government purchases. This perilous convergence of circumstances doesn't seem to faze the major processor-distributors or the USDA's Agricultural Marketing Service. But it is the key to several underreported embarrassments that are unlikely to go away any time soon. One of these is the mindset of nutritional policy-setters.

A 2021 report from the USDA's Economic Research Service treats the decline in milk-drinking as a serious health problem in the making and tries to pinpoint possible generational factors that might help account for it. It begins by pointing to the apparently increasing speed of the downturn and announcing, "About 90 percent of the U.S. population does not consume enough dairy products to meet Federal dietary requirements, and declining per capita consumption of fluid cow's milk prevents these individuals from consuming a diet more line in [sic] with those recommendations."[14]

Perhaps a more useful way of stating the issue would be "Not enough Americans drink enough milk to absorb the always-increasing industry output." And perhaps future ERS experts will ask which more urgently needs reexamining, the federal dietary requirements or consumers' waning enthusiasm for the milk channeled to them by the drinking-milk industry. As discussed in chapter 7, the idea of some minimum consumption target for milk got started during or just before World War I, when nutritional authorities were in a state of impassioned excitement over the very latest vitamin and mineral discoveries. The target amounts were never more than quasi-scientific guesses. How is it possible today to deplore some presumed dietary dereliction *shared by 90 percent of the population* without documenting the actual incidence of any ailments that it might be supposed to cause?

I am not suggesting that the authors of the report meant to surreptitiously recommend reducing the milk surplus by inspiring people to drink more. But their preconceptions about "enough" milk-drinking are scarcely appropriate at a moment when advisers on diet should be questioning whether existing federal guidelines adequately address the needs of nonwhite demographics or take into account the realities of the U.S. dairy industry.

As things now stand, chronic overproduction of milk is the single most serious problem of the industry and seems likely to remain so indefinitely. From time to time the situation stirs up awkward publicity and ineffectual would-be fixes. As president, Ronald Reagan inherited the fallout from some especially egregious surpluses that had built up in the late 1970s and impelled the Commodity Credit Corporation, in its role as stabilizer of agricultural prices (chapter 7), to buy up millions of pounds of unwanted milk that had been hastily turned into cheese and left to molder in government warehouses. The ensuing scandal inspired the Reagan administration to create the Dairy Termination Program, a plan by which dairy farmers would be paid to liquidate their herds and stay out of the milk business for at least five years. Unfortunately, any resulting cuts in the milk supply were offset by increased production by farmers who chose not to accept the buyout.[15]

The unique supply-and-demand problems of milk mean that an extraordinary amount of wastefulness is built into the system. Its combination of bulkiness and perishability sets it apart from all other major foods and severely restricts farmers' ability to make informed decisions—as opposed to guesswork—about maintaining a desired level of production. Almost as soon as milk travels from the cows into the bulk tank, the producer has to be assured that it will be pumped from the tank and delivered to the processor-distributor with as little loss of time as possible, to make room for the next tankful. The great size and unwieldiness of the marketing-order system, and the fact that cows cannot be turned on and off like machines, limit any farmer's flexibility. If one company decides to stop buying his or her milk or cut back on the amount it buys, it is horribly difficult to make other arrangements without a hitch. Selling off some cows to limit the damage may prove to be a mistake if demand goes up in a few months.

Because of this lack of leeway, the only short-term solution when demand goes down is to dump milk and—though compensatory arrangements exist in some cases—absorb the loss. The 2020 pandemic triggered a huge increase in the volume of milk dumped by dairy farmers because regular customers of the processor-distributors such as schools and restaurants were obliged to shut down and cancel their orders for long periods of time.[16]

EXPORTS AS SAFETY VALVE

But individual farmers' losses aren't seen as disastrous by industry policy-setters. They have found a more profitable, efficient answer to the national oversupply problem than hasty cheesemaking efforts and the Dairy Termination Program. The new safety valve is exports.

Needless to say, milk in its original form is not ideally exportable. But twentieth-century U.S. dairy industry researchers made great progress in abolishing the obvious disadvantages of the complete package and selling it as a large handful of more shelf-stable components. For instance, butter (though it can be exported as is) can be stored longer and under more variable conditions when it has been concentrated by removal of nearly all the residual buttermilk into the products called "butter oil" and "anhydrous butter." Both have more than 99 percent fat content instead of the 80 to 84 percent in most commercial butters. They have long been used in manufacturing some commercial versions of chocolate, ice cream, and shortbread. Cheese is also a perennial standby. A newer success story is whey, which for nearly a century has been one of the big stumbling blocks of the dairy industry.

People who have tried their hand at making a fresh cheese at home will understand the problem: whey is the aqueous (water-based) portion of milk, and cow's (as well as goat's) milk is usually more than 87 percent water. A gallon of milk—four quarts—turned into something like cottage cheese will leave you with an awkward disposal problem in the form of about three quarts of whey remaining after the curd separates and has been drained. If you decide to just throw it down the sink, you will be doing exactly what thousands of cheesemakers did for many decades, making whey into one of the most notorious industrial pollutants of waterways during the twentieth century.

Recently, however, the dairy industry has managed to convert the embarrassment into riches by evaporating the water from the whey and selling it in powdered form. In the United States, it has been marketed as a nutritional supplement (especially popular among bodybuilders and athletes, though facts are hard to distinguish from wishes). On both the domestic front and as an export, it is also nearly omnipresent in innumerable mass-produced foods—breads and other baked products, frozen desserts, coffee creamers, and various packaged sauces and dressings. Its uses go even further when "sweet" (nonfermented) and only lightly fermented whey are mined for the whey proteins as well as lactose, a valuable export in its own right when separated from the other whey components. In milk as it comes from an animal's mammary system, lactose is a crucial nutrient for newborns. If it hasn't been converted into lactic acid through fermentation, it can be recovered from whey and put to many uses, especially infant formulas (which must match the high lactose content of breast milk) and various commercial baked goods. As of 2019, the United States was the world's biggest exporter of whey.[17]

But the workhorse among today's dairy exports is powdered dried milk. This almost always has had the milkfat removed because without expensive precautions, the fat will go rancid in the heat of the usual dry-ing process. Today nonfat powdered dried milk finds its way around the world as a mainstay of U.S. food policy and global trade. An important precedent occurred during the postwar U.S. occupation of Japan, when millions of pounds of nonfat dry milk were cheaply sold to Japan as part of the school lunch programs devised by Supreme Commander of the Allied Powers Douglas MacArthur's advisers. Reconstituted by mixing with water, it was consumed as drinking-milk by schoolchildren every-where.[18] Eventually the easily manufactured substance proved to be an excellent way of coping with recurrent domestic milk surpluses. Many countries are also players in today's international dry milk trade; New Zealand outdoes all others in its grasp on the market. But the United States is steadily increasing its share.

In 2021, despite many supply chain difficulties caused by the 2020 pandemic, the United States was one of the top global exporters of milk products in general. Its next-door neighbors, Mexico and Canada, respectively accounted for $1,791 million and $917 million in sales. But more surprisingly, Southeast Asia ranked second to Mexico ($1,398 mil-lion) and China fourth ($708 million)[19]

I have already mentioned the Chinese government's new belief in milk's ability to create taller citizens and national greatness, as well as its unrewarding attempts to squeeze lactose-free milk out of genet-ically altered cows. China now is one of the largest global producers as well as importers of milk. Meanwhile, the same credulous attitudes have also been successfully nurtured in other Far Eastern nations where the overwhelming majority of people stop secreting lactase—and hence digesting lactose without difficulty—by puberty. How they came to think that they needed to consume a food presenting them with obvious digestive problems is, regrettably, no mystery. Campaigns by influential Western health-and-nutrition authorities and dairy indus-try representatives have convinced them of the need—ironically, even as reasons for questioning drinking-milk's reputation as a nutritional necessity for the entire human race have received increasing attention in the United States.

LACTASE NONPERSISTENCE:
GENETICALLY DETERMINED CONDITION
OR SALES OPPORTUNITY?

It is now more than fifty-five years since the seminal Johns Hopkins experiment by Pedro Cuatrecasas, Dean H. Lockwood, and Jacques R. Caldwell plainly showed that adult cessation of lactase secretion was common among Black Americans. The response of dietary authorities poorly served the Afro-American community—or indeed, any nonwhite Americans. The medical profession and the drinking-milk industry, as respectively trusted arbiters of and contributors to scientifically approved diets, were highly disconcerted by the news. Instead of grappling with the racial and cultural implications of the lactase persistence question, both these powers responded to lactase nonpersistence as if it were a newly discovered ailment, or perhaps allergy, named "lactose intolerance." That misinterpretation has never gone away. Milk processors quickly concocted a slew of new commercial products, advertised as being able to spare lactose-intolerance "victims" the sad consequences of milk deprivation. Nothing could better illustrate the lasting effects of indoctrination in the belief that failure to drink milk is somehow abnormal.

Products meant to help the lactose-intolerant by dosing milk with lactase produced by yeasts or fungi had unfortunate limitations. The problem was that the minute the enzyme hit the milk, it split lactose into the component sugars glucose and galactose, both of which are much sweeter than lactose. Together they produced a strangely sweet taste that some consumers got used to and others found off-putting. In any case, milk subjected to the process was advertised as the latest remedy for the "disorder." The off-flavors have since been slightly lessened if not fully eliminated; Lactaid, the best-known of the commercial reduced-lactose solutions to the supposed problem, is now as familiar as regular milk on supermarket dairy product shelves. Packets of lactase-containing supplements in capsule or tablet form are favored by some consumers.

To draw a hypothetical comparison: Suppose first, that people from a certain part of the world had been almost universally left-handed for several millennia and second, that after some centuries of assuming that this was the only possible state of affairs, they found the majority of other humans to be almost universally right-handed. If they had reacted by deciding that right-handedness was a deficiency in need of educational and technological fixes, they would have been no stupider or more conceited than the American-trained experts who tackled adult lactase nonpersistence with eyes wide shut.

The same distorted assumptions, along with the pursuit of profit that they inspired, are now expanding into global markets in an attempt to convince lactase-nonpersistent people in the Far East that there is something wrong with them.

In 2019 a market manager for DSM, the Dutch-based multinational maker of many products with both legitimate and fanciful nutritional claims, issued an online publicity release headed "Why Lactose-Free Is Going to Be Massive in Asia." Why, indeed? The reason turned to be, "There are likely to be at least forty times more people suffering from lactose intolerance in an Asian country like Vietnam than in a north European country like Denmark."[20]

Nobody except a very few infants congenitally unable to digest breast milk has ever "suffered from lactose intolerance" in the sense that people can suffer from migraine headaches or celiac disease. The most important role of lactase is in making the rich nutritional resource of lactose available to nursing babies until their digestive systems are mature enough to handle other foods. After that milestone, most of the world's children stop secreting lactase and do fine on diets that include either no dairy products at all or forms like yogurt or cheese.

Persuading consumers that everyone ought to enjoy the remarkable medical advantages of milk-drinking certainly makes lactose-free drinking-milk more marketable to more people. It does not make those benefits more real. The DSM release's further assertion that "82 percent of consumers polled in China believe that lactose-free dairy is healthier than regular dairy" proves nothing except the ignorance and credulity of the consumers in question—qualities that the Chinese government often capitalizes on in other political contexts and that Westerners should refrain from using in sales pitches designed to make people "in an Asian country like Vietnam" buy dubious nostrums. Campaigns like DSM's attempt to realize a "massive" Asian market for its lactase treatment of milk verge on greedy exploitations of genetic differences between races.

CALCIUM, OSTEOPOROSIS, AND UNCERTAIN KNOWLEDGE

Any survey of milk's nutritional merits is bound to touch on calcium, recognized almost from the outset of the twentieth century as having a crucial role in bone formation. The idea that children need to drink cow's milk sprang directly from the discovery that it is the most plentiful natural source of calcium. Most of the mineral is found linked with protein in the intricate casein micelles, though some also occurs dissolved in whey. Calcium's reported bone-building properties soon spurred public health officials to worry about whether Americans were getting "enough milk." World War II triggered a far-reaching attempt to establish the proper amounts of all significant nutrients, the Recommended Dietary Allowances (RDAs). First published in 1943, the RDA listings had the aura of scientific precision that laypeople often associate with official-looking numbers on paper. But they also came to be the object of fierce tussles among parties with their own dogs in the fight—farm producers, manufacturers, anticorporate protesters, and devotees of particular medical theories.

Today the RDAs are part of a larger, more sophisticated dietary-data system maintained by the National Academy of Medicine, but still function as government standards of reference for minimum and maximum advisable intakes of individual nutrients. And as always, milk is unusually problematic when it comes to evaluating experts' dietary advice.

The original calcium recommendations were, like the protein recommendations, an outgrowth of early twentieth-century concerns about

American schoolchildren's height and weight. Both were painstakingly measured at intervals, in the fear that children would grow up stunted without adequate intake of calcium and other minerals, vitamins, and protein. Perhaps this concern had at least some validity in a white American context. But being rooted in some of the same unrecognized race-based misconceptions that had lent milk the reputation of a universal superfood, it is a dubious fit with other contexts. That has historically been true in this country when twentieth-century white experts mulled over strategies for getting Black families to improve their calcium intake by drinking more milk, while wondering about their odd preference for buttermilk. It is true today, when increased milk consumption is being urged on people in the Far East with eager publicity about benefits like calcium.

A 1995 study in the *Hong Kong Medical Journal* sounded a warning against easy extrapolations from Western models. The authors pointed out that calcium recommendations for a population should be "estimated according to the efficiency of absorption, which may differ among different ethnic groups, particularly with different levels of dietary calcium intake." In a randomized experiment, they had administered specific daily doses of a calcium supplement (some children got a higher and some a lower dose) and an identical-looking placebo to thirty-four seven-year-olds, some living in Hong Kong and some in Guangdong province on the mainland. The Hong Kong children had had considerable exposure to Western dietary elements like meat, soft drinks, and in some cases milk. The dietary mainstays of the mainland children had remained relatively unchanged from a longtime Chinese pattern of "green vegetables, soy bean products, cereals, seeds, nuts, shells, and bone."

After six months on the supplements and the placebo, the authors found that the mainland children were absorbing significantly more of the added calcium than the Hong Kong children. In both, absorption rates were higher when the actual dose of calcium was lower. These results, they commented, cast doubt on the validity of an existing Food and Agriculture Organization/ World Health Organization recommendation of daily calcium intake for children: "This estimate was based on studies in Caucasian populations," whose absorption rate was much lower than those shown for Chinese children in the study (and also, they pointed out, those reported in Sri Lanka and India). They suggested, "The long tradition of having a low calcium intake in the Chinese diet has possibly led to Chinese developing a higher calcium absorption rate."[21]

Further evidence of puzzling twists and turns in the calcium story comes from statistics about the incidence of osteoporosis in different populations. In this country, gynecologists regularly cite the danger of hip fractures associated with lost bone mass as a reason for women to drink a great deal of milk both before and after menopause in order to be sure that they're getting enough calcium to maintain bone density. The eminent American nutritionist D. M. Hegsted was one of the first observers to cast doubt on the idea. In a study published in the *Journal of Nutrition* in 1986, he speculated that higher calcium consumption might actually *increase* the risk of osteoporotic fractures.[22] The authors of the Hong Kong study took note of his argument, observing that osteoporosis "was not found to be more common in Chinese, but the reverse—only one-third were affected compared with their American counterparts who had a much higher habitual calcium intake."[23]

Data supporting the apparently counterintuitive argument gradually accumulated. In 2012, *Osteoporosis International* published a summary of epidemiological evidence from sixty-three countries, showing that by far the highest incidences of hip fractures occur in Denmark, Sweden, Austria, and Norway—places with long traditions of milk-drinking, where adult lactase persistence is the norm.[24] Broadly speaking, the problem is strikingly worse in industrially developed than developing nations. Ethnic and racial differences are marked. A Norwegian study found that people born in Norway have five times greater risk of hip fractures than Norwegian residents born in Central and Southeast Asia.[25] In the United States, whites have the highest and Blacks the lowest incidences of hip fractures.[26] (Black women who do suffer fractures tend to have poorer outcomes than white women, though this undoubtedly reflects more limited access to medical care.)

In short, the medical advice that American women are likely to receive about dealing with osteopenia (somewhat reduced bone density) or preventing actual osteoporosis is very far from ideal. It shows a troubling reluctance to acknowledge how many unknowns now exist about calcium intake versus calcium absorption, or to relinquish assumptions about milk automatically building strong bones that clearly need some adjustment. Neither calcium supplements nor several glasses of milk a day can guarantee protection against osteoporosis and hip fractures. Researchers are a long way from understanding the factors responsible for differences in comparative statistics. While we wait for answers to extremely vexed questions, we can hope to see health and nutrition journalists more candidly accept that vexed questions exist. It is frustrating to see the grip on opinion that medical claims based on limited early evidence continue to exert despite the emergence of more and more counter-evidence.

NEW DIRECTIONS FOR DAIRYING?

The growth of the modern Western drinking-milk industry was fueled by some unfortunate scientific misconceptions, many of which are still being perpetrated. At the same time, the industry's rise was closely coupled with real scientific advances. It is in the interest of clear-headedness to disentangle them from each other—for instance, to discard the idea of drinking-milk from cows as an indispensable cornerstone of any healthful diet that was drilled into American schoolchildren for most of the twentieth century. Today that view is being assailed on all sides.

There is, for example, increasing competition from half a dozen kinds of plant-based products being marketed as milk. These strike me as being chiefly inspired by a culturally implanted conviction that pouring some chilled semi-flavorless white liquid into a glass, on one's cornflakes, or in one's coffee fills a genuine *need*. However, the standardized, feature-less cow's milk that they are meant to replace in the same uses scarcely deserves an impassioned defense. And it has to be said that notwithstanding problems like water-depleting almond orchards or elaborate cocktails of additives, they do not depend on pushing cows to punishing high-yield extremes before a premature death.

There is building indignation about the treatment of dairy animals, a driving force behind both the growing popularity of vegan "milks" and many consumers' willingness to pay more for cow's or goat's milk from small operations outside the commodity milk system. There is considerable political flak about the cumbersome and dysfunctional government price-support apparatus. There is even a certain amount of pushback against treating claims of drinking-milk's prodigious nutritional advantages as faultless scientific truth.

In sum, the long reign of milk mystique shows signs of being ripe for replacement by more realistic perspectives. And the time has come for these to include global perspectives—not arrogant visions of Western knowhow conquering markets on the far side of the planet, but an embrace of learning opportunities about the uses of milk from peoples who never consumed it in unfermented form. This does not mean banishing drinking-milk from the table of anybody who likes and can digest full-lactose milk. It means demoting it from a uniquely—and falsely—privileged position and making it simply one option among many others that have never before reached Western consumers.

My reason for saying that the time for global perspectives on milk consumption has come is that this is the first moment in the history of the United States as an independent nation at which observers can foresee adult lactase persistence eventually becoming a minority condition. In hindsight, that likelihood can be traced to the passage of the 1965 Hart-Celler Act, which abolished a restrictive older immigration quota system and for the first time permitted large numbers of people of non-British or non-Northwest European origin to legally immigrate to the United States. It took about forty years for students of population demographics to draw the inference spelled out in a 2008 Pew Research Center report: by 2050 the number of Americans descended from the formerly predominant stock will have grown only slightly, while those of more varied genetic origins will have sharply increased.[27] Subsequent reviews have confirmed the general drift of the report, while also indicating that the nation will become more multiracial as the percentage formed by people of unmixed white ancestry continues to decline.

Those changes, of course, are already being fueled by immigration—almost always, immigration from parts of the world where adult lactase persistence is rare. But some of those same areas have been great centers of dairying for millennia, and their cuisines make plentiful, resourceful use of fermented milk. I cannot think of a more promising next chapter in the modern American milk story.

Probably most Americans today are too young to remember what an eye-opening surprise yogurt was when it joined the lineup of everyday foods, or when goat's milk was a commercial rarity. Those two examples don't begin to hint at the enormous scope of dairy products that can start broadening our culinary horizons as immigration from many parts of Africa and Asia gathers steam. Already a Saudi-born Californian is trying to jump-start a U.S. camel's milk industry, and water buffalo farms in several states produce the extraordinarily rich milk that has historically been more popular in India than cow's milk (not to mention more esteemed for mozzarella cheese in Italy).

The stream of new arrivals from yogurt-making regions may also help to rescue yogurt from the bacteriological sameness of American brands dependent on a comparatively few standardized lab-grown cultures. In lands where it was the staff of life for millennia, different local versions were—though the situation is now changing fast—no more identical than different wines. East of the Mediterranean, from Syria to Iran, and also throughout the Balkans, members of the clan historically had particular refinements reflecting unique complexities in the makeup of the fermenting lactic acid bacteria. What would it be like to sample something close to the homemade *kissélo mléko* that Stamen Grigorov grew up on in Bulgaria? Or to experience the many qualities of "curd"—the usual Anglo-Indian word for yogurt—as it used to be made from zebu's or buffalo's milk in every part of the subcontinent, from the relatively cool north to the torrid south, before a few laboratory-grown bacterial strains smoothed out regional differences? How about persuading sheep and goat farm dairies to experiment with a version of the Sardinian *gioddu*? And why not resurrect some of the many kinds of fermented milk and cream—relatives of our cultured buttermilk and sour cream—that had their own attractions in the northern parts of the former Eastern Bloc, from East Germany far into Russia?

Perhaps the most exciting of the many potential contributions to the roster of new (in most Americans' experience) dairy products will come from Africa, with its long traditions of fermented milk. No continent historically was home to a greater number of milk-dependent societies, or to more inventive ways of exploiting lactic acid fermentation.[28] In Sudan, milk is fermented before being churned for butter; the residual buttermilk is drunk as *rob*. Ethiopian *ergo* is directly fermented rather than churned. Southern Ethiopia, however, is home to *ititu*, a member of the fascinating family of African "smoked milks."

The traditional fermenting vessel for milk throughout much of Africa is a calabash, which acquires a rich collection of lactic acid bacteria and other microorganisms through reuse over many batches. Smoked milk is produced by burning aromatic herbs or twigs and using the ashes to impregnate the inside of the gourd with a thin coating that communicates a smoky flavor to the milk as it ferments and apparently discourages pathogenic growth to some extent. *Ititu* seems to be the northernmost member of the tribe . Other versions of fermented milk that are often (though not always) smoked include the *mursik* and *kule naoto* of Kenya, *kivugoto* of Rwanda, and *amasi* of South Africa. *Amasi*, of which Nelson Mandela was a lifelong devotee, is now commercially manufactured (in smokeless versions, minus the calabash) from laboratory cultures and has a huge following among South Africans of all races and backgrounds. The Nigerian *nono* and Ghanaian *nunu*, which also used to be calabash-fermented, are other candidates for commercial production.

African agricultural and health ministries have been heavily propagandized by Western experts announcing that the road to prosperity and improved child nutrition depends on founding modern drinking-milk industries. But they also have an admixture of people who are interested in developing commercial versions of traditional fermented milk. There is no reason that these products couldn't attract a following in the United States, not only within but beyond growing African immigrant communities. Just as important: they may help to keep some very ancient legacies from being wiped out through ignorance.

BACK TO THE BEGINNING:
THE MICROBIAL HERITAGE

The grip of nineteenth- and early twentieth-century preconceptions about milk has proved remarkably hard to loosen, even among experts trying to research complex questions. A prime example has been the thinking of archaeologists and geneticists who study prehistoric human diets.

For many years, they worked from the assumption that the first domesticators of goats, sheep, and cattle must have drunk their milk fresh, like modern Westerners. After the 1965 experiment on white and Black subjects by Cuatrecasas, Lockwood, and Caldwell pointed the way toward a realization that adult lactase nonpersistence was the ancestral condition of humanity, the ground shifted to another thesis. The reasoning now was that the genetic quirk, or polymorphism, that allowed certain groups—especially Northwest Europeans—to digest full-lactose milk into adulthood must have conferred a decisive evolutionary advantage on anybody who possessed it.

Zooarchaeologists and paleogeneticists confidently repeated the evolutionary-advantage argument for some years. Concrete proof, however, turned out to be remarkably elusive. Different researchers proposed various timetables for the first appearances of the trait, while trying to explain exactly why the supposed advantage must have had a strong evolutionary impact—why it presumably allowed its possessors to survive to reproductive age more often than other people. Human remains that showed conclusive evidence of the crucial polymorphism earlier than a few thousand years ago were unexpectedly difficult to locate. In fact, the whole thesis began to look increasingly shaky.

In just the last few years, an entirely different interpretation appears to be taking shape. It began with researchers at the Max Planck Institute for the Science of Human History in Jena, Germany, becoming curious about how nomadic pastoralism had diffused along the Great Steppe of Eurasia in historic or prehistoric times. The Planck Institute investigators were also interested in a new tool of detection: the analysis of ancient dental plaque samples to detect evidence of people's diet as well as the makeup of an individual's microbiome. Eventually one of the lead researchers, Christina Warinner, recruited a team of colleagues to conduct an international expedition to Mongolia—not the Chinese province of Inner Mongolia, but the independent People's Republic of Mongolia, at the eastern end of the Great Steppe—in 2017. What they found in the far north of the country, close to Lake Khövsgöl, was a revelation in several ways.[29]

In the first place, the oldest human remains they were able to examine at archaeological sites showed evidence of milk consumption but not of lactase persistence. The current population is also about 95 percent lactase-nonpersistent. Yet these people are remnants of one of the most heavily milk-dependent societies on earth. In youth they had learned nearly innumerable ways of preparing the milk of cows, yaks, goats, sheep, camels, horses, and even reindeer through fermentation and various preservation techniques. The milk of each species had its own valued purposes and required its own special handling. The actual milking used to take place in the spring and summer grass season; people switched to a heavily meat-based diet in winter, when some crucial dairy item might remain frozen for months before being thawed out and used as a starter when warm weather. returned together with new milk.

The hosts of the Planck Institute's research team had never heard of dairy microbiology. They were puzzled when the scientists tried to explain the concept of lactic acid bacteria. But watching the skilled dairyists going about their work, the visitors saw more and more clearly that the entire surroundings teemed with unimaginably diverse microbial communities—the polar opposite of the pure strains carefully maintained by technicians under otherwise sterile conditions in factories that supply cultures to cheesemakers and yogurt-makers. The milk and the workers' hands were constantly in contact with permeable and textured surfaces like wooden and leather containers, felt and cloth garments, or the animals' hides, in startling contrast to the easy-to-sanitize glass, stainless steel, hard plastics, and disposable gloves that are necessary in a laboratory. The secret of their ability to extract the greatest possible nutritional benefit from the milk-centered diet of the warm months was microbial biodiversity, not microbial purity.

One outgrowth of the mission was a scholarly article issued in 2018 in the proceedings of the National Academy of Sciences as "Bronze Age Population Dynamics and the Rise of Dairy Pastoralism on the Eastern Eurasian Steppe." It is mostly concerned with evidence about just when dairying arrived in prehistoric Khövsgöl, but pointedly takes time out to acknowledge new research about other regions indicating—like the Mongolian example—that the first dairyists are unlikely to have been milk-drinkers: "Recent studies in Europe and the Near East have found that dairying preceded LP [lactase persistence] in these regions by at least 5,000 y [years], suggesting that LP may be irrelevant to the origins and early history of dairying."[30]

Just what does the Planck Institute's Khövsgöl investigation have to do with the story of modern milk? For answers, we may look to a project launched by Warinner and her colleagues, "Heirloom Microbes: The History and Legacy of Ancient Dairy Bacteria."[31] It aims to trace fermentation of milk by lactic acid bacteria as one of humanity's most ancient, most far-reaching accomplishments. Spontaneous fermentation in hot weather may have been the original trigger, but prehistoric peoples in far-flung regions of Eurasia and Africa developed resourceful technologies for maintaining stable communities of microbes and in the process making an indigestible food into a lifeline.

Living with herders in Khövsgöl during the summer of 2017, the Planck Institute team reached the frightening conclusion that irreplaceable local microbes are fast disappearing under the pressure to modernize Mongolia's dairy industry, and that the same threat is equally imminent elsewhere. The Heirloom Microbes project, which proposes to collect data from all dairying regions of the world, represents their effort to observe and record as much as they can of an endangered microscopic heritage and the human skills that have kept it alive through several millennia. It also has created an international alliance of archaeologists, geneticists, and microbiologists united in an effort to deploy their different abilities for the dual purpose of better understanding the past and working toward a better future for milk and people.

The milking story began with relationships between dairy animals and humans that were made possible by microbes. The headlong expansion of the drinking-milk trade into a gigantic industry has done much to obscure that knowledge. But today we stand a chance of once more drawing on it in a multiracial America where the ability to digest full-lactose milk is likely to be a minority rather than a majority condition and fermented milk can assume the key role that it had in the earliest ages of dairying.

ACKNOWLEDGMENTS

Two people deserve my thanks more than anyone else for helping bring this project to fruition.

When Jennifer Crewe first accepted my proposal in her capacity as director of Columbia University Press, we both saw it as a survey of today's raw milk wars. But somehow the book itself insisted on becoming something else: an unconventional history of a troubled mega-industry reflecting my conviction that milk is the world's most misunderstood food. It's my great good fortune that Jennifer wholeheartedly supported this change of direction and waited with heroic patience for the result.

The manuscript's other midwife has been my nephew Jorj—that is, George F. Bauer, Jr., my rock of Gibraltar in all things computer-related. I can't begin to count the number of times he patiently cleared up my cyber-missteps or rescued some chapter from out-and-out obliteration. He has been generosity incarnate.

The current book never would have existed without the help of the late Elisabeth Sifton, who encouraged me in a much earlier—though sadly, unsuccessful—attempt to tackle the subject of milk; and the late Judith Jones, who capably shepherded me through the writing of a cookbook dedicated to the culinary uses of milk.

We're lucky enough to live in a mini–golden age of research about many aspects of milk and dairying, in the United States and elsewhere. Among the scholars and writers who have helped to inspire or improve my own work are Miranda Brown, E. Melanie DuPuis, Jia-Chen Fu, Barbara Orland, William S. Rubel, Françoise Sabban, Kendra Smith-Howard, Deborah Valenze, and Andrea S. Wiley.

Heartfelt thanks to my indefatigable agent, Jane Dystel, and the team at Dystel, Goderich & Bourret.

Thanks also to the many friends and colleagues who have followed the progress of research and writing over several more years than I'd foreseen (the COVID-19 pandemic slowed things down considerably). Laura Shapiro courageously helped with some early brainstorming. I also had the pleasure of a stimulating exchange of ideas with Bronwen and Francis Percival at a formative stage of my thinking. Among other acts of generosity, Paul Freedman read about half the manuscript in an early draft and offered constructive advice. Others who read shorter bits or let me bounce ideas off them include Nancy Harmon Jenkins, Andrew Coe and Jane Ziegelman, Maricel Presilla, Michael Gray, Susan J. Talbutt, Regina Schrambling, and the late, much-missed Cara DeSilva.

Special thanks to Pedro Cuatrecasas for sharing with me his memories of the 1965 study at Johns Hopkins that provided the first published documentation of racial differences in the ability to digest lactase.

Wilhelm Knaus, Timo Sahi, and Mark G. Thomas kindly gave me access to publications of theirs through printouts or online links. I am indebted to helpful librarians at the New York Public Library, the Columbia University Libraries system, New York University's Bobst Library, the North Bergen (New Jersey) Public Library, the Bergen County (New Jersey) Cooperative Library System, and the Michigan State Law Library.

At Columbia University Press, I am grateful to the unfailingly helpful Sheniqua Larkin, Jennifer Crewe's assistant. Many thanks as well to the team that steered the manuscript through the production process: Susan Pensak; Marielle T. Poss; Zachary Friedman; Julia Kushnirsky, who designed the jacket; and Ben Kolstad of KnowledgeWorks Global Ltd., who has handled much of the heavy lifting.

NOTES

PREFACE

1. Anne Mendelson, *Milk: The Surprising Story of Milk Through the Ages* (New York: Knopf, 2008), viii.

INTRODUCTION

1. Pedro Cuatrecasas, personal communication, March 18, 2018.
2. Pedro Cuatrecasas, Dean H. Lockwood, and Jacques R. Caldwell, "Lactase Deficiency in the Adult: A Common Occurrence," *The Lancet* 285, no. 7375 (January 2, 1965): 14–18.
3. Nabil Sabri Enattah et al., "Identification of a Variant Associated with Adult-Type Hypolactasia," *Nature Genetics* 30 (January 14, 2002): 233–237.

1. MILK

1. Virginia H. Holsinger, "Lactose," in *Fundamentals of Dairy Chemistry*, 3rd ed., ed. Noble P. Wong, Robert Jenness, Mark Keeney, and Elmer H. Marth (New York: Van Nostrand Reinhold, 1988), 328. Lactase is also referred to in the scientific literature as β-D-galactosidase or lactase-phlorizin hydrolase (from its ability to break down a substance called phlorizin that is found in the bark of some trees). See also Andrea S. Wiley, entry "lactose intolerance" in *The Oxford Companion to Cheese*, ed. Catherine Donnelly (New York: Oxford University Press, 2016), 417–419.
2. David S. Newburg and Suzanne H. Neubauer, "Carbohydrates in Milk: Analysis, Quantities, and Significance," in *Handbook of Milk Composition*, ed. Robert G. Jensen (San Diego: Academic Press, 1995), 336–337.

3. The New Jersey cheesemaker Jonathan White, whose cows and calves live outdoors the year round, reports that he has found undigested grass in the stools of day-old calves; personal communication, July 7, 2021.

4. The term "microbial ecology" may have first been applied to the rumen by the bacteriologist Robert E. Hungate; see his paper "Microbial Ecology of the Rumen," *Bacteriology Reviews* 24 (1960), 353–364, https://journals.asm.org/doi/pdf/10.1128/br.24.4.353-364.1960.

5. James B. Russell and David B. Wilson, "Why Are Ruminal Cellulolytic Bacteria Unable to Digest Cellulose at Low pH?," *Journal of Dairy Science* 79, no. 8 (August 1996): 1503–1509, https://www.sciencedirect.com/science/article/pii/S0022030296765104.

6. Bronwen Percival and Francis Percival, *Reinventing the Wheel: Milk, Microbes, and the Fight for Real Cheese* (Oakland: University of California Press, 2017), 110.

7. John W. Sherbon, "Physical Properties of Milk," in *Fundamentals of Dairy Chemistry*, 3rd ed., ed. Noble P. Wong, Robert Jenness, Mark Keeney, and Elmer H. Marth (New York: Van Nostrand Reinhold, 1988), 411.

8. Gianaclis Caldwell, entry "flocculation" in *The Oxford Companion to Cheese*, ed. Catherine Donnelly (New York: Oxford University Press, 2016), 279.

2. FROM THE CRADLE OF DAIRYING TO THE ENGLISH MANOR

1. David W. Anthony, *The Horse, the Wheel, and Language: How Bronze-Age Riders from the Eurasian Steppes Shaped the Modern World* (Princeton, NJ: Princeton University Press, 2007), 197.

2. Andrew Sherratt, "Plough and Pastoralism: Aspects of the Secondary Products Revolution," in *Pattern of the Past: Studies in Honour of David Clarke*, ed. Ian Hodder, Glynn Isaac, and Norman Hammond (London: Cambridge University Press,1981), 277.

3. Sherratt, "Plough and Pastoralism, 261.

4. Paul Kindstedt, *Cheese and Culture: A History of Cheese and Its Place in Western Civilization* (White River Junction, VT: Chelsea Green Publishing, 2012), 28–35.

5. Barry Cunliffe, *By Steppe, Desert, and Ocean: The Birth of Eurasia* (Oxford: Oxford University Press, 2015), 454–466.

6. Homer, *The Iliad*, book IV, lines 1–5.

7. Herodotus, *The Histories*, book IV, chapter 2.

8. Strabo, *The Geography*, book VII, chapter 3, section 17; chapter 4, section 6.

9. Arminius (Armin) Vámbéry, *Travels in Central Asia* (London: John Murray, 1865; repr. Arno Press, 1970), 152.

10. Julius Caesar, *Gallic Wars*, Book IV, chapter 1; book VI, chapter 22.

11. Pliny the Elder, *Natural History*, book XI, chapter 96.

12. Tacitus, *Germania*, Chapter 23; Strabo, *The Geography*, Book IV, chapter 5, section 2.

13. Yuval Itan et al, "The Origins of Lactase Persistence in Europe," *PLoS Computational Biology*, August 28, 2009, https://journals.plos.org/ploscompbiol/article?id=10.1371/journal.pcbi.1000491.

14. Geoffrey Chaucer, *Works*, ed. F. N. Robinson, 2nd ed. (Cambridge, MA: Riverside Press,1957), 199 (*Canterbury Tales*, Fragment VII, lines 2821–2846).

15. *Monasticon Anglicanum: A New Edition*, compiled by W. Dugdale, ed. John Caley, Henry Ellis, and Bulkeley Bandinel (London: James Bohn, 1846), vol. I, 517, https://books.google.com/books?id=61ZVAAAAcAAJ&pg=PA517.

16. *Walter of Henley's Husbandry, Together with an Anonymous Seneschaucie and Robert Grosseteste's Rules*, trans. and ed. Elizabeth Lamond (London: Longmans, Green, and Co, 1890), 112–113, https://archive.org/details/walterhenleyshu01cunngoog/page /n4/mode/2up.

17. Robert Greene and Thomas Lodge, *A Looking Glasse for London and England*, in *The Plays and Poems of Robert Greene*, ed. J. Churton Collins (Oxford, Clarendon Press, 1905), vol. 1, 155 (Act I, scene 3, lines 352–355), https://archive.org/details/plays poemsrober01greegoog/page/n176/mode/2up.

3. THE RISE OF DRINKING-MILK

1. *Thomas Platter's Travels in England*, trans. and ed. Clare Williams (London: Jonathan Cape, 1937), 150, https://archive.org/details/in.ernet.dli.2015.506933/page/n5/mode/2up.

2. James Shirly, *Hide Park, a Comedy* (London: Thomas Coles for Andrew Crook, 1637), unpaginated, The Fourth Act.

3. Gervase Markham, *Cheape and Good Husbandry for the Well-Ordering of All Beasts, and Fowles, and for the Generall Cure of Their Diseases* (London: Printed by T[homas] S[nodham] for Roger Jackson, 1614), Book I, 43.

4. *The Diary of Samuel Pepys: Daily Entries from the 17th Century London Diary*, https://www.pepysdiary.com/diary/1669/04/25/.

5. *The Diary of Samuel Pepys*, https://www.pepysdiary.com/diary/1663/06/10/, https://www.pepysdiary.com/diary/1666/06/17/, https://www.pepysdiary.com/diary/1668/05/20/, https://www.pepysdiary.com/diary/1668/05/27/.

6. *The Diary of Samuel Pepys*, https://www.pepysdiary.com/diary/1666/07/15/

7. *The Diary of Samuel Pepys*, https://www.pepysdiary.com/diary/1668/05/20

8. *The Diary of Samuel Pepys*, https://www.pepysdiary.com/diary/1667/05/15/

9. George Cheyne, *The English Malady: Or, a Treatise of Nervous Diseases of all Kinds* (London, S. Powell, 1733; reprint, Scholars' Facsimiles & Reprints, 1976), 224.

10. Cheyne, *The English Malady*, 229–230.

11. Thomas Sydenham, *Tractatus de Podagra et Hydrope* (London: R.N. 1683), 75–76, https://books.google.com/books?id=WndmAAAAcAAJ. For a later English translation, see *The Works of Thomas Sydenham, M.D. on Acute and Chronic Diseases*, ed. George Wallis (London: G.G.J. and J. Robinson, W. Otridge, S. Hayes, and E. Newbery. 1788), 223–225, https://babel.hathitrust.org/cgi/pt?id=mdp.39015029957506.

12. Cheyne, *The English Malady*, 231, 249.

13. George Cheyne, *The Natural Method of Curing the Diseases of the Body, and the Disorders of the Mind Depending on the Body*, 5th ed. (London: Dan. Browne, R. Manby, J. Whiston and B. White, and A. Strahan, 1753), 126, https://archive.org/details/naturalmethodofc1753chey/.

14. Cheyne, *The Natural Method of Curing*, 128–129.

15. *The Letters of Doctor George Cheyne to Samuel Richardson* (1733–1743), ed. Charles F. Mullett (Columbia, MO: 1943), 127.

16. Deborah Valenze, *Milk: A Local and Global History* (New Haven, CT: Yale University Press, 2011), 110–115.

17. John Wesley, *Primitive Physick: Or, an Easy and Natural Method of Curing Most Diseases*, 9th ed. (London: W. Strahan, 1761), xiii, xviii, https://books.google.com /books?id=fLEUAAAAQAAJ.

18. J. H. Plumb, "The New World of Children," in *The Birth of a Consumer Society: The Commercialization of Eighteenth-Century England*, ed. Neil McKendrick, John Brewer, and J. H. Plumb (London: Europa Publications, 1982), 310.

19. Cheyne, *The English Malady*, 310.

20. Walter Harris, *A Treatise of the Acute Diseases of Infants*, trans. John Martyn (London: Thomas Astley, 1742), 24, 31, 56, https://books.google.com/books?id=LQplAAAAcAAJ.

21. William Cadogan, *An Essay upon Nursing*, 4th ed. (London: J. Robert, 1750), 35, https:// books.google.com/books?id=Ay5cAAAAQAAJ.

22. Samuel Latham Mitchill, "The Doctrine of Septon," Appendix 3 in *A Scientist in the Early Republic: Samuel Latham Mitchill, 1764–1831*, ed. Courtney Robert Hall (New York: Russell and Russell, 1962, reissued 1967), 136.

23. Walter Scott, *The Heart of Mid-Lothian*, chap. 47.

24. A. F. M. Willich, *Lectures on Diet and Regimen* (New-York: T. and J. Swords, 1801), 234, https://babel.hathitrust.org/cgi/pt?id=nyp.33433011660473.

25. Joseph Clarke, "Observations on the Properties Commonly Attributed by Medical Writers to HUMAN MILK," in *The Transactions of the Royal Irish Academy* (Dublin: George Bonham, 1788), 183–185, https://babel.hathitrust.org/cgi/pt?id=pst.000060071798.

26. Sir John Sinclair, *The Code of Health and Longevity* (Edinburgh: Arch. Constable & Co., 1807), vol. I, 275n, https://babel.hathitrust.org/cgi/pt?id=nyp.33433004142059.

4. SETTING THE STAGE FOR PASTEURIZATION

1. Robert M. Hartley, *Historical, Scientific and Practical Essay on Milk as an Article of Human Sustenance* (New York: Jonathan Leavitt, 1842), 108.

2. Hartley, *Historical, Scientific and Practical Essay on Milk*, 145–146.

3. Hartley, *Historical, Scientific and Practical Essay on Milk*, 156–157.

4. Hartley, *Historical, Scientific and Practical Essay on Milk*, 257.

5. Hartley, *Historical, Scientific and Practical Essay on Milk*, 335.

6. Hartley, *Historical, Scientific and Practical Essay on Milk*, 77–78.

7. Advertisements for Borden's Condensed Milk and Alden & Woodhull's Concentrated Milk, *Frank Leslie's Illustrated Newspaper*, May 22, 1858, 399. For an account of Leslie's strategy, see Jennifer E. Moore, "Ours Has Been No Pleasing Task: Sensationalism in Frank Leslie's Campaign Against Swill Milk," in *Sensationalism: Murder, Mayhem, Mudslinging, Scandals, and Disasters in 19th-Century Reporting*, ed. David B. Sachsman and David W. Bulla (New Brunswick, NJ: Transaction Publishers, 2013), 127–140.

8. For an account of the interest in extracts and chemical proxies meant to avoid the inefficiencies of unmodified foodstuffs, see the chapter "Milk in the Nursery, Chemistry in the Kitchen," in Deborah Valenze, *Milk: A Local and Global History* (New Haven, CT: Yale University Press, 2011), 153–177.

9. Joe B. Frantz, *Gail Borden: Dairyman to a Nation* (Norman: University of Oklahoma Press, 1951), 201–221.

10. Advertisement in *The Lancet General Advertiser*, December 18, 1852 (advertising section follows p. 584), https://books.google.com/books?id=6RhAAAAAcAAJ&pg=PA560 -IA8&lpg=PA560-IA8&dq=Lancet+%2B+December+18,+1852+%2B+%22Lancet +General+Advertiser.

11. James Caird, *English Agriculture in 1850–51* (London: Longman, Brown, Green, and Longmans, 1852), 234–235, https://babel.hathitrust.org/cgi/pt?id=wu.89047222195&vie w=1up&seq=268.

12. Frantz, *Gail Borden*, 226–229.

13. Text of Borden's patent: https://patentimages.storage.googleapis.com/9d/d3/12/bf443 d33f791e4/US15553.pd.

14. Frantz, *Gail Borden*, 238–240.

15. New York Academy of Medicine, "Report on Condensed Milk, by the Section on Materia Medica and Botany," November 4, 1857, p. 5, https://collections.nlm.nih.gov /bookviewer?PID=nlm:nlmuid-101203722-bk#page/6/mode/2up.

16. *Brooklyn Daily Eagle*, April 30, 1858, 11, https://www.newspapers.com/clip/27453470 /home-delivery-condensed-milk/. John Mullaly, in *The Milk Trade of New York and Vicinity* (New York: Fowler and Wells, 1853), 95, estimated that milk could be supplied to establishments such as hotels by direct contract with farmers for three or four cents a quart, "which is about twenty per cent. less than they could purchase it from the [notoriously untrustworthy] milk dealers in the city," https://babel.hathitrust.org/cgi /pt?id=loc.ark:/13960/t8mc9kw2f&view=2up&seq=98&skin=2021.

17. *Frank Leslie's Illustrated Newspaper*, May 22, 1858, 399.

18. X. A. Willard, "The American Milk-Condensing Factories and Condensed Milk Manufacturers," in *Journal of the Royal Agricultural Society of England*, 2nd series, vol. 8 (London: John Murray, 1872), 103–152. Borden's sanitary rules are on pp. 112–113, https://babel.hathitrust.org/cgi/pt?id=hvd.32044089548515.

19. Thirty-Seventh Congress of the United States, *An Act to Establish a Department of Agriculture*, May 1, 1862, https://www.nal.usda.gov/topics/act-establish-department -agriculture; *An Act Donating Public Lands to the several States and Territories which may provide Colleges for the Benefit of Agriculture and the Mechanic Arts*, July 2, 1862, https://www.nal.usda.gov/topics/morrill-land-grant-college-act.

20. *The Philadelphia merchants' & manufacturers' business directory for 1856–57* (Philadelphia: Griswold & Co., 1856), 97, https://babel.hathitrust.org/cgi/pt?id=uiug .30112089222431&view=1up&seq=143&skin=2021; R. J. Griesbach, *150 Years of Research at the United States Department of Agriculture: Plant Introduction and Breeding* (Washington, DC: U.S. Department of Agriculture, Agricultural Research Service, 2013), 4, https://www.ars.usda.gov/ARSUserFiles/oc/np/150YearsofResearchatUSDA/150Years ofResearchatUSDA.pdf.

21.   F. Ratchford Starr, *Farm Echoes* (New York: Orange Judd, 1883).

22.   Gervase Markham, *Countrey Contentments, Book 2: The English Hus-wife.* (London: John Beale for Roger Jackson,1615; rept. Theatrum Orbis Terrarum Ltd. and Da Capo Press, 1973), 109.

23.   Charles Dickens, *The Mystery of Edwin Drood*, chapter 22.

24.   Starr, *Farm Echoes*, 88; "Echo Farm Supplement," *The Cultivator & Country Gentleman*, 42, no. 1259 (March 8, 1877): 161–164, https://books.google.com/books?id =ZadMAAAAYAAJ&pg=PA164&lpg=PA164&dq=%22Echo+Farm%22+%2B+muslin.

25.   Crusoe [pseud.], "The Jerseys at Echo Farm," *Wallace's Monthly* 4, no. 1 (February 1878): 7–8, https://books.google.com/books?id=18ICAAAAYAAJ&pg=PA1&lpg=PA1&dq =%22Wallace%27s+Monthly%22+%2B+February+1878%22. Butter at $1.25 a pound is cited in an advertisement for the Cooley Creamer in *The Cultivator and Country Gentleman* 49, no. 1632 (May 8, 1884): 407, https://books.google.com/books?id=urfZ96MqWzYC &pg=PA407&lpg=PA407&dq=%22Cooley+Creamer%22+%2B+Cultivator.

26.   Starr, *Farm Echoes*, 97; "Improvements at Echo Farm," *Cultivator and Country Gentleman* 45 no. 1423 (May 6, 1880): 300, https://babel.hathitrust.org/cgi/pt?id=osu .32435057780538&view=1up&seq=308&skin=2021&size=125.

27.   Starr, *Farm Echoes*, 98–100.

28.   "Improvements at Echo Farm."

29.   John Mullaly, *The Milk Trade in New York and Vicinity* (New York: Fowlers and Wells, 1853), 95, https://babel.hathitrust.org/cgi/pt?id=loc.ark:/13960/t8mc9kw2f&view =2up&seq=99&skin=2021.

30.   Martin Wilckens, *Nordamerikanische Landwirtschaft: Erfahrungen und Anschauungen gesammelt auf einer Studienreise im Jahre 1889* (Tübingen: H. Laupp'schen Buchhand-lung, 1890), 193, https://babel.hathitrust.org/cgi/pt?id=uiug.30112076102455.

31.   J. Cheston Morris, "On Milk Supply in Large Cities," *The Boston Medical and Surgical Journal* 110 no. 14 (April 3, 1884): 315–317, https://books.google.com/books ?vid=HARVARD:32044103050498.

32.   For Atwater's early efforts, see T. Swann Harding, *Two Blades of Grass: A History of Scientific Development in the U.S. Department of Agriculture* (Norman: University of Oklahoma Press, 1947), 174–176 and 220–224; and Alan I. Marcus, *Agricultural Science and the Quest for Legitimacy: Farmers, Agricultural Colleges, and Experiment Stations, 1870–1890* (Ames: Iowa State University Press, 1985), 72–77.

33.   Hatch Act of 1887: *The Statutes at Large of the United States of America from December, 1885, to March, 1887*, 440–442, https://tile.loc.gov/storage-services/service/ll/llsl//llsl -c49/llsl-c49.pdf.

34.   1889 act granting Department of Agriculture Cabinet status: *The Statutes at Large of the United States of America from December, 1887, to March, 1889*, 659, https://tile.loc .gov/storage-services/service/ll/llsl//llsl-c50/llsl-c50.pdf.

35.   W. O. Atwater, "Economy of Food," *Good Housekeeping* 19 no. 4 (October 1894): 145–149, https://books.google.com/books?id=Rco2AQAAMAAJ&pg=PA145&lpg=PA145&dq =%22W.O.+Atwater%22+%2B+milk+%2B+economical.

36. Morris, "On Milk Supply in Large Cities," 317.

37. Constitution of the American Public Health Association (Cambridge, MA: H.O. Houghton and Company), xiii–xv, https://www.ncbi.nlm.nih.gov/pmc/articles /PMC2272676/pdf/pubhealthpap00028-0002.pdf.

38. Walter De F. Day, statement in *Annual report of the Board of the Health Department of the City of New York, Report on Vital Statistics*, January 1, 1880, 212, https://archive .org/details/annualreportofbo1878newy/page/1/mode/1up.

39. Philip Van Ingen, "The History of Child Welfare Work in the United States," in *A Half Century of Public Health: Jubilee Historical Volume of the American Public Health Association*, ed. Mazÿck Porcher Ravenel (New York: American Public Health Association, 1921, rept. Arno Press and the New York Times, 1970), 290.

40. For a description of the situation as viewed by a contemporary, see John Spargo, *The Common Sense of the Milk Question* (New York: Macmillan, 1908), 1–45.

41. I have not been able to trace the first appearance of this phrase, but it certainly was given currency by *Hoard's Dairyman*. It was familiar enough by 1898 for Hoard to joshingly refer to it at a meeting of the Wisconsin Dairymen's Association; see *Twenty-Sixth Annual Report of the Wisconsin Dairymen's Association* (Madison, WI: Democrat Printing Company, State Printer, 1898), 6–7, https://books.google .com/books?id=AvXNAAAAMAAJ&pg=PA7&lpg=PA7&dq=%22Wisconsin +Dairymen%27s+Association%22+%2B+%22foster+mother%22.

42. "The Dairy and the World Food Problem": Address by Herbert Hoover at the National Milk and Dairy Farm Exposition, New York City, May 23, 1918 (Washington, DC: Government Printing Office, 1918), 3–4, https://archive.org/details/dairyworldfoodproohoov.

43. A. Jacobi, "Infant Diet: A Paper Read Before the Public Health Association of New York" (New York: Putnam, 1873), 21–22, https://books.google.com/books?hl=en&lr =&id=nvBbAAAAcAAJ&oi=fnd&pg=PA1&ots=WQKnGVSXyM&sig =t9xEiZ9anew2_e9qvAYkeM2YCOE#v=onepage&q&f=false.

44. The Soxhlet extractor is still an indispensable piece of apparatus, available from any laboratory supply company.

45. F. Soxhlet, "Ueber Kindermilch und Säuglings-Ernährung," in *Münchener Medizinische Wochenschrift*, 33rd year, nos. 15 and 16 (April 13 and April 20, 1886): 253—256 and 276–278, https://babel.hathitrust.org/cgi/pt?id=chi.78903947.

46. Henry Koplik, "The History of the First Milk Depot or Gouttes de Lait with Consultations in America," *Journal of the American Medical Association* 63, no. 18 (October 31, 1914): 1574–1575. "*Gouttes de Lait*" was the name of a similar program in France, https://ia600708.us.archive.org/view_archive.php?archive=/28/items/crossref-pre -1923-scholarly-works/10.1001%252Fjama.1914.02570170065028.zip&file=10.1001%252 Fjama.1914.02570180060016.pdf.

47. Spargo, *The Common Sense of the Milk Question*, 235.

48. Henry Koplik, "The Administration of Sterilized Milk in Dispensaries," in *The New York Medical Journal* 54 (January 31, 1891): 123–124, https://babel.hathitrust.org/cgi/pt?id =nnc2.ark:/13960/t98656z8m.

49. Nathan Straus, "Pure Milk or Poison?," address to the Milk Conference held at the New York Academy of Medicine, November 20, 1906, published in Lina Gutherz Straus, *Disease in Milk: The Remedy Pasteurization: The Life Work of Nathan Straus*, 2nd ed. (New York: E. P. Dutton, 1917, rept. Arno Press, 1977), 212–213.

5. PASTEURIZATION

1. Carl W. Hall and G. Malcolm Trout, *Milk Pasteurization* (Westport, CT: AVI Publishing Company, 1968), 1.
2. S. Josephine Baker, *Fighting for Life* (New York: Macmillan, 1939; rept. New York Review Book Classics, 2013), 127.
3. Fesca's pasteurizer is illustrated in *Rudolph von Wagner's Jahres-Bericht über die Leistungen der chemischen Technologie, 1882* (Leipzig: Verlag von Otto Wigand, 1883): 917, https://babel.hathitrust.org/cgi/pt?id=uc1.b2985056&view=2up&seq=14&skin=2019. For a description of Fjord's pasteurizer with illustrations, see C. O. Jensen, *Essentials of Milk Hygiene*, trans. and amplified by Leonard Pearson (New York: Lippincott, 1907), 131–133, https://www.google.com/books/edition/Essentials_of_Milk_Hygiene /e8BAAAAYAAJ?hl=en&gbpv=1&printsec=frontcover.
4. H. Bitter, "Versuche über das Pasteurisiren der Milch," *Zeitschrift für Hygiene* 8 (December 1890): 240–286, https://zenodo.org/record/2156316#.Ya4X3i-B21F.
5. Charles E. North, "Milk and Its Relation to Public Health," in *A Half Century of Public Health: Jubilee Historical Volume of the American Public Health Association*, ed. Mazÿck Porcher Ravenel (New York: American Public Health Association, 1921, rept. Arno Press and the New York Times, 1970), 274.
6. Arno Dosch, "The Pasteurized Milk Fraud," *Pearson's Magazine* 24, no. 6 (December 1910): 721–729, https://babel.hathitrust.org/cgi/pt?id=njp.32101064078734.
7. *New York Medical Journal* 85 no. 3 (March 1907): 458, https://babel.hathitrust.org/cgi /pt?id=iau.31858044865271.
8. The standard history of Coit's Medical Milk Commissions is Manfred J. Waserman, "Henry L. Coit and the Certified Milk Movement in the Development of Modern Pediatrics," *Bulletin of the History of Medicine* 46 no. 4 (July–August 1972): 359–390.
9. Rowland Godfrey Freeman, "The Sterilization of Milk at Low Temperatures," *The Medical Record: A Weekly Journal of Medicine and Surgery* 42 (July 2, 1892): 8–10, https://babel.hathitrust.org/cgi/pt?id=coo.31924056973203.
10. Adrian Naoun et al., "*Mycobacterium tuberculosis* H37RV Induces Gene Expression of PDE4A and PDE7A In Human Macrophages," *UTSA Journal of Undergraduate Research and Scholarly Works* 7 (December 1010): 2, https://provost.utsa.edu /undergraduate-research/journal/files/vol7/JURSW.v7.11.Naoun.pdf.
11. John Spargo, *The Common Sense of the Milk Question* (New York: Macmillan, 1908), 129–131.

12. M. J. Rosenau, *The Milk Question* (Boston: Houghton Mifflin, 1912), 99.

13. United States Supreme Court, October Term 1905, 199 U.S. 552: The People of the State of New York *ex rel.* Lieberman v. Van De Carr, decided December 11, 1905, https://casetext.com/case/lieberman-v-van-de-carr.

14. For the text of the 1908 Chicago tuberculin ordinance, see *Journal of the House of Representatives of the 46th General Assembly of the State of Illinois* (Springfield: Illinois State Journal Co., State Printers, 1909), 378–379. The state legislature planned to hand over the issue of overriding the Chicago tuberculin test mandate to a joint investigative committee, 379–380, https://babel.hathitrust.org/cgi/pt?id=uiuo.ark:/13960/t2m66d115.

15. David de Sola Pool, "Nathan Straus," in "Special Articles," *American Jewish Yearbook* 33 (September 12, 1931, to September 30, 1932/5692): 137, http://www.ajcarchives.org/AJC_DATA/Files/1931_1932_5_SpecialArticles.pdf.

16. Julie Miller, "To Stop the Slaughter of the Babies: Nathan Straus and the Drive for Pasteurized Milk, 1893–1920," *New York History: Quarterly Journal of the New York State Historical Association* 74 no. 2 (April 1993): 158–184. Miller incorrectly reports the dates of his term as park commissioner as 1889 to 1893; for the correct dates, see https://www.nycgovparks.org/about/history/commissioners#Department_of_Parks.

17. Andrew Carnegie, "Wealth," *North American Review* 148 no. 391 (June 1889): 653–664.

18. Some of Straus's charitable efforts during the Panic of 1893 are described in Lina Gutherz Straus, *Disease in Milk, The Remedy Pasteurization: The Life Work of Nathan Straus* (New York: Dutton, 1917, rept. Arno Press, 1977; hereafter *"Disease in Milk"*), 119, though dates in this compilation of documents are sometimes muddled. Typical of the positive newspaper coverage are the *New York Times* reports: "Where the Poor Can Buy Coal: Mr. Nathan Straus's Praiseworthy Scheme Underway," January 22, 1893, 11; "Selling Coal to the Poor: More Than Ten Tons Disposed of at Mr. Straus's Station," January 23, 1893, 8; and "Mr. Straus's Happy Idea: The Cold Snap Increases the Demand Largely," February 5, 1893, 3.

19. My reconstruction of the milk depot's history and Straus's involvement is chiefly based on the collection of Nathan Straus papers and newspaper clippings in the Manuscripts and Archives Division of the New York Public Library (hereafter "Straus papers") and *Disease in Milk.*

20. Letter from Alexander Kinkaid to Nathan Straus, May 10, 1893; and "Pure Milk at Cost Price," *New York World*, June 2, 1893, Straus papers. See also Rowland Godfrey Freeman, "The Straus Milk Charity of New York City," *Archives of Pediatrics* 14, no. 11 (November 1897): 838–844, https://books.google.com/books?id=SRNHAAAAYAAJ&pg=PA838&lpg=PA838&dq=%22A.L.+Kinkead%22+%2B+milk.

21. Kinkaid to Straus, May 10 and May 15, 1893; "Pure Milk at Cost Price," Straus papers. The *New York Times* coverage is again typical: "Milk Depot for the Poor," May 30, 1893; "May be Fed for 8 Cents a Day," June 2, 1893; "Good Milk for the Poor," June 21, 1893.

22. Nathan Straus, 'Helping People to Help Themselves," *North American Review* 158, no. 450 (May 1894): 542–553.

23. Edwin G. Burrows and Mike Wallace, *Gotham: A History of New York City to 1898* (New York: Oxford University Press, 1999), 1193; David C. Hammack, *Power and Society: Greater New York at the Turn of the Century* (New York: Russell Sage Foundation, 1982), 149–150; *The Review of Reviews*, American ed., 10, no. 5 (November 1894): 467–471, https://books.google.com/books?id=tCDnhF5feCQC&pg=PA470&lpg=PA470&dq =Straus+%2B+Tammany+%2B+withdrew.

24. "To Vindicate Park Officials," *New York Times*, May 17, 1895, 3.

25. Nathan Straus, "Letter to the Mayors of the Principal Cities of the United States and Canada," June 8, 1895, *Disease in Milk*, 185–186.

26. Nathan Straus, "How to Reduce Infant Mortality (Letter sent to the Presidents of the Health Boards of American cities and Canada)," *Disease in Milk*, 187–193.

27. Straus, "Letter to the Mayors," 185.

28. Straus, "How to Reduce Infant Mortality," 193.

29. In 1883 F. Ratchford Starr firmly declined to jump on the much-touted "ensilage" band-wagon until experts had finished establishing the scientific facts; F. Ratchford Starr, *Farm Echoes* (New York: Orange Judd, 1883), 76. But in another twenty years the state and federal agricultural bureaucracies, along with agriculture-school professors, would be solidly behind it.

30. *Disease in Milk*, 227, 255, 256.

31. Nathan Straus, "Milk Pasteurization: An Economic and Social Duty," *Disease in Milk*, 229–239.

32. Lina Straus to Annie Nason, January 15, 1910, Straus papers. A form letter about Nathan's illness had been issued to the press by the family the previous day. The *New York Sun* broke the story on January 17 ("Nathan Straus a Sick Man: Serious Nervous Breakdown Follows Lakewood Fight," Straus papers). The story of Straus's involvement with the Lakewood Preventorium is summarized in Cynthia A. Connolly, *Saving Sickly Children: The Tuberculosis Preventorium in American Life, 1909–1970* (New Brunswick, NJ: Rutgers University Press, 2008), 53–59. The Straus papers at the New York Public Library reveal more of the mounting dissensions leading up to his breakdown.

33. "A City Newspaper on the Tuberculin Test," *The Pacific Dairy Review* 12, no. 24 (July 9, 1908): 7, https://books.google.com/books?id=Gws-AQAAMAAJ&pg=RA1-PA7 &lpg=RA1-PA7&dq=%22New+York+Herald%22+%2B+tuberculin. The anonymous writer attributes the story to the well-known dairy journalist Valancey E. Fuller in another trade periodical, *The Practical Dairyman*.

34. "Tuberculin Cast Aside as Fad in New Hampshire," *New York Herald*, May 25, 1908, Straus papers. Unless otherwise noted, all subsequent newspaper items about the Herald's anti-tuberculin and anti-pasteurization campaigns are, except for *New York Times* citations, from the Straus papers, which include voluminous newspaper clippings.

35. "The Herald Campaign Against Advertising Dictation," *Printers' Ink* 68, no. 3 (July 21, 1909): 21, https://books.google.com/books?id=F7I9AQAAMAAJ&pg=RA2-PA21 &lpg=RA2-PA21&dq=%22New+York+Herald%22+%2B+%22pasteurized+milk %22+%2B+%22Nathan+Straus%22.

36. "Get Thin on Pasteurized Milk," *Wenatchee* (Washington State) *Daily World*, May 4, 1909, https://chroniclingamerica.loc.gov/data/batches/wa_american_ver02/data/sn86 072041/00237286479/1909050401/0231.pdf.

37. "Raw Milk Resists Bacteria," *The Milk Reporter* 26, no. 8 (August 1910): 1, https:// books.google.com/books?id=N-dIAAAAYAAJ&pg=RA7-PA1&lpg=RA7-PA1&dq =%22New+York+Herald%22+%2B+raw+milk+%2B+germicidal.

38. Milton J. Rosenau and George W. McCoy, "The Germicidal Property of Milk," in *Milk and Its Relation to the Public Health*, Hygienic Laboratory Bulletin No. 41 (Washington, DC: Government Printing Office, 1908), 447–476, https://books.google .com/books?id=hBzQAAAAMAAJ&pg=PA472&lpg=PA472&dq=%22cholera +bacillus%22+%2B+%22raw+milk%22.

39. "The Herald Campaign."

40. "Objectionable Bacteria Found in Pasteurized Milk Served at Penny-a-Glass Booths in New York Parks, Scientists Say," *New York Herald*, August 7, 1910. This was the lead article of the *Sunday Herald*, followed the next day by another front-page exposé focusing on the condition of "loose" milk sold in grocery stores: "Investigation of Pasteurized Milk Dispensed from Cans Points to the Urgent Need of Sanitary Reform in Methods," August 8, 1910. It contained a shorter coda: "'Heated Milk' Sold, in All Conditions." Throughout August, Bennett's milk-purity commandos kept up the attack on pasteurization, and Straus as its champion, from both New York headquarters and the *Herald's* overseas bureaus.

41. "Objectionable Bacteria Found."

42. "'Heated Milk' Sold."

43. The *New York American*'s story, cabled from Berlin on August 24, appeared September 25 as "Straus Gives Up Pasteurization Stations in New York."

44. "Milk Depots to Go, Straus Repeats," *New York Times*, September 5, 1910.

45. "Straus Gives Up Pasteurization Stations in New York," *New York American*; for Board of Health budget figure, see *The Encyclopedia of New York*, 2nd ed., ed. Kenneth T. Jackson (New Haven, CT: Yale University Press, 2010), 188.

46. "Mr. Straus' Lifesaving Work," *Brooklyn Daily Eagle*, August 26, 1910.

47. "Dr. Wiley Praises Straus," *New York Times*, September 9, 1910.

48. "Cooper Union Rings with Straus Praises," *New York Times*, October 9, 1910.

49. *Disease in Milk*, 296–297.

50. "Great Tribute Paid to Nathan Straus," *New York Times*, February 1, 1911.

51. *Disease in Milk*, 296–297.

52. "City Milk Depots to Be Opened Soon," *New York Times*, January 28, 1911.

53. Edwin O. Jordan, "The Municipal Regulation of Milk Supply," *Journal of the American Medical Association* 61, no. 26, 2288 (December 27, 1913): 3, https://babel.hathitrust.org /cgi/pt?id=mdp.39015082605323&view=1up&seq=2297&skin=2021; S. Henry Ayers, The Present Status of the Pasteurization of Milk, United States Department of Agriculture Bulletin No. 342 (Washington, DC: Government Printing Office, 1916), 3. https://www .google.com/books/edition/Department_Bulletin/TRcQh6SA_TgC?hl=en&gbpv=1 &dq=%22The+Present+Status+of+the+Pasteurization+of+Milk%22&pg=PA2&printsec =frontcover.

54. United States Census Bureau, 1920 Census, vol. 1, chap. 1: Number and Distribution of Inhabitants, p. 47, https://www2.census.gov/library/publications/decennial/1920/volume-1/41084484v1ch1.pdf.

55. Rosenau, *The Milk Question*, 150, 185.

56. Horatio Newton Parker, *City Milk Supply* (New York: McGraw-Hill, 1917), 364.

57. Waserman, "Henry L. Coit and the Certified Milk Movement," 380–383.

58. "Medical News: New York," *Journal of the American Medical Association* 64, no. 9 (February 27, 1915): 752, https://ia600708.us.archive.org/view_archive.php?archive=/28/items/crossref-pre-1923-scholarly-works/10.1001%252Fjama.1915.02570280038011.zip&file=10.1001%252Fjama.1915.02570350044022.pdf The Dr. Park in question is William H. Park, Director of Laboratories, New York City Department of Health.

59. "Statement by the Medical Milk Commission of Essex County, New Jersey, Relative to the Problem of Bovine Tuberculosis," *Archives of Pediatrics* 32 (February 1915): 115–123, https://books.google.com/books?id=jeJFAAAAYAAJ&pg=PA122&lpg=PA122&dq=Fairfield+Dairy,+New+Jersey+%2B+tuberculin+test.

60. *Disease in Milk*, 344.

61. "Straus Milk Plant Is Offered to City," *New York Times*, January 5, 1919.

62. "10,000 at Funeral of Nathan Straus," *New York Times*, January 14, 1931; David de Sola Pool, "Nathan Straus."

63. Spargo, *The Common Sense of the Milk Question*, 248–249, 264–265.

6. SOUR MILK, BRIEFLY RETHOUGHT

1. 61st Congress, 3rd Session, Senate Document No. 863: "Report of a Special Committee Appointed by the Washington Chamber of Commerce to Investigate the Milk Situation in. the District of Columbia" (Washington, DC: Government Printing Office,1911), 115, https://books.google.com/books?id=5tdGAQAAIAAJ&pg=PA1&lpg=PA1&dq=61st+Congress,+3rd+Session,+%22Milk+Situation+in+the+District+of+Columbia%22.

2. John Grieve, "An Account of the Method of Making a Wine, Called by the Tartars Koumiss; with Observations on Its Use in Medicine," *Transactions of the Royal Society of Edinburgh*, vol. I (Edinburgh: J. Dickson, 1788), 178, https://books.google.com/books?id=TDEeAQAAMAAJ&pg=PA25&lpg=PA25&dq=Dr.+John+Grieve+%2B+koumiss+%2B+Transactions.

3. Grieve, "An Account of the Method of Making a Wine," 184–185.

4. For more on Postnikov's effort, see the project "Canvas Empire: A Spatial History of the Russian Empire," by Kelly O'Neill, https://scalar.fas.harvard.edu/imperiia/kumiss-cures.

5. United States Patent Office, U.S. Patent 117,889, August 8, 1871, Victor Apollinaris Jagielski, "Improvement in Dietetic Compounds from Milk," https://patentimages.storage.googleapis.com/oo/f6/d6/ec4e72c177629c/US117889.pdf; Victor Jagielski, *Koumiss and Its Use in Medicine* (Chicago: A. Arend, 1874), https://books.google.com/books?id=leQrAQAAMAAJ&printsec=frontcover&source=gbs_ge_summary_r&cad=0#v=onepage&q&f=false.

6. The most thorough account of Garfield's shooting and subsequent medical ordeal is Candice Millard, *Destiny of the Republic: A Tale of Madness, Medicine, and the Murder of a President* (New York: Doubleday, 2011).

7. Robert Reyburn, "Clinical History of the Case of President James Abram Garfield." This account, by one of the attending physicians, was serialized in the *Journal of the American Medical Association* in seven installments beginning on March 24, 1894, and ending on May 5, 1894. Reference is to a version self-published by Reyburn in one volume, https://babel.hathitrust.org/cgi/pt?id=chi.37460527&view=1up&seq=9&skin=2021, p. 43.

8. "Koumiss," *Scientific American* 45, no. 10, new series (September 3, 1881): 144, https://books.google.com/books?id=XyozAQAAMAAJ&pg=PA144&lpg=PA144&dq=koumiss+%2B+treatment+%2B+President+Garfield.

9. *The Letters of Mark Twain and Joseph Hopkins Twichell,* ed. Harold K. Bush, Steve Courtney, and Peter Messent (Atlanta: University of Georgia Press, 2017), 113–114.

10. Mary F. Henderson, *Diet for the Sick* (New York: Harper & Brothers, 1885), 31–38.

11. Fannie Merritt Farmer, *The Boston Cooking-School Cook Book* (Boston: Little, Brown, 1896, rept. Levin Associates, 1996), 496; Fannie Merritt Farmer, *Food and Cookery for the Sick and Convalescent,* rev. ed. (Boston: Little, Brown, 1915), 81.

12. Samuel Purchas, *Hakluytus Posthumus, or Purchas His Pilgrimages: Containing a History of the World in Sea Voyages and Land Travells by Englishmen and Others,* vol. 9 (Glasgow: James McLehose and Sons, 1905), 379, https://archive.org/details/hakluytusposthum09purc/page/n7/mode/2up.

13. W. Eton, *A Survey of the Turkish Empire,* 2nd ed. (London: T. Cadell and W. Davies, 1799), 240–241, https://books.google.com/books?id=fjMOAAAAQAAJ&printsec=frontcover&source=gbs_ge_summary_r&cad=0#v=onepage&q&f=false.

14. J. Griffiths, *Travels in Europe, Asia Minor, and Arabia* (London: T. Cadell, W. Davies, and Peter Hill, 1805), 113, https://archive.org/details/39020025955355-travelsineurope/page/n9/mode/2up.

15. *A Hand-Book for Travellers in the Ionian Islands, Greece, Turkey, Asia Minor, and Constantinople* (London: John Murray, 1840), viii, https://archive.org/details/b22020822/page/n19/mode/2up.

16. *Handbook for Travellers in Asia Minor, Transcaucasia, Persia, etc.,* ed. Charles Wilson (London: John Murray, 1895), 13, https://babel.hathitrust.org/cgi/pt?id=hvd.32044024585200&view=1up&seq=33&skin=2021.

17. "Matzoon, or Fermented Cows' Milk," paper by Dr. Dadirrian presented at a meeting of the New York Academy of Medicine, June 18, 1885, *The Medical Record* 28 no. 1 (July 2, 1885): 24–25, https://babel.hathitrust.org/cgi/pt?id=chi.78915934&view=1up&seq=34&skin=2021.

18. Advertisement with registered trademark, *Medical and Surgical Register of the United States* (Detroit, MI: R.L. Polk, 1890), 755, https://babel.hathitrust.org/cgi/pt?id=uiug.30112071223207&view=1up&seq=738&skin=2021.

19. Dadirrian v. Yacubian et al. (1898), https://cite.case.law/f/90/812/; Dr. Dadirrian & Sons Co., Plaintiff, v. William Hauenstein, Defendant, The Miscellaneous Reports of the Cases Decided in the Courts of Record in the State of New York, vol. 37

(Albany: James B. Lyon, 1902), 25, https://books.google.com/books?id=5G4LAAAAYAAJ
&pg=PA23&lpg=PA23&dq=Hauenstein+%2B+matzoon.

20. *The Federal Reporter* 80 (June–July, 1897), Dadirrian v. Gullian et al., 986–988, https://books
.google.com/books?id=KnsnhQfZBdsC&pg=PA987&lpg=PA987&dq=Dadirrian
+%2B+lebben.

21. H. W. Conn and W. M. Esten, "The Comparative Growth of Different Species of Bacteria
in Normal Milk," *Fourteenth Annual Report of the Storrs Agricultural Experiment Station*,
Storrs, CT, 1901, 14, https://babel.hathitrust.org/cgi/pt?id=ucw.ark:/13960/t2h717827
&view=2up&seq=4&skin=2021.

22. Conn and Esten, "The Comparative Growth of Different Species," 15.

23. J. Allan Downie and J. Peter W. Young, "The ABC of Symbiosis," *Nature* 412 (August 9,
2001): 597, https://www.nature.com/articles/35088167?proof=t.

24. Herbert C. Friedmann, "Escherich and Escherichia," *Advances in Applied Microbiology* 60 (2006): 133–196, reissued in *EcoSalPlus* 6 no 1 (2014), https://journals.asm.org
/doi/10.1128/ecosalplus.ESP-0025-2013.

25. Ernst Moro, "Ueber den Bacillus acidophilus n. spec.: Ein Beitrag zur Kenntnis
der normalen Darmbacterien des Säuglings," *Jahrbuch für Kinderheilkunde und
Physische Erziehung*, vol. 52 (Berlin: Verlag von S. Karger, 1900), 38–55, https://books
.google.com/books?id=WNZDAQAAMAAJ&pg=PA39&lpg=PA39&dq=%22Ernst
+Moro%22+%2B+%22Ueber+den+Bacillus+acidophilus+n.spec.%22.

26. Henry Tissier, *Recherches sur la flore intestinale de nourrisons (Etat normal et
pathologique)* (Paris: Georges Carré et C. Naud, 1900), 85–96, https://archive.org
/details/BIUSante_TPAR1900x529/page/n3/mode/2up.

27. Henry Tissier, "Etude d'une variété d'infection intestinale," *Annales de l'Institut
Pasteur*, 19me année, no. 5 (May, 1905): 273, 297, https://babel.hathitrust.org/cgi
/pt?id=uc1.b3749555&view=2up&seq=314&skin=2021.

28. Robert P. Hudson, "Theory and Therapy: Ptosis, Stasis, and Autointoxication,"
Bulletin of the History of Medicine 63 no.3 (Fall 1989): 396–397, https://www.jstor
.org/stable/44447619?read-now=1&refreqid=excelsior%3A77c6bad31e38a8f6d386257
dca717828&seq=1#metadata_info_tab_contents.

29. "Russia Mourns the Death of Metchnikoff," *American Review of Reviews* 54
(September 1916): 331, https://babel.hathitrust.org/cgi/pt?id=hvd.hn46be&view=1up
&seq=13&skin=2019.

30. Stamen Grigorov, "Etude sur un lait fermenté comestible. Le 'Kissélo-mléko' de Bulgarie,"
Revue médicale de la Suisse romande, 25 année, no. 10 (October 20, 1905): 714–721,
https://babel.hathitrust.org/cgi/pt?id=hvd.hn46be&view=1up&seq=13&skin=2019.

31. Elie Metchnikoff, *Quelques Remarques sur le Lait Aigri* (Paris: E. Rémy, 1908), 21, 25–27,
https://hal-pasteur.archives-ouvertes.fr/pasteur-00724105v2/document.

32. Luba Vihanski, *Immunity: How Elie Metchnikoff Changed the Course of Modern Medicine* (Chicago: Chicago Review Press, 2016), 162–163.

33. Vihanski, *Immunity*, 178.

34. Advertisement for Zoolak, *New York Times*, April 22, 1906, 23.

35. Walter L. Kulp and Leo F. Rettger, "Comparative Study of Lactobacillus acidophilus
and Lactobacillus bulgaricus," *Journal of Bacteriology* 9, no. 4 (July 1924): 357–395,

https://babel.hathitrust.org/cgi/pt?id=mdp.39015023787578&view=2up&seq=10&skin=2021.

36. Leo F. Rettger and Harry A. Cheplin, "Bacillus Acidophilus and Its Therapeutic Application," *Archives of Internal Medicine* 29, no. 3 (March 1922): 357–367, https://babel.hathitrust.org/cgi/pt?id=uiug.30112039493264&view=2up&seq=10&skin=2021.

37. Grigorov, "Etude sur un lait fermenté," 721.

38. See, for example, *Kansas Agitator*, May 19, 1905, https://chroniclingamerica.loc.gov/lccn/sn83040052/1905-05-19/ed-1/seq-3/.

39. Harold McGee, *On Food and Cooking: The Science and Lore of the Kitchen*, rev. ed. (New York: Scribner, 2004), 48.

40. Philippe Marteau et al., "Effect of the Microbial Lactase (*EC* 3.2.1.23) Activity in Yoghurt on the Intestinal Absorption of Lactose: An In Vivo Study in Lactase-Deficient Humans," *British Journal of Nutrition* 64 (1990): 71–79: https://www.cambridge.org/core/services/aop-cambridge-core/content/view/C8B73A84123B0F13C0FC874FA1036430/S000711459000085Xa.pdf.

41. The principle of "community" stability is usefully summarized in Sandor Ellix Katz, *The Art of Fermentation* (White River Junction, VT: Chelsea Green, 2012).

42. Nicholas Kopeloff, *Man vs. Microbes* (New York: Knopf, 1930), 132–135; Chester Linwood Roadhouse and James Lloyd Henderson, *The Market Milk Industry* (New York: McGraw-Hill, 1950), 427–430.

43. S. Josephine Baker, *Fighting for Life* (New York: Macmillan, 1939, rept. New York Review Books, 2013), 250.

44. Henry G. Piffard, "The Milk Problem," *New York Medical Journal* 85, no. 17 (April 27, 1907): 773–778, https://archive.org/details/newyorkmedicaljo8519unse/page/n787/mode/2up.

45. Henry G. Piffard, "A Study of Sour Milks," *New York Medical Journal* 87, no. 1 (January 4, 1908): 1–8, https://archive.org/details/newyorkmedicaljo8719unse/page/n9/mode/2up.

46. Piffard, "A Study of Sour Milks," 6–7.

47. Piffard, "A Study of Sour Milks," 8.

48. "Topics of the Times," *New York Times*, January 8, 1908, 8.

49. J. H. Kellogg, *The Battle Creek Sanitarium System: History, Organization, Methods* (Battle Creek, MI: Modern Medicine, 1908), 13, https://books.google.com/books?id=GUoJAAAAIAAJ&printsec=frontcover&source=gbs_ge_summary_r&cad=0#v=onepage&q&f=false.

50. Howard Markel, *The Kelloggs: The Battling Brothers of Battle Creek* (New York: Pantheon, 2017), 170.

51. *The Gospel of Health* 3, no. 7 (July 1899): 127, https://documents.adventistarchives.org/Periodicals/GOH/GOH18990701-V03-07.pdf.

52. J. H. Kellogg, "A Remarkable Discovery," *Good Health* 42, no. 11 (November 1907): 612–613, https://archive.org/details/good-health-volume-42-issue-11-november-1st-1907/page/n41/mode/2up.

53. Advertisement, "Friendly Germs for Sale by Mail," *New York Times*, November 24, 1907, The Times's Special Dispatches, 3.

54. *Collier's: The National Weekly*, January 4, 1908, 7.

55.   J. H. Kellogg, *The Uses of Water in Health and Disease* (Battle Creek, MI: Modern Medicine, 1876), https://babel.hathitrust.org/cgi/pt?id=loc.ark:/13960/t16m4f692&view=1up&seq=7&skin=2021.

56.   Kellogg, *The Battle Creek Sanitarium System*, 117–121, https://babel.hathitrust.org/cgi/pt?id=nyp.33433011428764&view=1up&seq=7&skin=2021.

57.   J. H. Kellogg, *Colon Hygiene* (Battle Creek, MI: Good Health Publishing), 169–174, 188–191, https://babel.hathitrust.org/cgi/pt?id=mdp.39015064546305&view=1up&seq=449&skin=2021.

58.   J. H. Kellogg, *Autointoxication or Intestinal Toxemia* (Battle Creek, MI: Modern Medicine Publishing, 1918), 134, 136, https://babel.hathitrust.org/cgi/pt?id=osu.32435081594095&view=1up&seq=335&skin=2021.

59.   Kellogg, *Colon Hygiene*, 370–388.

60.   Kellogg, *Autointoxication or Intestinal Toxemia*, 125–171, 196.

61.   J. H. Kellogg, *The New Dietetics: What to Eat and How* (Battle Creek, MI: Modern Medicine Publishing, 1921), 299–304, https://archive.org/details/newdietetics whaookellgoog/page/298/mode/2up?ref=ol&view=theater.

62.   For a detailed account of Kellogg's involvement with soy foods, see William Shurtleff and Akiko Aoyagi, "Dr. John Harvey Kellogg and Battle Creek Foods: Work with Soy" (Lafayette, CA: Soy Info Center, 2004), https://www.soyinfocenter.com/HSS/john_kellogg_and_battle_creek_foods.php.

63.   Kellogg's soy acidophilus patent: United States Patent Office, US Patent 1,982,994, "Method of Making Acidophilus Milk," December 4, 1934, https://patentimages.storage.googleapis.com/d2/a5/d9/e2d65fba2f0297/US1982994.pdf

64.   Markel, *The Kelloggs*, 332.

65.   Jia-Chen Fu, *The Other Milk: Reinventing Soy in Republican China* (Seattle: University of Washington Press, 2018).

66.   Kellogg, *Colon Hygiene*, 173.

67.   United States Patent Office, John Harvey Kellogg, of Battle Creek, Michigan; "Flaked Cereals and Process of Preparing Same," specification forming part of Letters Patent No. 558, 303, dated April 14, 1896, https://patentimages.storage.googleapis.com/54/89/59/6d9aad382846f0/US558393.pdf.

68.   R. H. Aders Plimmer, "On the Presence of Lactase in the Intestines of Animals and on the Adaptation of the Intestine to Lactose," *The Journal of Physiology* 35 (December 29, 1906): 20–31, https://physoc.onlinelibrary.wiley.com/doi/pdf/10.1113/jphysiol.1906.sp001178.

7. MILK FOR THE MASSES

1.   United States Congressional Serial Set, vol. 9922: *Report of the Federal Trade Commission on. the Sale and Distribution of Milk Products, Connecticut and Philadelphia Milksheds*, Appendix: Transcripts of Testimony, 255https://books.google.com/books?id=brpGAQAAIAAJ&pg=PA255&lpg=PA255&dq=%22We+will+identify+them+in+the+record+as+Chinese+puzzles%22.

2. E. Melanie DuPuis, *Nature's Perfect Food: How Milk Became America's Drink* (New York: New York University Press, 2002), 107.

3. *Report of the Mayor's Committee on Milk, City of New York* (New York, December 1917), 12–13, https://babel.hathitrust.org/cgi/pt?id=uc1.b4501356&view=1up&seq=5.

4. *Report of the Mayor's Committee on Milk*, 18–19.

5. *Report of the Mayor's Committee on Milk*, 20.

6. M. J. Rosenau, *The Milk Question* (Boston: Houghton Mifflin, 1912), 243–246.

7. Rosenau, *The Milk Question*, 245–246.

8. "The Dairy and the World Food Problem": Address by Herbert Hoover, United States Food Administrator, at the National Milk and Dairy Farm Exposition, New York City, May 25, 1918 (Washington, DC: Government Printing Office, 1918), 7, 11.

9. "The Dairy and the World Food Problem," 10, 7.

10. "The Dairy and the World Food Problem," 4, 13.

11. "The Dairy and the World Food Problem," 7, 8, 13.

12. Kenneth W. Bailey, *Marketing and Pricing of Milk and Dairy Products in the United States* (Ames: Iowa State University Press, 1997), 111.

13. DuPuis, *Nature's Perfect Food*, 198–200.

14. *National Dairy Council: An Organization—Not for Profit—to Advance Dairying, Agriculture and Soil Fertility* (Chicago: Office of the Council, 1916), foreword, n.p., https://babel.hathitrust.org/cgi/pt?id=coo.31924002926131&view=2up&seq=20&skin=2021.

15. *National Dairy Council*, 14, 26, 31–32, 35.

16. The State of Illinois, *First Annual Report of the Department of Agriculture*, July 1, 1917 to June 30, 1918, 25–30, https://books.google.com/books?id=W_M2AQAAIAAJ&pg=RA1-PA28&lpg=RA1-PA28&dq=Illinois+%2B+"Campaign+for+the+Dairy+Cow".

17. "Mayor Will Drink Milk for a Week," *New York Times*, June 5, 1921, 25.

18. *Report of the Mayor's Committee on Milk*, 73.

19. *Report of the Mayor's Committee on Milk*, 73–75.

20. Rosenau, *The Milk Question*, 242.

21. United States Department of Agriculture, *Yearbook 1922* (Washington, DC: Government Printing Office, 1923), 316, fig. 37, https://archive.org/details/yoa1922/page/317/mode/2up.

22. United States Department of Agriculture, *Yearbook 1922*, 317, Fig. 38.

23. Rosenau, *The Milk Question*, 242.

24. Rosenau, *The Milk Question*, 251.

25. Henry E. Alvord, "Dairy Development in the United States," in *Yearbook of the United States Department of Agriculture, 1899* (Washington, DC: Government Printing Office, 1900), 398, https://books.google.com/books?id=Dnz_IpgNjsIC&pg=PA381&lpg=PA381&dq=%22Henry+E.+Alvord%22+%2B+%22Dairy+Development+in+the+United+States%22.

26. C. H. Hapgood, "Cow Milking Apparatus," U.S. Patent 1,787,152, December 30, 1930, https://patentimages.storage.googleapis.com/ae/be/b0/576bfa053123ff/US1787152.pdf.

27. Sheila Hibben, *The National Cookbook: A Kitchen Americana* (New York: Harper & Brothers, 1932), 218–219.

28. *The Picayune's Creole Cook Book*, 2nd ed. (New Orleans: The Picayune, 1924; rept. New York: Dover Editions, 1971), 199–200.

29. Leslie C. Frank, "A State-Wide Milk Sanitation Program," *Public Health Reports* 39, no. 45 (November 7, 1924): 2767, https://www.ncbi.nlm.nih.gov/pmc/articles/PMC1975986/pdf/pubhealthrepor1902537-0001.pdf.

30. Frank, "A State-Wide Milk Sanitation Program," 2769–2770, 2780–2782.

31. Frank, "A State-Wide Milk Sanitation Program," 2780–2783.

32. Frank, "A State-Wide Milk Sanitation Program," 2770.

33. "Report of the Committee on Uniform Standard Milk Ordinance, Conference of State and Territorial Health Officers, 1926," *Public Health Reports* 41, no. 31 (July 30, 1926): 1575, 1603.

34. "Report of the Committee on Uniform Standard Milk Ordinance," 1579.

35. *Public and Local Acts of the Legislature of the State of Michigan, Passed at the Regular Session of 1947* (Lansing, MI: Franklin De Kleine, State Printers, 1947), 459–461, Act No. 291, https://babel.hathitrust.org/cgi/pt?id=mdp.39015034782576&view=page&seq=491&skin=2021.

36. Irene Till, "Milk: The Politics of an Industry," in Walton Hamilton et al, *Price and Price Policies* (New York: McGraw-Hill, 1938), 445.

37. Till, "Milk," 447.

38. Till, "Milk," 457.

39. Till, "Milk," 452.

40. Till, "Milk," 438, 439.

41. Till, "Milk," 524.

42. Alden C. Manchester, *The Public Role in the Dairy Economy: Why and How Governments Intervene in the Milk Business* (Boulder, CO: Westview Press, 1983), 24.

43. John D. Black, *The Dairy Industry and the AAA* (Washington, DC: Brookings Institution, 1935), 73, 78–80.

44. *Steagall Commodity Credit Act*, http://nationalaglawcenter.org/wp-content/uploads/assets/farmbills/steagall1941.pdf.

45. *Agricultural Act of 1948*, http://nationalaglawcenter.org/wp-content/uploads/assets/farmbills/1948.pdf; Agricultural Act of 1949, https://28xeuf2otxva18q7lx1uemec-wpengine.netdna-ssl.com/wp-content/uploads/assets/farmbills/1949.pdf.

46. See the chapter "Federal Milk Marketing Orders" in Bailey, *Marketing and Pricing of Milk*, 109–14.

47. American Dairy Products Institute, "Milk Pricing 101," *ADPI Intelligence*, 4, no. 6, summary, https://www.adpi.org/Portals/0/Academy/Milk%20Pricing%20101.pdf.

48. *Hearings Before the Committee on Banking and Currency*, United States Senate, Seventy-ninth Congress, Second Session, on S. 2028, vol. 1, April 15–May 1, 1946 (Washington, DC: Government Printing Office, 1946), 725, figures from National Cooperative Milk Producers Federation, https://books.google.com/books?id=a5FFAQAAMAAJ&pg=PA725&lpg=PA725&dq=1945+%2B+total+US+milk+production+%2B+%22122,219,000,000+pounds%22.

49. Don P. Blayney, *The Changing Landscape of U.S. Milk Production*, USDA Statistical Bulletin No. 978, June 2002, p. 6, table 3, https://www.ers.usda.gov/webdocs/publications/47162/17864_sb978_1_.pdf?v=41056.

50. USDA *Census of Agriculture*, 1940, vol. 3, General Report, part 7: Livestock and Livestock Products, 572.

51. United States Department of Agriculture, Bureau of Agricultural Economics, *The Dairy Situation: Farm Production, Disposition, and Income from Milk, 1944–45, and Miscellaneous Statistics*, September 1946 (DS 177), 10 and 23. https://books.google.com /books?id=H8ZGAQAAIAAJ&pg=PP1&lpg=PP1&dq=%22Farm+Production,+Disposition, +and+Income+from+Milk,+1944+-45%22; Blayney, *Changing Landscape*, p. 2, table 1.

52. Blayney, *Changing Landscape*, 22 (appendix table 2).

53. Figures are from Blayney, *Changing Landscape*, p. 22, appendix table 2, and p. 2, table 1.

54. Charles E. North, "The Milk Industry and the War," *American Journal of Public Health* 9, no. 4 (April 1919): 266, https://www.ncbi.nlm.nih.gov/pmc/articles/PMC1362434/pdf /amjphealth00212-0019.pdf.

8. TECHNOLOGY IN OVERDRIVE I

1. Joel G. Winkjer, "Cooperative Bull Associations," *Farmers' Bulletin 993* (Washington, DC: United States Department of Agriculture, July 1918), https://naldc.nal.usda.gov /download/5421129/PDF.

2. R. H. Foote, "The History of Artificial Insemination: Selected Notes and Notables," *Journal of Animal Science* 80 (January 2, 2002): 3–6, https://www.asas.org/docs/default -source/midwest/mw2020/publications/footehist.pdf?sfvrsn=59da6c07_0; Michael D. Smith, Rodney D. Geisert, and John J. Parrish, "Reproduction in Domestic Ruminants During the Past 50 Years: Discovery to Application," *Journal of Animal Science* 96 no. 7 (July 2018): 2952–2970, https://www.ncbi.nlm.nih.gov/pmc/articles/PMC6095338/.

3. Chad Dechow, "U.S. Breed Composition Has Been Slowly Shifting," *Hoard's Dairyman* (July 15, 2015), 469.

4. For a description of the process, see "Embryo Transfer in the Dairy Herd," Mississippi State University Extension Publication No. P2682, 1–6, https://extension.msstate.edu /sites/default/files/publications/publications/p2682_web.pdf.

5. Michael L. O'Connor and Jana L. Peters, "Artificial Insemination Technique," Penn State Extension (July 2, 2012), https://extension.psu.edu/artificial-insemination-technique.

6. Xiang-Peng Yue, Chad Dechow, and Wan-Shen Liu, "A Limited Number of Y Chromosomes Is Present in North American Holsteins," *Journal of Dairy Science* 98, no. 4 (April 2015): 2738–2745, https://www.sciencedirect.com/science/article/pii /S0022030215000727; M. C. Lucy, "Reproductive Loss in High-Producing Dairy Cattle: Where Will It End?," *Journal of Dairy Science* 84, no. 6 (June 2001): 1277–1293, https://pubmed.ncbi.nlm.nih.gov/11417685/.

7. United States Census: *Urban Area Facts*, https://www.census.gov/programs-surveys /geography/guidance/geo-areas/urban-rural/ua-facts.html.

8. R. M. Washburn, *Productive Dairying*, 2nd ed. (Philadelphia: Lippincott, 1922), 36, https://books.google.com/books?id=qOAqAQAAMAAJ&pg=PA42&lpg=PA42&dq =cows+%2B+%22dairy+type%22+%2B+%22less+flesh%22.

9.   Washburn, *Productive Dairying*, 33.

10. "Breeds of Dairy Cattle," Circular 543, University of Illinois College of Agriculture Extension Service in Agriculture and Home Economics (Urbana, December 1942), 24, 34, https://core.ac.uk/download/pdf/10200452.pdf.

11. Henry E. Alvord, "Breeds of Dairy Cattle," U.S. Department of Agriculture Farmers' Bulletin No. 106 (Washington, DC: Government Printing Office, 1899), 26, 32, https://babel.hathitrust.org/cgi/pt?id=uiug.30112019279394&view=1up&seq=1&skin=2021.

12. Kelli Boylan, "Selz-Pralle Dairy Does Things Right," *Progressive Dairyman* (February 22, 2018), https://www.progressivedairy.com/topics/a-i-breeding/selz-pralle-dairy-does-things-right; Ashley Yager, "Wisconsin's Leading Production Ladies: Ever-Green-View Etax-ET," *Wisconsin Holstein News* 89, no. 4 (April 2017): 22, https://issuu.com/wiholstein/docs/april17wiholsteinnews.

13. Don P. Blayney, *The Changing Landscape of U.S. Milk Production*, United States Department of Agriculture Statistical Bulletin No. 978 (June 2002), 2, table 1, https://downloads.usda.library.cornell.edu/usda-esmis/files/h989r321c/7d279w693/f7624g40c/mkpr0222.pdf; USDA milk production figures as of February 23, 2020, released by National Agricultural Statistics Service, https://www.nass.usda.gov/Publications/Todays_Reports/reports/mkpr0220.pdf.

14. Barbara Orland, "Turbo-Cows: Producing a Competitive Animal in the Nineteenth and Early Twentieth Centuries," in *Industrializing Organisms: Introducing Evolutionary History*, ed. Susan R. Schrepfer and Philip Scranton (New York: Routledge, 2004), 167–189.

15. A. C. McCandlish, L. S. Gillette, and H. H. Kildee, "Influence of Environment and Breeding in Increasing Dairy Production—II," Agricultural Experiment Station, Iowa State College of Agriculture and Mechanic Arts, Bulletin No. 188 (March 1919), https://books.google.com/books?id=bCsnAQAAMAAJ&pg=PA65&lpg=PA65&dq=%22A.C.+McCandlish,L.S.+Gillette,+and+H.H.+Kildee%22.

16. Meggan Hain, "Answering Tough Questions About Cow-Calf Separation," *HD Notebook* (Hoard's Dairyman blog), May 12, 2021, https://hoards.com/blog-30175-answering-tough-questions-about-cow-calf-separation.html; Jennifer Bentley et al., "The Newborn Calf & Colostrum Management," Iowa State University Extension and Outreach, https://www.extension.iastate.edu/dairyteam/files/page/files/FINAL_Newborn%20calves%20%26%20Colostrum%20management.pdf.

17. Drought conditions may shorten the nursing period for beef calves. See Kris Ringwall, "How Early Is Too Early to Wean?," in Ohio BEEF Cattle Letter, Ohio State University Extension Beef Team, https://u.osu.edu/beef/2017/07/05/how-early-is-too-early-to-wean/.

18. Bovine Alliance on Management and Nutrition (BAMN), "A Guide to Calf Milk Replacers: Types, Use and Quantity," https://www.aphis.usda.gov/animal_health/nahms/dairy/downloads/bamn/BAMN08_GuideMilkRepl.pdf.

19. Andrew C. McCandlish, *The Feeding of Dairy Cattle* (New York: Wiley, 1922), 178–199, http://reader.library.cornell.edu/docviewer/digital?id=chla2758853#page/285/mode/1up.

20. McCandlish, *The Feeding of Dairy Cattle*, 34–35, 54–56, 265.

21. Ric R. Grummer, Doug G. Marshek, and A. Hayirli, "Dry Matter Intake and Energy Balance in the Transition Period," *Veterinary Clinics of North America and Food Animal Practice* 20 (December 2004): 447–470.

22. Howard D. Tyler and M. E. Ensminger, *Dairy Cattle Science*, 4th ed. (Upper Saddle River, NJ: Pearson/Prentice Hall, 2006), 389.

23. Tyler and Ensminger, *Dairy Cattle Science*, 394.

24. James E. Nocek, "Bovine Acidosis: Implications on Laminitis," *Journal of Dairy Science* 80, no. 5 (May 1997): 1005–1028, https://www.journalofdairyscience.org/article/S0022 -0302(97)76026-0/pdf; G. R. Oetzel, "Understanding the Impact of Subclinical Ketosis," paper delivered at the 24th Florida Ruminant Symposium, February 5–6, 2013, https:// animal.ifas.ufl.edu/apps/dairymedia/rns/2013/2_oetzel.pdf.

25. G. M. Jones and T. M. Bailey, Jr., "Understanding the Basics of Mastitis," Virginia Polytechnic Institute and State University, Cooperative Extension Publication No. 404–233, https://vtechworks.lib.vt.edu/bitstream/handle/10919/48392/404-233 _pdf.pdf?sequence=1.

26. Alvord, "Breeds of Dairy Cattle," 157, 163.

27. Michael Osmundson, "From 1950 to Present: The Evolution of 'Dairy Character,' " *Progressive Dairy*, January 17, 2014, https://www.progressivedairy.com/topics/a-i-breeding /from-1950-to-present-the-evolution-of-dairy-character.

28. Alvord, "Breeds of Dairy Cattle"; "Facts About Holstein Cattle," Holstein USA, https:// ww.holsteinusa.com/holstein_breed/holstein101.html?tab=2#TabbedPanels1.

29. Blayney, *The Changing Landscape*, 22, appendix table 2.

30. Blayney, *The Changing Landscape*, p. 6, table 3; United States Census Bureau, *Statistical Abstracts of the United States, 2001*: Section 17 (Agriculture), p. 543, table 842, https:// www.census.gov/prod/2002pubs/01statab/agricult.pdf.

31. *Report of the Mayor's Committee on Milk, City of New York* (New York: December, 1917), 73–75.

32. Blayney, *The Changing Landscape*, 8, table 5a.

33. James M. MacDonald, Jerry Cessna, and Roberto Mosheim, "Changing Structure, Financial Risks, and Government Policy for the U.S. Dairy Industry," United States Department of Agriculture, Economic Research Report No. 205 (March 2016), 7–8, figures 1 and 2, https://www.ers.usda.gov/webdocs/publications/45519/56833_err205 _errata.pdf?v=8453.8. See also James M. MacDonald, Jonathan Law, and Roberto Mosheim, "Consolidation in U.S. Dairy Farming," United States Department of Agriculture, Economic Research Report No. 274 (July 2020), 11n, https://www.ers.usda.gov /webdocs/publications/98901/err-274.pdf.

34. Tyler and Ensminger, *Dairy Cattle Science*, 116–121.

35. Tyler and Ensminger, *Dairy Cattle Science*, 217.

36. Kenneth W. Bailey, *Marketing and Pricing of Milk and Dairy Products in the United States* (Ames: Iowa State University Press, 1997), 175–176.

37. Jud Heinrichs and Alanna Kmicikewycz, "Total Mixed Rations for Dairy Cows," Penn State Extension (May 5, 2016), https://extension.psu.edu/total-mixed-rations-for -dairy-cows.

38. Tyler and Ensminger, *Dairy Cattle Science*, 98.

39. MacDonald et al., "Consolidation in U.S. Dairy Farming," 12–18, 40. For representative journalistic coverage of the new mega-dairy farms' environmental impact, see Lynne Terry, "While Small Dairy Farms Shut Down, This Mega-Dairy Is Shipping Milk to

China," *Civil Eats*, November 27, 2018, https://civileats.com/2018/11/27/while-small
-dairy-farms-shut-down-this-mega-dairy-is-shipping-milk-to-china/; Debbie Weingarten and Tony Davis, "A Mega-Dairy Is Transforming Arizona's Aquifer and Farming Lifestyles," *High Country News*, August 1, 2021, https://www.hcn.org/issues/53.8
/agriculture-a-mega-dairy-is-transforming-arizonas-aquifer-and-farming-lifestyles;
Debbie Weingarten, "'There are ghosts in the land': How US Mega-Dairies Are Killing
Off Small Farms," *The Guardian* (US ed.), June 1, 2021, https://www.theguardian.com
/environment/2021/jun/01/there-are-ghosts-in-the-land-how-us-mega-dairies-are
-killing-off-small-farms; Bradley W. Park, "Requiem for a Mega-Dairy: Bills Seek
Moratorium on Supersize Dairy Farms in Oregon," Oregon Public Broadcasting, January
28, 202,1 https://www.opb.org/article/2021/01/27/mega-dairy-oregon-moratorium/.

40.   Andrea Nüsse, "Tausende Liter Wasser für einen Liter Milch, *Der Tagesspiegel*, May 10,
2002, https://www.tagesspiegel.de/gesellschaft/panorama/tausende-liter-wasser-fuer-einen
-liter-milch/311198.html.

41.   Kelly McEvers, "The Cost of Making Milk in the Desert," *NPR Weekend Edition*, Sunday,
June 14, 2009, https://www.npr.org/templates/story/story.php?storyId=105381728;
"A Tour to Al-Safi Dairy Farm in Al Kharj Around Riyadh," https://lifeinsaudiarabia.
net/a-tour-to-al-safi-dairy-farm-in-a/; "California Dairies: Protecting Water Quality:
A Primer for Consultants, Local Government Agencies, and Lending Institutions,"
University of California Agriculture and Natural Resources Publication 21630, https://
anrcatalog.ucanr.edu/pdf/21630e.pdf.

42.   Okeyo Mwai et al., "African Indigenous Cattle: Unique Genetic Resources in a
Rapidly Changing World," *Asian-Australasian Journal of Animal Sciences* 28, no. 7
(July 2015): 911–921, https://www.animbiosci.org/journal/view.php?doi=10.5713/ajas
.15.0002R.

43.   Andrew Rice, "A Dying Breed," *New York Times Magazine*, January 27, 2008; see interview with the Ugandan farmer Jackson Sezibwa, https://www.nytimes.com/2008/01/27
/magazine/27cow-t.html.

44.   Dale E. Bauman et al., "Responses of High-Producing Dairy Cows to Long-Term
Treatment with Pituitary Somatotropin and Recombinant Somatotropin," *Journal of
Dairy Science* 68, no. 6 (June 1985): 1352–1362, https://www.journalofdairyscience.org/
article/S0022-0302(85)80972-3/pdf.

45.   The American Cancer Society declined to endorse claims about heightened cancer
risk: American Cancer Society, "Recombinant Bovine Growth Hormone," https://
www.cancer.org/cancer/cancer-causes/recombinant-bovine-growth-hormone.html
#references.

46.   DealBook, "Eli Lilly to Buy Monsanto's Dairy Cow Hormone for $300 Million," *New
York Times*, August 20, 2008.

47.   Dale E. Bauman, "Bovine Somatotropin: Review of an Emerging Animal Technology,"
Journal of Dairy Science 75, no. 12 (December 1992): 3432–3451, https://www.journalof
dairyscience.org/article/S0022-0302(92)78119-3/pdf.

48.   The U.S. and Canadian responses are compared and contrasted in Lisa Nicole Mills,
*Science and Social Context: The Regulation of Recombinant Bovine Growth Hormone in
North America* (Montreal: McGill-Queen's University Press, 2002).

49. Peter Singer, *Animal Liberation: A New Ethics for Our Treatment of Animals* (New York: New York Review of Books/Random House, 1975).

50. W. M. Rauw et al., "Undesirable Side Effects of Selection for High Production Efficiency in Farm Animals: A Review," *Livestock Production Science* 56 (October 1998): 15–33, https://www.journalofdairyscience.org/article/S0022-0302(92)78119-3/pdf.

51. Wilhelm Knaus, "Dairy Cows Trapped Between Performance Demands and Adaptability," *Journal of the Science of Food and Agriculture* 89, no. 7 (May 2009): 1107–1114. Article kindly forwarded to me by Professor Knaus.

52. Knaus, "Dairy Cows Trapped," 1109.

53. L. B. Hansen, "Consequences of Selection for Milk Yield from a Geneticist's Viewpoint," *Journal of Dairy Science* 83, no. 5 (May 2000): 1145–1150, https://www.journalof dairyscience.org/article/S0022-0302(00)74980-0/pdf.

54. John F. Oncken, "Cross Country: Giving red Holsteins Their Due," *The Capital* [Madison, WI] *Times*, April 21, 2011, https://madison.com/ct/business/cross_country /cross-country-giving-red-holsteins-their-due/article_861a98e2-6c63-11e0-a336 -001cc4c002e0.html.

55. Heather Smith Thomas, "ProCROSS Dairy Genetics Experiences Rapid Growth," *American Dairyman*, October 15, 2020, https://www.americandairymen.com/articles /procross-dairy-genetics-experiences-rapid-growth.

56. B. J. Heins, L. B. Hansen, and A. J. Seykora, "Production of Pure Holsteins Versus Crossbreds of Holstein with Normande, Montbeliarde, and Scandinavian Red," *Journal of Dairy Science* 89, no. 7 (July 1, 2006): 2799–2804, https://www.journalofdairyscience .org/article/S0022-0302(06)72356-6/fulltext#relatedArticles; B. J. Heins, L. B. Hansen, and A. J. Seykora, "Fertility and Survival of Pure Holsteins Versus Crossbreds of Holsteins with Normande, Montbeliarde, and Scandinavian Red," *Journal of Dairy Science* 89, no. 12 (December 2006): 4944–4951.

57. U.S. Food and Drug Administration, *Code of Federal Regulations*, Title 21, chapter I, sub-chapter B—Food for Human Consumption, section 131.110(a), https://www.accessdata .fda.gov/scripts/cdrh/cfdocs/cfcfr/CFRSearch.cfm?CFRPart=131&showFR=1.

58. Rice, "A Dying Breed."

59. Chad Dechow, "Holstein Lineages Trace Back to Two Bulls," *Hoard's Dairyman*, October 25, 2019, https://hoards.com/article-26608-holstein-lineages-trace-back-to -two-bulls.html; Maureen O' Hagan, "From Two Bulls, Nine Million Dairy Cows," *Scientific American*, June 20, 2019, https://www.scientificamerican.com/article/from -two-bulls-nine-million-dairy-cows/; Sarah Zhang, "The Dairy Industry Lost $420 Million from a Flaw in a Single Bull," *The Atlantic*, October 31, 2016, https://www .theatlantic.com/health/archive/2016/10/the-dairy-industry-lost-420-million-from-a -flaw-in-a-single-bull/505616/.

60. "Holsteins Born at Penn State to Improve Genetic Diversity Are 'Udderly' Amazing," *Penn State News*, May 21, 2018, https://www.psu.edu/news/research/story/holsteins -born-penn-state-improve-genetic-diversity-are-udderly-amazing/; Christy Achen, "Flashback Friday: What 1960's Holstein Genetics Look Like Today," *Hoard's Dairyman*, June 29, 2018, https://hoards.com/blog-23429-flashback-friday-what-1960s-holstein -genetics-look-like-today.html.

61. VikingGenetics advertisement, "Breed Naturally Healthy Cows," https://www.vikinggenetics.com/dairy.

62. Michael Laris, "Herd Round the World," *Washington Post*, June 30, 2002, https://www.washingtonpost.com/archive/politics/2002/06/30/herd-round-the-world/31b57773-5eb6-4032-9bd9-3b8924719657/.

63. World Wide Sires, "Global Impact: The Revolution of an Industry," https://issuu.com/wwsires/docs/05_16_hi_insert_eng.

64. Les Hansen, "The Impact of Genomics on Rapid Increase of Inbreeding of Holsteins," *Progressive Dairy*, April 17, 2020, https://www.progressivedairy.com/topics/a-i-breeding/the-impact-of-genomics-on-rapid-increase-of-inbreeding-of-holsteins.

65. Andrew Martin and *Tribune* national correspondent, "Wisconsin Dairy Feels Squeeze," *Chicago Tribune*, December 24, 2004, https://www.chicagotribune.com/news/ct-xpm-2004-12-24-0412240218-story.html; Beth Newhart, "Are Idaho and Texas the Future of US Dairy?," *Dairy Reporter*, August 27, 2019, https://www.dairyreporter.com/Article/2019/08/27/Are-Idaho-and-Texas-the-future-of-US-dairy.

9. TECHNOLOGY IN OVERDRIVE II

1. *Report of the 1916 New York State "Wicks Committee,"* quoted in *Report of the Mayor's Committee on Milk, City of New York* (New York, December 1917), 27–28.

2. Stefan Pilz et al., "Rationale and Plan for Vitamin D Food Fortification: A Review and Guidance Paper," *Frontiers in Endocrinology* 9 (July 17, 2018); scroll to History of Vitamin D Food Fortification, https://www.ncbi.nlm.nih.gov/pmc/articles/PMC6056629/.

3. G. Malcolm Trout, *Homogenized Milk: A Review and Guide* (East Lansing: Michigan State College Press, 1950), 5–10. "Gaulin Homogenizer" is still the trade name for a line of American homogenizers descended from Gaulin's original.

4. United States Patent Office, A. Gaulin, of Paris, France, "System for Intimately Mixing Milk," Letters Patent No. 756,953, patented April 12, 1904, https://patentimages.storage.googleapis.com/f5/ca/60/3331d44840d3cc/US756953.pdf.

5. Trout, *Homogenized Milk*, 61–68.

6. The claims for homogenized milk's superior digestibility were based on the theory that cows' milk arriving in the stomach presented obstacles to digestion because it formed a comparatively hard, tough curd. Experts had established that homogenized milk had a lower "curd tension" than unhomogenized milk, meaning that it formed a softer curd. See Trout, *Homogenized Milk*, 30–35.

7. See entry "homogenization" in *The Oxford Companion to Cheese*, ed. Catherine Donnelly (New York: Oxford University Press, 2016), 360–361. The lower curd tension of homogenized milk also interferes with proper curd formation for aged or ripened cheeses.

8. Raymond B. Becker, *Dairy Cattle Breeds: Origin and Development* (Gainesville: University of Florida Press, 1973), 223.

9. Mark Kurlansky, *Milk! A 10,000-Year Food Fracas* (New York: Bloomsbury, 2018), 190.

10. B. L. Herrington, *Milk and Milk Processing* (New York: McGraw-Hill, 1948), 174.

11. Trout, *Homogenized Milk*, 100–103.

12. A thoughtful survey of Keys's diet-heart hypothesis and its reception in the medical community is Todd Olszewski, "The Causal Conundrum: The Diet-Heart Debates and the Management of Uncertainty in American Medicine," *Journal of the History of Medicine and Allied Sciences* 70, no. 2 (April 2015): 218–249.

13. *Dietary Goals for the United States*, prepared by the staff of the Select Committee on Nutrition and Human Needs, United States Senate (Washington, DC: U.S. Government Printing Office, February, 1977).

14. *Dietary Goals for the United States—Supplemental Views*, prepared by the staff of the Select Committee on Nutrition and Human Needs, United States Senate (Washington, DC: U.S. Government Printing Office, November, 1977).

15. *Dietary Goals for the United States—Supplemental Views*, 623.

16. *Dietary Goals for the United States*, 2d ed., prepared by the staff of the Select Committee on Nutrition and Human Needs, United States Senate (Washington, DC: U.S. Government Printing Office, December, 1977), 4, item 5 (changed from version on page 13, item 4 of 1st ed.).

17. Ralph Selitzer, *The Dairy Industry in America* (New York: Dairy & Ice Cream Field and Books for Industry, 1976), 78–83.

18. Lincoln M. Lampert, *Modern Dairy Products*, 3d ed. (New York: Chemical Publishing Company, 1975), 13, table 1.3.

19. *Code of Federal Regulations*, 7, Parts 210 and 220, "National School Lunch Program and School Breakfast Program: Nutrition Standards for All Foods Sold in School as Required by the Healthy, Hunger-Free Kids Act of 2010," Interim Final Rule, *Federal Register* 78, no. 125 (Friday, June 28, 2013): 39069, https://www.govinfo.gov/content/pkg/FR-2013-06-28/pdf/2013-15249.pdf.

20. John Lloyd and James Cheyne, "The Origins of the Vaccine Cold Chain and a Glimpse of the Future," *Vaccine* 35, no. 17 (April 9, 2017): 2115–2120, https://www.sciencedirect.com/science/article/pii/S0264410X17300476?via%3Dihub.

21. Leslie C. Frank, "A State-Wide Milk Sanitation Program," *Public Health Reports* 39, no. 45 (November 1924): 2782, 2783, https://www.ncbi.nlm.nih.gov/pmc/articles/PMC1975986/pdf/pubhealthreporig02537-0001.

22. Mark Bushnell, "Then Again: Bulk Milk Tanks Altered the Family Farm Way of Life," *VTDigger*, January 13, 2019, https://vtdigger.org/2019/01/13/bulk-milk-tanks-altered-family-farm-way-life/.

23. Noel Stocker, "Progress in Farm-to-Plant Bulk Milk Handling," U.S. Department of Agriculture, Farmer Cooperative Service Circular 8 (November 1954), iv–v, https://ia903002.us.archive.org/13/items/progressinfarmto08stoc/progressinfarmto08stoc.pdf; Agricultural Experiment Station of the Alabama Polytechnic Institute, Circular No. 120, June, 1957, "Questions and Answers about Bulk Milk Tanks," https://aurora.auburn.edu/bitstream/handle/11200/1921/1117CIRC.pdf?sequence=1.

24. Chester Linwood Roadhouse and James Lloyd Henderson, *The Market Milk Industry* (New York: McGraw-Hill, 1950), 325–330.

25. National Dairy Development Board for Efficient Dairy Plant Operation, *Technews*, no. 46 (September–October 2003), "Control of Post Process Contamination of Milk," https://www.dairyknowledge.in/sites/default/files/technews_46.pdf.

26. Charles V. Morr and Ronald L. Richter, "Chemistry of Processing," in *Fundamentals of Dairy Chemistry*, 3d ed., ed. Noble P. Wong (New York: Van Nostrand Reinhold, 1988), 741.

27. Robert A. Wright, "Plastic Is New Entry in Battle of the Milk Bottles," *New York Times*, August 2, 1964.

28. Selitzer, *The Dairy Industry in America*, 365–368.

29. National Dairy Development Board for Efficient Dairy Plant Operation, *Technews*, no. 52 (September–October 2004), "Biofilms in Dairy Plants," https://www.dairy knowledge.in/sites/default/files/technews_52.pdf.

30. Amy C. Lee Wong, "Biofilms in Food Processing Environments," *Journal of Dairy Science* 81, no. 10 (October 1998): 2765–2770, https://www.journalofdairyscience.org /article/S0022-0302(98)75834-5/pdf.

31. Catherine W. Donnelly, "Listeria Monocytogenes: A Continuing Challenge," *Nutrition Reviews* 59, no. 6 (June 2001): 183–194, https://academic.oup.com/nutritionreviews /article/59/6/183/1934329.

32. Lisa Schnirring, "Sheep Among Many Suspects in Farm Listeria Probe," University of Minnesota Center for Infectious Disease Research and Policy (CIDRAP), October 5, 2011, https://www.cidrap.umn.edu/news-perspective/2011/10/sheep-among -many-suspects-farm-listeria-probe.

33. For a comprehensive summary of the issues, see Anna Rovid Spickler, fact sheet "Listeriosis," Center for Food Security & Public Health, Iowa State University College of Veterinary Medicine, May, 2019, https://www.cfsph.iastate.edu/Factsheets/pdfs /listeriosis.pdf.

34. R. B. Elliott et al., "Type 1 (Insulin-Dependent) Diabetes Mellitus and Cow Milk: Casein Variant Consumption," *Diabetologia* 42 (1999): 292–296, https://link.springer .com/content/pdf/10.1007/s001250051153.pdf.

35. Keith Woodford, *Devil in the Milk: Illness, Health, and the Politics of A1 and A2 Milk* (White River Junction, VT: Chelsea Green Publishing, 2007), 21–22.

36. Daniela Küllenberg de Gaudry et al., "Milk A1 β-Casein and Health-Related Outcomes in Humans: A Systematic Review," *Nutrition Reviews* 77, no. 5 (May 2919): 278–306, https://academic.oup.com/nutritionreviews/article/77/5/278/5307073.

37. Rosalie Marion Bliss, "Transgenic Cows Resist Mastitis-Causing Bacteria," USDA Agricultural Research Service, April 4, 2005, https://www.ars.usda.gov/news-events /news/research-news/2005/transgenic-cows-resist-mastitis-causing-bacteria/.

38. Shefali Sharma and Zhang Rou, "China's Dairy Dilemma: The Evolution and Future Trends of China's Dairy Industry," Institute for Agriculture and Trade Policy, February 2014, 15–16, https://www.iatp.org/sites/default/files/2017-05/2017_05_03_Dairy Report_f_web.pdf.

39. Office of War Information, Washington, DC, "Vice President Henry G. [*sic*] Wallace's Address Before the Free World Association," May 8, 1942, http://www.ibiblio.org/pha /policy/1942/1942-05-08a.html. See also Hilary A. Smith, "Good Food, Bad Bodies:

Lactose Intolerance and the Rise of Milk Culture in China," in *Moral Foods: The Construction of Nutrition and Health in Modern Asia*, ed. Angela Ki Che Leung and Melissa L. Caldwell (Honolulu: University of Hawai'i Press, 2019), 262–284.

40. Bee Wilson, *First Bite: How We Learn to Eat* (New York: Basic Books, 2015), 222–225; Katarzyna J. Cwiertka, *Modern Japanese Cuisine: Food, Power and National Identity* (London: Reaktion Books, 2006), 157.

41. Sharma and Zhang, "China's Dairy Dilemma," 13.

42. "Genetically Engineered, Low-Lactose Dairy Calf Bred in China," Xinhua, June 11, 2012, http://www.china.org.cn/china/2012-06/11/content_25621439.htm.

43. Xiaohu Su et al., "Production of Microhomologous-Mediated Site-Specific Integrated LacS Gene Cow Using TALENs," *Theriogenology* 119 (October 1, 2018): 282–288, https://www.sciencedirect.com/science/article/abs/pii/S0093691X18305016.

44. Götz Laible et al., "Increased Gene Dosage for β- and κ-Casein in Transgenic Cattle Improves Milk Composition Through Complex Effects," *Nature: Scientific Reports* 6 (November 23, 2016), https://www.nature.com/articles/srep37607.

45. Charles Choi, "ATryn, on Old MacDonald's Pharm," *Scientific American*, September 2006, reposted January 10, 2009, https://www.scientificamerican.com/article/atryn-pharming-goats-transgenic/; Rodney Joyce, "Human Gene in Cow's Milk Part of MS Treatment Test," Reuters, August 24, 1999, https://www.iatp.org/news/human-gene-in-cows-milk-part-of-ms-treatment-test.

10. REVIVING THE RAW MILK CAUSE

1.   Otto Carqué, *Rational Diet: An Advanced Treatise on the Food Question* (Los Angeles: Times-Mirror Press, 1923), 450, https://babel.hathitrust.org/cgi/pt?id=ucbk.ark:/28722/h2wj94&view=1up&seq=9&skin=2021.

2.   A thoughtful recent history of naturopathy, and its relationships with other contemporary alternative medical movements, is Susan E. Cayleff, *Nature's Path: A History of Naturopathic Healing in America* (Baltimore, MD: Johns Hopkins University Press, 2016).

3.   Bernarr Macfadden, *The Miracle of Milk: How to Use the Milk Diet Scientifically at Home* (New York: Macfadden Publications, 1923), 61–62, 72, https://babel.hathitrust.org/cgi/pt?id=coo.31924003432584&view=1up&seq=126&skin=2021.

4.   Macfadden, *The Miracle of Milk*, 103, 108.

5.   Elizabeth Fee, "Signing the US Medicare Act: A Long Political Struggle," *The Lancet: Perspectives: The Art of Medicine* 386 (July 25, 2015): 332–333, https://www.thelancet.com/pdfs/journals/lancet/PIIS0140-6736(15)61400-3.pdf.

6.   *Time* magazine, May 11, 1925, https://content.time.com/time/subscriber/article/0,33009,728468,00.html *Time Magazine*, May 11, 1925].

7.   Justia US Law, Public Citizen v. Heckler, 653 F. Supp. 1229 (D.D.C. 1987), https://law.justia.com/cases/federal/district-courts/FSupp/653/1229/2400650/.

8.   M. G. Enig et al., "Isomeric Trans Fatty Acids in the U.S. Diet" (abstract), *Journal of the American College of Nutrition* (October 1990), National Library of Medicine, https://pubmed.ncbi.nlm.nih.gov/2258534/.

9.   F. A. Kummerow, letter to Senator George McGovern, May 31, 1977, in *Dietary Goals for the United States—Supplemental Views*, prepared by the staff of the Select Committee on Nutrition and Human Needs, United States Senate (Washington, DC: U.S. Government Printing Office, November 1977),138.

10. Ronald P. Mensink and Martijn B. Katan, "Effect of Dietary Trans Fatty Acids on High-Density and Low-Density Lipoprotein Cholesterol Levels in Healthy Subjects," *New England Journal of Medicine* 323 (August 16, 1990): 439–445, https://www.nejm.org/doi/full/10.1056/nejm199008163230703.

11. CDC Newsroom, "Obesity Continues Climb Among American Adults," press release, October 4, 2000, https://www.cdc.gov/media/pressrel/r2k1004a.htm.

12. A useful historical survey is Ann F. La Berge, "How the Ideology of Low Fat Conquered America," *Journal of the History of Medicine and Allied Sciences* 63, no. 2 (April 2008): 139–177, https://academic.oup.com/jhmas/article/63/2/139/772615.

13. Nina Teicholz, *The Big Fat Surprise: Why Butter, Meat, and Cheese Belong in a Healthy Diet* (New York: Simon & Schuster, 2014), 247.

14. Weston A. Price, *Nutrition and Physical Degeneration*, 8th ed. (La Mesa, CA: Price-Pottenger Foundation, 2008). The book was originally published in 1939 by the New York medical publisher Paul B. Hoeber with the subtitle *A Comparison of Primitive and Modern Diets and Their Effects*, https://www.ecoboerderij-dehaan.nl/images/Tekstbestanden/Nutrition_and_Physical_Degeneration_-_Dr_Weston_A_Price_1939.pdf.

15. *New York Times*, March 5, 1994, letter to the editor ("Before You Take the Vegetarian Vow") from Sally W. Fallon and Mary G. Enig.

16. Sally Fallon with Pat Connolly and Mary G. Enig, *Nourishing Traditions: The Cookbook That Challenges Politically Correct Nutrition and the Diet Dictocrats* (San Diego: ProMotion Publishing, 1995). Second edition lists Sally Fallon with Mary G. Enig (Brandywine, MD: New Trends Publishing, 1999). All citations refer to second edition.

17. Geoffrey Morell, ND, J.p. https://heal.me/geoffrey-morell-naturopathic-doctor-energy-healer.

18. Fallon, *Nourishing Traditions*, back cover blurb.

19. Edward Howell, *The Status of Food Enzymes in Digestion and Metabolism* (Chicago: National Enzyme Company, 1946), 6, https://babel.hathitrust.org/cgi/pt?id=uc1.b4139489&view=1up&seq=1&skin=2021.

20. Fallon, *Nourishing Traditions*, 591.

21. Fallon, *Nourishing Traditions*, 576.

22. Gerald L. Geison, *The Private Science of Louis Pasteur* (Princeton, NJ: Princeton University Press, 1995), uses Pasteur's private laboratory notebooks to document frequent sleight of hand in his extrapolations from concrete data to eventual hypotheses.

23. In a *Nourishing Traditions* sidebar, pp. 146–47, Fallon Morell's close colleague Tom Valentine treats the microzyma theory and Béchamp's reported rebuttal of Pasteur's germ theory as facts.

24. Gerald Geison firmly rejects this claim: *The Private Science of Louis Pasteur*, 275.

25. Thomas S. Cowan and Sally Fallon Morell, *The Contagion Myth: Why Viruses (Including "Coronavirus") Are Not the Cause of Disease* (New York: Skyhorse Publishing, 2020).

26. R. Fuller, "A Review: Probiotics in Man and Animals," *Journal of Applied Bacteriology* 66 (1989): 365–378.

27. Dana Goodyear, "Raw Deal: California Cracks Down on an Underground Gourmet Club," *New Yorker*, April 23, 2012, https://www.newyorker.com/magazine/2012/04/30/raw-deal.

28. Hon. Ron Paul of Texas, in the House of Representatives, Wednesday, January 28, 2009, "Introduction of Legislation Allowing Interstate Shipment of Unpasteurized Milk," *Congressional Record*, Daily Edition, 155, no. 17, https://www.congress.gov/congressional-record/2009/01/28/extensions-of-remarks-section/article/E160-6.

29. Representative Thomas Massie "Representatives Massie & Pingree Introduce Bipartisan Bill to Allow Interstate Traffic of Raw Milk," press release, Washington, July 30, 2021, https://massie.house.gov/news/documentsingle.aspx?DocumentID=395374.

30. Farm to Consumer Legal Defense Fund, "Interactive Map," https://www.farmtoconsumer.org/raw-milk-nation-interactive-map/.

31. Not recent but still useful is the survey of emergent food-borne illnesses in Nicols Fox, *Spoiled: The Dangerous Truth About a Food Chain Gone Haywire* (New York: Basic Books, 1997).

32. See Fox, *Spoiled*, 217–260, for a detailed chronology of the Jack in the Box outbreak.

33. Bill Marler, blog, "Brianne Kiner—The 1993 Jack in the Box E. Coli Outbreak," https://billmarler.com/key_case/jack-in-the-box-e-coli-outbreak.

34. In *The Raw Milk Revolution: Behind America's Emerging Battle Over Food Rights* (White River Junction, VT: Chelsea Green Publishing, 2009), David E. Gumpert gives a detailed account of Chris Martin's illness and the later legal fallout, 24–33 and 132–152.

35. Chloe Sorvino, "This Secretive Billionaire Makes the Cheese for Pizza Hut, Domino's and Papa John's," *Forbes*, June 12, 2017, https://www.forbes.com/sites/chloesorvino/2017/05/23/james-leprino-exclusive-mozzarella-billionaire-cheese-pizza-hut-dominos-papa-johns/?sh=7c1a42594958.

36. Sheehan's written testimony to legislatures is updated from time to time to cite recent documentation of illnesses spread through raw milk, but the basic message has been repeated almost verbatim since 2006. A 2013 submission to the Nevada State Assembly is a representative sample. See https://www.leg.state.nv.us/Session/77th2013/Exhibits/Assembly/HHS/AHHS578I.pdf.

37. Linda Bren, "Got Milk? Make Sure It's Pasteurized," *FDA Consumer: The Magazine of the U.S. Food and Drug Administration* 38 no. 5 (September–October 2004): 29–31, https://foodsafety.wisc.edu/assets/pdf_Files/milk_pasteurized.pdf.

38. An Associated Press dispatch by Paul Elias circulated the news of the crackdown to many newspapers across the country on June 12, 2008. For a typical item, see https://www.montereyherald.com/2008/06/12/officials-crack-down-on-unpasteurized-milk/.

39. Thomas Bartlett, "The Raw Deal: The FDA Says It's Dangerous. Selling It Is Illegal. So Why Does an Avid Band of Devotees Swear by the Virtues of Unpasteurized Milk?," *Washington Post Lifestyle Magazine*, October 1, 2006, https://www.washingtonpost.com/archive/lifestyle/magazine/2006/10/01/the-raw-deal-span-classbankheadthe-fda-says-its-dangerous-selling-it-is-illegal-so-why-does-an-avid-band-of-devotees-swear-by-the-virtues-of-unpasteurized-milk-span/a519b231-cff2-4c98-9ea1-b708fe602904/.

40. Gumpert, in *The Raw Milk Revolution*, chronicles many episodes in the first decade of the WAPF-led campaign for raw milk in useful detail.

41. Solenne Costard et al., "Outbreak-Related Disease Burden Associated with Consuming Unpasteurized Cow's Milk and Cheese, United States, 2009–2014," Centers for Disease Control and Prevention, *Emerging Infectious Diseases* 23, no. 6 (June 2017), https://wwwnc.cdc.gov/eid/article/23/6/15-1603_article.

42. See description of BactoScan™ from a Canadian dairy industry think tank: https://lactanet.ca/en/how-does-a-bactoscan-work/.

43. Marion Nestle, *Food Politics: How the Food Industry Influences Nutrition and Health* (Berkeley: University of California Press, 2002), 238–239.

11. THE FUTURE

1. Jim Goodman, "Perdue to Small Farmers: Stop Whining, Your Demise Is Inevitable," *Wisconsin Examiner*, October 3, 2019, https://wisconsinexaminer.com/2019/10/03/perdue-to-small-farmers-stop-whining-your-demise-is-inevitable/.

2. Don P. Blayney, *The Changing Landscape of U.S. Milk Production*, United States Department of Agriculture Statistical Bulletin No. 978 (June 2001), p. 6, table 3, https://www.ers.usda.gov/webdocs/publications/47162/17864_sb978_1_.pdf?v=41056.

3. *Market Intel*, "USDA Report: U.S. Dairy Farm Numbers Continue to Decline," February 26, 2021, https://www.fb.org/market-intel/usda-report-u.s.-dairy-farm-numbers-continue-to-decline.

4. Debbie Weingarten, "America's Dairy Farms Are in Crisis and the Farm Bill Won't Help," *Talk Poverty*, June 7, 2018, https://talkpoverty.org/2018/06/07/americas-dairy-farms-crisis-farm-bill-wont-help/.

5. Henrich Brunke and Crystel Stanford, "Commodity Profile: Dairy Products," Agricultural Marketing Resource Center, Agricultural Issues Center, University of California at Davis, November 2003, https://aic.ucdavis.edu/profiles/dairy.pdf; "Cheese Industry Profile," Agricultural Marketing Resource Center, November, 2021, https://www.agmrc.org/commodities-products/livestock/dairy/cheese-industry-profile.

6. Estimate is from the website of the American Cheese Society (2020), https://www.cheesesociety.org/industry-data/.

7. Lloyd M. Smith, "Trends in Consumption of Dairy Foods," *Journal of Dairy Science* 65 (1982), https://www.journalofdairyscience.org/article/S0022-0302(82)82217-0/pdf; International Dairy Foods Association, "American Dairy Consumption Reaches All-Time High; Cheese, Butter and Yogurt Continue to Drive Growth for Dairy Industry," press release, September 14, 2020, https://www.idfa.org/news/american-dairy-consumption-reaches-all-time-high-cheese-butter-and-yogurt-continue-to-drive-growth-for-dairy-industry.

8. See the website https://www.rawmilkinstitute.org/.

9. Raw Milk Institute (RAWMI), "Common Standards," https://www.rawmilkinstitute.org/common-standards.

10. Cookson Beecher, "Farmers, Advocates Launch Raw Milk Institute," *Food Safety News*, September 28, 2011, https://www.foodsafetynews.com/2011/09/farmers-advocates-launch-raw-milk-institute/.

11. Max K. Hinds and William F. Johnstone, *Dairy Economics Handbook*, USDA Agriculture Handbook No. 138, Federal Extension Service, November 1958, p. 8, https://books.google.com/books?id=TXmH062_wNoC&pg=PA7&lpg=PA7&dq=per+capita+milk+consumption+%2B+1945+-+1950.

12. Agricultural Economic Insights (AEI), "US Dairy Consumption in 9 Charts," February 23, 2020, https://aei.ag/2020/02/23/u-s-dairy-consumption-trends-in-9-charts/; Jim Dickrell, "Per Capita Dairy Consumption: A Tale of Two Commodities," *Dairy Herd Management News*, October 28, 2020, https://www.dairyherd.com/news-news/business/capita-dairy-consumption-tale-two-commodities.

13. USDA, Bureau of Agricultural Economics, "Milk Cows and Production on Farms," February 15, 1946, https://downloads.usda.library.cornell.edu/usda-esmis/files/05741r719/pr76f6007/d504rp05m/MilkProdDa-02-15-1946.pdf; Blayney, *The Changing Landscape*, 2, table 1; *Market Intel*, "USDA Report: U.S. Dairy Farm Numbers."

14. Hayden Stewart et al., "Examining the Decline in U.S. Per Capita Consumption of Fluid Cows' Milk, 2003–18," USDA Economic Research Service, Economic Research Report No. (ERR-300), October 2021, https://www.ers.usda.gov/publications/pub-details/?pubid=102446.

15. General Accounting Office, Report to Congressional Requesters, "Dairy Termination Program: A Perspective on Its Participants and Milk Production," May 31, 1988, https://www.gao.gov/assets/rced-88-157.pdf.

16. Jim Cornall, "US Dairy Farmers Dumping Milk Due to Coronavirus Situation," *Dairy Reporter*, April 6, 2020, https://www.dairyreporter.com/Article/2020/04/06/US-dairy-farmers-dumping-milk-due-to-coronavirus-situation.

17. U.S. Dairy Export Council, Why U.S. Whey Protein, n.d., accessed September 7, 2022, https://www.thinkusadairy.org/products/whey-protein-and-ingredients/why-us-whey.

18. Katarzyna J. Cwiertka, *Modern Japanese Cuisine: Food, Power and National Identity* (London: Reaktion, 2006), 157–158. See also comment on Japan as a market for U.S. milk surpluses in a report prepared for Secretary of Agriculture Orville L. Freeman in 1962, W. B. Dickinson Jr., "Milk Surpluses," *Editorial Research Reports 1962*, 1 (1962), https://library.cqpress.com/cqresearcher/document.php?id=cqresrre1962050200.

19. Daniel Workman, "Top Milk Exporting Countries," https://www.worldstopexports.com/top-milk-exporting-countries/.

20. https://www.dsm.com/food-beverage/en_US/insights/insights/dairy/why-lactose-free-is-going-to-be-massive-in-asia.html.

21. S. S. F. Leung et al., "The Calcium Absorption of Chinese Children in Relation to Their Intake," *Hong Kong Medical Journal* 1, no. 1 (March 1995): 58–62, https://www.hkmj.org/system/files/hkm9503p58.pdf.

22. D. M. Hegsted, "Calcium and Osteoporosis," *Journal of Nutrition* (November 1986): 2316–2319. Andrea S. Wiley has called attention to the "calcium paradox" in *Re-imagining Milk* (New York: Routledge, 2011), 80.

23. Leung et al., "The Calcium Absorption of Chinese Children," 58.

24. J. Kanis et al., "A Systematic Review of Hip Fracture Incidence and Probability of Fracture Worldwide," *Osteoporosis International* (2012), https://www.ncbi.nlm.nih.gov /pmc/articles/PMC3421108/.

25. G. Aamodt et al., "Ethnic Differences in Risk of Hip Fracture in Norway: A NOREPOS Study," *Osteoporosis International* (2020), https://www.ncbi.nlm.nih.gov/pmc/articles /PMC7360634/.

26. Marc G. Hochberg, "Racial Differences in Bone Strength," *Transactions of the American Clinical and Climatological Association* 118 (2007): 305–315, https://www.ncbi.nlm.nih .gov/pmc/articles/PMC1863580/.

27. Jeffrey S. Passel and D'Vera Cohn, "U.S. Population Projections: 2005–2050," *Pew Research Center Report*, February 11, 2008, https://www.pewresearch.org/hispanic/2008 /02/11/us-population-projections-2005-2050/.

28. For a partial list of African fermented milk products, see Silvana Mattiello et al., "Typical Dairy Products in Africa from Local Animal Resources," *Italian Journal of Animal Science* 17, no. 3 (2018): https://www.tandfonline.com/doi/full/10.1080 /1828051X.2017.1401910. A remarkable account of smoked milk products among the Samburu people of Kenya is William Rubel, Jane Levi, and Elly Loldepe, "*Keata Kule Lorien*: Finding the ideal balance within the smoke-cured fresh and fermented milk of Northern Kenya's Samburu," in *Cured, Fermented and Smoked Foods: Proceedings from the Oxford Symposium on Food and Cookery 2010*, ed. Helen Saberi (Totnes, Devon: Prospect Books, 2011), 278–287.

29. Virginia Gewin, "What Mongolia's Dairy Farmers Have to Teach Us About the Hidden History of Microbes," *Sapiens Anthropology Magazine* 6 (February 2020), https://www .sapiens.org/archaeology/dairying-history-microbes/.

30. Choongwon Jeong et al., "Bronze Age Population Dynamics and the Rise of Dairy Pastoralism on the Eastern Eurasian Steppe," *PNAS* (November 27, 2018), https://www .pnas.org/content/115/48/E11248.

31. "Heirloom Microbes" project, http://christinawarinner.com/research-2/research-h/.

SELECT BIBLIOGRAPHY

Adams, Mark. *Mr. America: How Muscular Millionaire Bernarr Macfadden Transformed the Nation Through Sex, Salad, and the Ultimate Starvation Diet.* New York: HarperCollins, 2009.

Alvord, Henry E. "Breeds of Dairy Cattle." U.S. Department of Agriculture Farmers' Bulletin No. 106. Washington, DC: Government Printing Office, 1899.

Alvord, Henry E. "Dairy Development in the United States." In *Yearbook of the United States Department of Agriculture, 1899.* Washington, DC: Government Printing Office, 1900.

Anthony, David W. *The Horse, the Wheel, and Language: How Bronze-Age Riders from the Eurasian Steppes Shaped the Modern World.* Princeton, NJ: Princeton University Press, 2007.

Apple, Rima D. *Mothers & Medicine: A Social History of Infant Feeding, 1890–1950.* Madison: University of Wisconsin Press, 1987.

Apple, Rima D. *Vitamania: Vitamins in American Culture.* New Brunswick, NJ: Rutgers University Press, 1996.

Atkins, Peter W. *Liquid Materialities: A History of Milk, Science, and the Law.* Burlington, VT: Ashgate, 2010.

Bailey, Kenneth W. *Marketing and Pricing of Milk and Dairy Products in the United States.* Ames, IA: Iowa State University Press, 1997.

Baker, S. Josephine. *Fighting for Life.* New York: Macmillan, 1939. Reprint, New York: New York Review Books, 2013.

Bauman, Dale E. "Bovine Somatotropin: Review of an Emerging Animal Technology." *Journal of Dairy Science* 75, no. 12 (July 1992): 3432–3451.

Bauman, Dale E., Philip J. Eppard, Melvin J. DeGeeter, and Gregory M. Lanza. "Responses of High-Producing Dairy Cows to Long-Term Treatment with Pituitary Somatotropin and Recombinant Somatotropin 1,2." *Journal of Dairy Science* 68, no. 6 (June 1985): 1352–1362.

Bayless, Theodore M., and Norton S. Rosensweig. "A Racial Difference in Incidence of Lactase Deficiency: A Survey of Milk Intolerance and Lactase Deficiency in Healthy Adult Males." *Journal of the American Medical Association* 197, no. 12 (September 19, 1966): 138–142.

Becker, Raymond B. *Dairy Cattle Breeds: Origin and Development.* Gainesville: University of Florida Press, 1973.

Beecher, Cookson. "Farmers, Advocates Launch Raw Milk Institute." *Food Safety News,* September 28, 2011.

Bitter, H. "Versuche über das Pasteurisieren der Milch." *Zeitschrift für Hygiene* 8 (1890): 240–282.

Blayney, Don P. "The Changing Landscape of U.S. Milk Production." *USDA Statistical Bulletin no. 978* (June 2002).

Bogucki, Peter. "The Spread of Early Farming in Europe." *American Scientist* 84, no 3 (May 1996): 242–253.

Cadogan, William. *An Essay upon Nursing,* 4th ed. London: J. Roberts, 1750.

Caird, James. *English Agriculture in 1850–51,* 2nd ed. London: Longman, Brown, Green, and Longmans, 1852.

Cayleff, Susan E. *Nature's Path: A History of Naturopathic Healing in America.* Baltimore, MD: Johns Hopkins University Press, 2016.

Cheyne, George. *The English Malady: Or, a Treatise of Nervous Diseases of All Kinds.* London: S. Powell, 1733. Reprint, New York: Scholars' Facsimiles and Reprints, 1976.

Cheyne, George. *The Natural Method of Curing the Diseases of the Body, and the Disorders of the Mind,* 5th ed. London: Dan. Browne, R. Manby, J. Whiston, B. White, and A. Strahan, 1753.

Clarke, Joseph, "Observations on the Properties Commonly Attributed by Medical Writers to HUMAN MILK." *The Transactions of the Royal Irish Academy.* Dublin: George Bonham, 1788, 171–186.

Conn, H. W., and W. M. Esten. "The Comparative Growth of Different Species of Bacteria in Normal Milk." *Fourteenth Annual Report of the Storrs Agricultural Experiment Station.* Storrs, CT, 1901.

Cuatrecasas, Pedro, Dean H. Lockwood, and Jacques R. Caldwell. "Lactase Deficiency in the Adult: A Common Occurrence." *The Lancet* 285, no. 7375 (January 2, 1965): 14–18.

Cunliffe, Barry. *By Steppe, Desert, and Ocean: The Birth of Eurasia.* Oxford: Oxford University Press, 2015.

Czaplicki, Alan. "'Pure Milk Is Better Than Purified Milk': Pasteurization and Milk Purity in Chicago, 1908–1916." *Social Science History* 31, no. 3 (Fall 2007): 411–433.

Dadirrian, Markar Gevork. "Matzoon, or Fermented Cow's Milk." *The Medical Record: A Weekly Journal of Medicine and Surgery* 28, no. 1 (July 4, 1885): 24–25.

Dechow, Chad. "U.S. Breed Composition Has Been Slowly Shifting." *Hoard's Dairyman,* July 15, 2015, 469.

Dechow, C. D., W. S. Liu, L. W. Specht, and H. Blackburn. "Reconstitution and Modernization of Lost Holstein Male Lineages Using Samples from a Gene Bank." *Journal of Dairy Science* 103, no. 5 (May 2020): 4510–4516.

Donnelly, Catherine W. "Listeria Monocytogenes: A Continuing Challenge." *Nutrition Reviews* 59, no. 6 (June 2001): 183–194.

Donnelly, Catherine, ed. *The Oxford Companion to Cheese.* New York: Oxford University Press, 2016.

Dosch, Arno. "The Pasteurized Milk Fraud." *Pearson's Magazine* 24, no. 6 (December 1910): 721–729.

Duffy, John. *A History of Public Health in New York City, 1866–1966.* New York: Russell Sage Foundation, 1968.

Duffy, John. *The Sanitarians: A History of American Public Health.* Urbana: University of Illinois Press, 1990.

DuPuis, E. Melanie. *Nature's Perfect Food: How Milk Became America's Drink.* New York: New York University Press, 2002.

Enattah, Nabil Sabri, Timo Sahi, Erkki Savilahti, Joseph D. Terwilliger, Leena Peltonen, and Irma Järvelä. "Identification of a Variant Associated with Adult-Type Hypolactasia." *Nature Genetics* 30 (February 2002): 233–237.

Estabrook, Barry. "A Tale of Two Dairies." *Gastronomica* 10, no. 4 (Winter 2010): 48–52.

Estabrook, Barry. "A Tale of Two Dairy Farms." *The Atlantic*, August 10, 2010.

Fallon, Sally, with Pat Connolly and Mary G. Enig. *Nourishing Traditions: The Cookbook That Challenges Politically Correct Nutrition and the Diet Dictocrats.* San Diego: ProMotion Publishing, 1995.

Fallon, Sally, with Mary S. Enig. *Nourishing Traditions: The Cookbook That Challenges Politically Correct Nutrition and the Diet Dictocrats.* Revised 2nd ed. Brandywine, MD: New Trends Publishing, 1999.

Foote, R. H. "The History of Artificial Insemination: Selected Notes and Notables." *Journal of Animal Science* 80, e-suppl. 2 (January 1, 2002): 1–10.

Fox, Nicols. *Spoiled: The Dangerous Truth About a Food Chain Gone Haywire.* New York: Basic Books, 1997.

Frank, Leslie C. "A State-Wide Milk Sanitation Program." *Public Health Reports* 39, no. 45 (November 7, 1924): 2765–2887.

Frantz, Joe B. *Gail Borden: Dairyman to a Nation.* Norman: University of Oklahoma Press, 1951.

Freeman, Rowland Godfrey. "On the Sterilization of Milk at Low Temperatures." *The Medical Record: A Weekly Journal of Medicine and Surgery* 42 (July 2, 1892): 8–10.

Freidberg, Susanne. *Fresh: A Perishable History.* Cambridge, MA: Belknap Press of Harvard University Press, 2009.

Fuller, R. "Probiotics in Man and Animals." *Journal of Applied Bacteriology* 55, no. 5 (May 1989): 365–378.

Geison, Gerald L. *The Private Science of Louis Pasteur.* Princeton, New Jersey: Princeton University Press, 1995.

Gewin, Virginia. "What Bacterial Cultures Reveal About Ours." *Sapiens Anthropology Magazine*, February 6, 2020.

Goodyear, Dana. "Raw Deal: California Cracks down on an Underground Gourmet Club." *New Yorker*, April 23, 2012.

Grieve, John. "An Account of the Method of Making a Wine, Called by the Tartars KOUMISS; with Observations on Its Use in Medicine." *Transactions of the Royal Society of Edinburgh*, vol. 1, 178–190. Edinburgh: J. Dickson, 1788.

Griffiths, J. *Travels in Europe, Asia Minor, and Arabia.* London and Edinburgh: T. Cadell, W. Davies, and Peter Hill, 1805.

Grigorov, Stamen. "Etude sur un lait fermenté comestible. Le 'Kissélo-mléko' de Bulgarie." *Revue médicale de la Suisse romande*, XXXv année, no. 10 (October 20, 1905): 714–721.

Grummer, Ric R., Doug G. Marshek, and A. Hayirli. "Dry Matter Intake and Energy Balance in the Transition Period." *Veterinary Clinics of North America and Food Animal Practice* 20 (December 2004): 447–470.

Guerrini, Anita. *Obesity and Depression in the Enlightenment: The Life and Times of George Cheyne.* Norman: Oklahoma University Press, 2000.

Gumpert, David E. *Life, Liberty, and the Pursuit of Food Rights: The Escalating Battle over Who Decides What We Eat.* White River Junction, VT: Chelsea Green, 2013.

Gumpert, David E. *The Raw Milk Revolution: Behind America's Emerging Battle over Food Rights.* White River Junction, VT: Chelsea Green, 2009.

Hall, Carl W., and G. Malcolm Trout. *Milk Pasteurization.* Westport, CT: AVI, 1968.

Hansen, Les. "The Impact of Genomics on Rapid Increase of Inbreeding in Holsteins." *Progessive Dairy*, April 17, 2020.

Hansen, L. B., J. B. Cole, G. D. Marx, and A. J. Seykora. "Productive Life and Reasons for Disposal of Holstein Cows Selected for Large Versus Small Body Size." *Journal of Dairy Science* 82, no. 4 (April 1999): 795–801.

Harris, Walter. *A Treatise of the Acute Diseases of Infants.* Trans. John Martyn. London: Thomas Astley, 1742.

Hartley, Robert M. *Historical, Scientific and Practical Essay on Milk as an Article of Human Sustenance.* New York: Jonathan Leavitt, 1842.

Hayes, Denis, and Gail Boyer Hayes. *Cowed: The Hidden Impact of 93 Million Cows on America's Health, Economy, Politics, Culture, and Environment.* New York: Norton, 2015.

Heinrichs, Jud, and Alanna Kmicikewycz. "Total Mixed Rations for Dairy Cows." Penn State Extension, May 5, 2016.

Heins, B. J., L. B. Hansen, A. J. Seykora. "Production of Pure Holsteins Versus Crossbreeds of Holstein with Normande, Montbeliarde, and Scandinavian Red." *Journal of Dairy Science* 89, no. 7 (July 1, 2006): 2799–2804.

Henderson, Mary F. *Diet for the Sick.* New York: Harper & Brothers, 1885.

Herrington, B. L. *Milk and Milk Processing.* New York: McGraw-Hill, 1948.

Hoover, Herbert. "The Dairy and the World Food Problem: Address at the National Milk and Dairy Farm Exposition, New York City, May 25, 1918." Washington, DC: Government Printing Office, 1918.

Howell, Edward. *The Status of Food Enzymes in Digestion and Metabolism.* Chicago: National Enzyme Company, 1946.

Itan, Yuval, Bryony L. Jones, Catherine J. E. Ingram, Dallas M. Swallow, and Mark G. Thomas. "A Worldwide Correlation of Lactase Persistence Phenotype and Genotypes." *Evolutionary Biology* 10, no. 1 (2010): 1–11.

Jagielski, Victor. *Koumiss and Its Use in Medicine*. London: Chapman, 1870.

Jensen, Robert G., ed. *Handbook of Milk Composition*. San Diego: Academic Press, 1995.

Jeon, Choongwon, Shevan Wilkin, Tsend Amgalantugs, Abigail S. Bouwman, William Timothy Treal Taylor, Richard W. Hagan, Sabri Bromage, Soninkhishig Tsolmon, Christian Trachsel, Jonas Grossman, Judith Littleton, Cheryl A. Makarewicz, John Krigbaum, Marta Burri, Ashley Scott, Ganmaa Davaasambuu, Joshua Wright, Franziska Irmer, Erdene Myagmar, Nicole Boivin, Martine Robbeets, Frank J. Rühli, Johannes Krause, Bruno Frohlich, Jessica Hendy, and Christina Warinner. "Bronze Age Population Dynamics and the Rise of Dairy Pastoralism on the Eastern Eurasian Steppe." *PNAS* 115, no. 48. Published online November 5, 2018.

Jones, G. M., and T. M. Bailey, Jr. "Understanding the Basics of Mastitis." *Virginia Cooperative Extension Publication 404-233* (May 1, 2009).

Kanis, J. A., A. Odén, E. V. McCloskey, H. Johansson, D. A. Wahl, C. Cooper, and IOF Working Group on Epidemiology and Quality of Life. "A Systematic Review of Hip Fracture Incidence and Probability of Fracture Worldwide." *Osteoporosis International* 23, no. 9 (September 2012): 2239–2256.

Kardashian, Kirk. *Milk Money: Cash, Cows, and the Death of the American Dairy Farm*. Durham: University of New Hampshire Press, 2012.

Katz, Sandor Ellix. *The Art of Fermentation: An In-Depth Exploration of Essential Concepts and Processes from Around the World*. White River Junction, VT: Chelsea Green, 2012.

Kellogg, J. H. *Autointoxication or Intestinal Toxemia*. Battle Creek, MI: Modern Medicine Publishing, 1918.

Kellogg, J. H. *The Battle Creek Sanitarium System: History, Organization, Methods*. Battle Creek, MI: Modern Medicine Publishing, 1908.

Kellogg, J. H. *The Battle Creek Sanitarium System: History, Organization, Methods*. 2nd ed. Battle Creek, MI: Modern Medicine Publishing, 1913.

Kellogg, J. H. *Colon Hygiene*. Battle Creek, MI: Good Health Publishing, 1916.

Kellogg, J. H. *The New Dietetics: What to Eat and How*. Battle Creek, MI: Modern Medicine Publishing, 1921.

Kindstedt, Paul S. *Cheese and Culture: A History of Cheese and Its Place in Western Civilization*. White River Junction, VT: Chelsea Green, 2012.

Kindstedt, Paul S., and Tsetsgee Ser-Od. "Survival in a Climate of Change: The Origins and Evolution of Nomadic Dairying in Mongolia." *Gastronomica*, no. 3 (Fall 2019): 20–28.

Klinkenborg, Verlyn. "Holstein Dairy Cows and the Inefficient Efficiencies of Modern Farming." *New York Times*, January 5, 2004.

Knaus, Wilhelm. "Dairy Cows Trapped Between Performance Demands and Adaptability." *Journal of the Science of Food and Agriculture* 89, no. 7 (May 2009): 1107–1114.

Koplik, Henry. "The History of the First Milk Depot or Gouttes de Lait with Consultations in America." *Journal of the American Medical Association* 63, no. 18 (October 31, 1914): 1574–1575.

Kulp, Walter L., and Leo F. Rettger. "Comparative Study of Lactobacillus Acidophilus and Lactobacillus Bulgaricus." *Journal of Bacteriology* 9, no. 4 (July 1924): 357–394.

Kurlansky, Mark. *Milk! A 10,000-Year Food Fracas*. New York: Bloomsbury, 2018.

La Berge, Ann F. "How the Ideology of Low Fat Conquered America." *Journal of the History of Medicine and Allied Sciences* 63, no. 2 (April 2008): 139–177.

Lampert, Lincoln M. *Modern Dairy Products: Composition, Food Value, Processing, Testing, Imitation Dairy Products.* 3rd ed. New York: Chemical Publishing Company, 1975.

Laudan, Rachel. *Cuisine and Empire: Cooking in World History.* Berkeley: University of California Press, 2013.

Leonardi, Michela, Pascale Gerbault, Mark G. Thomas, and Joachim Burger. "The Evolution of Lactase Persistence in Europe: A Synthesis of Archaeological and Genetic Evidence." *International Dairy Journal* 22 (2012): 88–97.

Leung, S. S. F., W. T. K. Lee, J. C. Y. Cheng, and S. Fairweather-Tait. "The Calcium Absorption of Chinese Children in Relation to Their Intake." *Hong Kong Medical Journal* 1, no. 1 (March 1995): 58–62.

Levenstein, Harvey. *Fear of Food: A History of Why We Worry About What We Eat.* Chicago: University of Chicago Press, 2012.

Levenstein, Harvey. *Paradox of Plenty: A Social History of Eating in Modern America.* New York: Oxford University Press, 1993.

Levenstein, Harvey. *Revolution at the Table: The Transformation of the American Diet.* New York: Oxford University Press, 1988.

Lytton, Timothy D. *Outbreak: Foodborne Illness and the Struggle for Food Safety.* Chicago: University of Chicago Press, 2019.

MacDonald, James M., Jerry Cessna, and Roberto Mosheim. "Changing Structure, Financial Risks, and Government Policy for the U.S. Dairy Industry." United States Department of Agriculture, Economic Research Service. Economic Research Report No. 205 (March 2016).

MacDonald, James M., Jonathan Law, and Roberto Mosheim. "Consolidation in U.S. Dairy Farming." United States Department of Agriculture, Economic Research Service. Economic Research Report No. 274 (July 2020).

MacDonald, James M., Erik O'Donoghue, William D. McBride, Richard F. Nehring, Carmen L. Sandretto, and Roberto Mosheim. "Profits, Costs, and the Changing Structure of Dairy Farming." United States Department of Agriculture, Economic Research Service. Economic Research Report No. 47 (September 2007).

Macfadden, Bernarr. *The Miracle of Milk: How to Use the Milk Diet Scientifically at Home.* New York: Macfadden Publications, 1923.

Manchester, Alden C. *The Public Role in the Dairy Economy: Why and How Governments Intervene in the Milk Business.* Boulder, CO: Westview, 1983.

Manchester, Alden C., and Don P. Blayney. "Milk Pricing in the United States." U.S. Department of Agriculture, Market and Trade Economics Division, Economic Research Service. Agriculture Information Bulletin No. 761 (February 2001).

Marcus, Alan I. *Agricultural Science and the Quest for Legitimacy: Farmers, Agricultural Colleges, and Experiment Stations, 1870–1890.* Ames: Iowa State University Press, 1985.

Markel, Howard. *The Kelloggs: The Battling Brothers of Battle Creek.* New York: Pantheon, 2017.

McCandlish, Andrew C. *The Feeding of Dairy Cattle.* New York: John Wiley & Sons, 1922.

McGee, Harold. *On Food and Cooking: The Science and Lore of the Kitchen.* 2nd ed. New York: Scribner, 2004.

Meckel, Richard A. *Save the Babies: American Public Health Reform and the Prevention of Infant Mortality, 1850–1929.* Baltimore, MD: Johns Hopkins University Press, 1990.

Mendelson, Anne. "'In Bacteria Land'": The Battle over Raw Milk." *Gastronomica* 11, no. 1 (Spring 2011): 35–43.

Mendelson, Anne. *Milk: The Surprising Story of Milk Through the Ages.* New York: Knopf, 2008.

Mensink, R. P., and M. B. Katan. "Effect of Dietary Trans Fatty Acids on High-Density and Low-Density Lipoprotein Cholesterol Levels in Healthy Subjects." *New England Journal of Medicine* 323, no. 7 (August 16, 1990): 439–445.

Miller, Julie. "To Stop the Slaughter of the Babies: Nathan Straus and the Drive for Pasteurized Milk, 1893–1920." *New York History* 74 no. 2 (April 1993): 159–184.

Mills, Lisa Nicole. *Science and Social Context: The Regulation of Recombinant Bovine Growth Hormone in North America.* Montreal: McGill-Queen's University Press, 2002.

Moro, Ernst." Ueber den Bacillus acidophilus n. spec.: Ein Beitrag zur Kenntnis der normalen Darmbacterien des Säuglings." *Jahrbuch für Kinderheilkunde* 52 (1900): 38–55.

Morris, J. Cheston. "On Milk Supply in Large Cities." *Boston Medical and Surgical Journal* 110 no. 14 (April 3, 1884): 315–317.

Mullaly, John. *The Milk Trade of New York and Vicinity.* New York: Fowlers and Wells, 1853.

Nestle, Marion. *Food Politics: How the Food Industry Influences Nutrition and Health.* Berkeley: University of California Press, 2002.

Nocek, James E. "Bovine Acidosis: Implications on Laminitis." *Journal of Dairy Science,* 80 (1997): 1005–1028.

North, Charles E. "Milk and Its Relation to Public Health." In *A Half Century of Public Health,* ed. Mazÿck Porcher Ravenel, 236–289. New York: American Public Health Association, 1921. Reprint, New York: Arno Press and the New York Times, 1970.

Nüsse, Andrea. "Tausende Liter Wasser für einen Liter Milch." *Der Tagesspiegel,* May 10, 2002.

Oetzel, G. R. "Understanding the Impact of Subclinical Ketosis." Paper delivered at 24th Florida Ruminant Symposium, February 5, 2013.

O'Hagan, Maureen. "From Two Bulls, Nine Million Dairy Cows." *Scientific American,* June 20, 2019.

Olszewski, Todd M. "The Causal Conundrum: The Diet-Heart Debates and the Management of Uncertainty in American Medicine." *Journal of the History of Medicine and Allied Sciences* 70, no. 7 (April 2015): 218–249.

Orland, Barbara. "Turbo-Cows: Producing a Competitive Animal in the Nineteenth and Early Twentieth Centuries." In *Industrializing Organisms: Introducing Evolutionary History,* ed. Susan R. Schrepfer and Philip Scranton, 167–189. New York: Routledge, 2004.

Osmundson, Michael. "From 1950 to Present: The Evolution of 'Dairy Character.'" *Progressive Dairy,* January 17, 2014.

Pepys, Samuel. *The Diary of Samuel Pepys: Daily Entries from the 17th Century London Diary.* Website maintained by Phil Gyford, text based principally on *The Diary of Samuel Pepys M.A. F.R.S.,* ed. Henry B. Wheatley. London: George Bell & Sons, 1893. https://www.pepysdiary.com/diary/.

Percival, Bronwen, and Francis Percival. *Reinventing the Wheel: Milk, Microbes, and the Fight for Real Cheese.* Oakland: University of California Press, 2017.

Piffard, Henry. "The Milk Problem." *New York Medical Journal* 85, no. 17 (April 27, 1907): 773–778.

Piffard, Henry G. "A Study of Sour Milks." *New York Medical Journal* 87, no. 1 (January 4, 1908): 1–8.

Plumb, J. H. "The New World of Children." In *The Birth of a Consumer Society: The Commercialization of Eighteenth-Century England,* ed. Neil McKendrick and J. H. Plumb, 286–315. London: Europa Publications, 1982.

Price, Catherine, *Vitamania: Our Obsessive Quest for Nutritional Perfection.* New York: Penguin, 2015.

Price, Weston A. *Nutrition and Physical Degeneration.* 8th ed. La Mesa, CA: Price-Pottenger Nutrition Foundation, 2008.

Rauw, W. M., E. Kanis, E. N. Noordhuizen-Stassen, and F. J. Grommers. "Undesirable Side Effects of Selection for High Production Efficiency in Farm Animals: A Review." *Livestock Production Science* 56 (1998): 15–33.

Report of the Mayor's Committee on Milk. City of New York. December, 1917.

Rettger, Leo F., and Harry A. Cheplin. "Bacillus Acidophilus and Its Therapeutic Application." *Archives of Internal Medicine* 29 no. 3 (March 1922): 357–367.

Reyburn, Robert. *Clinical History of the Case of President James Abram Garfield,* reprinted from *Journal of the American Medical Association,* March 24–May 5, 1894. Self-published by Reyburn at the office of the American Medical Association, 1894.

Rice, Andrew. "A Dying Breed: A Cautionary Tale of Well-Intentioned Development." *New York Times Magazine,* January 27, 2008, 43–47.

Roadhouse, Chester Linwood, and James Lloyd Henderson. *The Market Milk Industry.* New York: McGraw-Hill, 1950.

Rosenau, M. J. *The Milk Question.* Boston: Houghton Mifflin, 1912.

Rosenau, M. J., and George W. McCoy, "The Germicidal Property of Milk." In *Milk and Its Relation to the Public Health,* Hygienic Laboratory Bulletin No. 41, 449–476. Washington, DC: Government Printing Office, 1908.

Rubel, William, Jane Levi, and Elly Loldepe. "*Keata Kule Lorien*: Finding the Ideal Balance Within the Smoke-Cured Fresh and Fermented Milk of Northern Kenya's Samburu." In *Cured, Fermented and Smoked Foods: Proceedings from the Oxford Symposium on Food and Cookery 2010,* ed. Helen Saberi. Totnes, Devon: Prospect, 2011, 278–287.

Russell, James B., and David B. Wilson. "Why Are Ruminal Cellulytic Bacteria Unable to Digest Cellulose at Low pH?" *Journal of Dairy Science* 79, no. 8 (August 1996): 1503–1509.

Sahi, Timo. "Hypolactasia and Lactase Persistence: Historical Review and the Terminology." *Scandinavian Journal of Gastroenterology* 29, suppl. 202 (1994): 1–6.

Schlebecker, John T., and Andrew W. Hopkins. *A History of Dairy Journalism in the United States, 1810–1950.* Madison: University of Wisconsin Press, 1957.

Ségurel, Laure, and Céline Bon. "On the Evolution of Lactase Persistence in Humans." *Annual Review of Genomics and Human Genetics* 18 (2017): 297–319.

Selitzer, Ralph. *The Dairy Industry in America.* New York: Dairy & Ice Cream Field and Books for Industry Division of Magazines for Industry, 1976.

Sharma, Shefali, and Zhang Rou. "China's Dairy Dilemma: The Evolution and Future Trends of China's Dairy Industry." Institute for Agriculture and Trade Policy, February 2014.

Sherratt, Andrew. "Plough and Pastoralism: Aspects of the Secondary Products Revolution." In *Pattern of the Past: Studies in Honour of David Clarke*, ed. I. Hodder, G. Isaac, and N. Hammond, 261–305. Cambridge: Cambridge University Press, 1981.

Singer, Peter. *Animal Liberation: A New Ethics for Our Treatment of Animals*. New York: Random House/New York Review of Books, 1975.

Smith, Hilary A. "Good Food, Bad Bodies: Lactose Intolerance and the Rise of Milk Culture in China." In *Moral Foods: The Construction of Nutrition and Health in Modern Asia*, ed. Angela Ki Che Leung and Melissa L. Caldwell. Honolulu: University of Hawai'i Press, 2019, 262–284.

Smith-Howard, Kendra. *Pure and Modern Milk: An Environmental History Since 1900*. New York: Oxford University Press, 2014.

Soxhlet, F. "Ueber Kindermilch und Säuglings-Ernährung." *Münchener Medizinische Wochenschrift*. Jahrgang 33 nos. 15 and 16 (April 13 and April 20, 1886): 253–256 and 276–278.

Spickler, Anna Rovid. Fact Sheet: "Listeriosis." Center for Food Security & Public Health, Iowa State University College of Veterinary Medicine, May 2019.

Starr, F. Ratchford, *Farm Echoes*. New York: Orange Judd, 1883.

Stocker, Noel. *Progress in Farm-to-Plant Bulk Milk Handling*. US. Department of Agriculture, Farmer Cooperative Service Circular No. 8, November 1954.

Storhaug, Christian Løvold, Svein Kjetil Fosse, and Lars T. Fadnes. "Country, Regional, and Global Estimates for Lactose Malabsorption in Adults: A Systematic Review and Meta-Analysis." *Lancet Gastroenterology & Hepatology* 2, no. 10 (October 1, 2017): 738–746.

Straus, Lina. *Disease in Milk: The Remedy Pasteurization: The Life Work of Nathan Straus*. 2nd ed. New York: E.P. Dutton, 1917. Reprint, New York: Arno Press, 1977.

Su, Xiaohu, Shenyuan Wang, Guanghua Su, Zhong Zheng, Jiaqi Zhang, Yunlong Ma, Zonzheng Liu, Huanmin Zhou, Yanru Zhang, and Li Zhang. "Production of Microhomologous-Mediated Site-Specific Integrated LacS Gene Cow Using TALENs." *Theriogenology* 119 (October 1, 2018): 282–288.

Szilagyi, Andrew, Catherine Walker, and Mark G. Thomas. "Lactose Intolerance and Other Related Food Sensitivities." In *Lactose: Evolutionary Role, Health Effects, and Applications*, ed. Marcel Paques and Cordula Lindner, 113–153. London: Academic Press, 2019.

Taubes, Gary. *Good Calories, Bad Calories: Challenging the Conventional Wisdom on Diet, Weight Control, and Disease*. New York: Knopf, 2001.

Teicholz, Nina. *The Big Fat Surprise: Why Butter, Meat, and Cheese Belong in a Healthy Diet*. New York: Simon & Schuster Paperbacks, 2014.

Thirsk, Joan. *Food in Early Modern England: Phases, Fads, Fashions, 1500–1760*. London: Hambledon Continuum, 2006.

Thomas, Heather Smith. "ProCROSS Dairy Genetics Experiences Rapid Growth." *American Dairymen*, October 15, 2020.

Till, Irene. "Milk: The Politics of an Industry." In *Price and Price Policies*, ed. Walton Hamilton, Mark Adams, Albert Abrahamson, Irene Till, George Marshall, and Helen Everett Meiklejohn, 431–524. New York: McGraw-Hill, 1938.

Tissier, Henry. "Etude d'une variété d'infection intestinale chez le nourisson." *Annales de l'Institut Pasteur*, 19me année. Paris: Masson et Cie, May, 1905, 273–297.

Tissier, Henry. *Recherches sur la flore intestinale normale et pathologique du nourisson*. Paris: Georges Carré et C. Naud, 1900.

Trout, G. Malcolm. *Homogenized Milk: A Review and Guide*. East Lansing: Michigan State College Press, 1950.

Tyler, Howard D., and M. E. Ensminger. *Dairy Cattle Science*. 4th ed. Upper Saddle River, NJ: Pearson Prentice Hall, 2006.

Valenze, Deborah. *Milk: A Local and Global History*. New Haven, CT: Yale University Press, 2011.

Velten, Hannah. *Cow*. London: Reaktion, 2007.

Vihanski, Luba. *Immunity: How Elie Metchnikoff Changed the Course of Modern Medicine*. Chicago: Chicago Review Press, 2016.

Walker, Catherine, and Mark G. Thomas. "The Evolution of Lactose Digestion." In *Lactose: Evolutionary Role, Health Effects, and Applications*, ed. Marcel Paques and Cordula Lindner, 1–35. London: Academic Press, 2019.

Waserman, Manfred J. "Henry L. Coit and the Certified Milk Movement in the Development of Modern Pediatrics." *Bulletin of the History of Medicine* 46 no. 4 (July–August 1972): 359–390.

Washburn, R. M. *Productive Dairying*. 2nd ed. Philadelphia: Lippincott, 1922.

Weingarten, Debbie. "America's Dairy Farms Are in Crisis, and the Farm Bill Won't Help." talkpoverty, June 7, 2018. https://talkpoverty.org/2018/06/07/americas-dairy-farms-crisis -farm-bill-wont-help/.

Weingarten, Debbie. "There Are Ghosts in the Land: How US Mega-Dairies Are Killing Off Small Farms." *The Guardian*, June 1, 2021.

Whorton, James C. *Inner Hygiene: Constipation and the Pursuit of Health in Modern Society*. New York: Oxford University Press, 2000.

Whorton, James C. *Nature Cures: The History of Alternative Medicine in America*. New York: Oxford University Press, 2002.

Wiley, Andrea S. *Cultures of Milk: The Biology and Meaning of Dairy Products in the United States and India*. Cambridge, MA: Harvard University Press, 2014.

Wiley, Andrea S. *Re-imagining Milk*. New York: Routledge, 2011.

Willard, X. A. "The American Milk-Condensing Factories and Condensed Milk Manufacture." *Journal of the Royal Agricultural Society of England* 8, no. 2 (1872): 103–152.

Wolf, Jacqueline H. *Don't Kill Your Baby: Public Health and the Decline of Breastfeeding in the Nineteenth and Twentieth Centuries*. Columbus: The Ohio State University Press, 2001.

Wong, Noble P., ed. *Fundamentals of Dairy Chemistry*. 3rd ed. New York: Van Nostrand Reinhold, 1988.

Woodford, Keith. *Devil in the Milk: Illness, Health, and the Politics of A1 and A2 Milk*. White River Junction, VT: Chelsea Green, 2007.

Yong, Ed. *I Contain Multitudes: The Microbes Within Us and a Grander View of Life*. New York: HarperCollins/Ecco, 2016.

Yue, Xiang-Peng, Chad Dechow, and Wan-Sheng Liu. "A Limited Number of Y Chromosome Lineages Is Present in North American Holsteins." *Journal of Dairy Science* 98, no. 4 (April 2015): 2738–2745.

INDEX

adult lactase nonpersistence (also called "lactose intolerance"), 16–17; dissimilar racial distributions of trait first demonstrated by Cuatrecasas-Lockwood-Caldwell experiment, 2, 3; majority condition worldwide, 4; prevalent among nonwhite Americans, 3

adult lactase persistence (also called "lactose tolerance"), dissimilar racial distributions of trait unrecognized during formative period of modern Western nutritional science, 5–6; majority condition among white people of northwest European descent, 4, 30; trait conferred by novel polymorphism appearing in prehistoric Europe, 46

Agricultural Adjustment Act of (1933), 199–200

Agricultural Adjustment Administration (AAA), 200

agricultural schools and experiment stations, 8, 9; and Hatch Act, 91–92; and Morrill Act, 84

Agriculture Acts of 1948 and 1949, 205, 223

Alabama Milk Ordinance (1924), 194–97

Albert Fesca & Co., 105–6

alkaline phosphatase (ALP), 288

allergies, as autoimmune condition, 290–91; and raw milk, 290

allopathic medicine, 274–76, 288

Al-Safi Dairy Company, 227, 229

Alvord, Henry E., 192

American Association for the Study and Prevention of Infant Mortality, 133

American Medical Association, 276, 302

American Heart Association, 279–81

American Public Health Association, 94–95, 302

animal domestication, 33–35; of cattle, 34–35; of 40; of horses, 33–34, 39–41; of sheep and goats, 34–35

Anthony, David W., 34

antibiotics, 218, 292

Aoyagi, Akiko, 173

artificial insemination (AI), 208–10, 213–14, 230, 233; and genomic sequencing, 237–38

artificial vagina, 208

aseptic packaging, 258

Atwater, Wilbur O., 90–92, 179

aurochsen, 35, 208

autointoxication, 155–56, 167–68, 171

Babcock, Richard Fayerweather, 186

Bacillac, 157, 164

Bacillus acidophilus. See Lactobacillus acidophilus

Bacillus bifidus. See Bifidobacteria

Bacillus bulgaricus. See Lactobacillus bulgaricus

Bacillus coli communis. See Escherichia coli

Baker, S. Josephine, 105, 163

batch pasteurization, 106, 129, 132, 133, 198, 246, 297

Batchelder, Nahum J., 125

Batten, William, 55

Battle Creek Sanitarium ("San"), 166–67, 170–71, 173

Bauman, Dale E., 230

Béchamp, Antoine, 289

Beecher, Cookson, 320

Bennett, James Gordon, Jr., attacks Nathan Straus, 126–29, 132; opposition to milk pasteurization, 126; opposition to tuberculin testing, 125–26. See also New York Herald

Bernard, Claude, 289

beta-lactoglobulin, 273

Bifidobacteria, 151, 163, 293

biofilms, 260–62

birthrate, early twentieth-century decline in, 97

Bitter, Heinrich,106

Bliss, Doctor Wilbur, 144–45

Borden, Gail, Jr., and condensed milk patent, 80; and milk sanitation protocols, 82; and swill milk scandal, 81; and wartime orders for U.S. Army, 81–82. See also Moore, Edward Duke

Bos bovis, 35

Bos primigenius, 35

Bouchard, Charles, 155

bovine genetics. See artificial insemination

breakfast cereals, and milk consumption, 174–75

breastfeeding, early twentieth-century decline in, 97

breast milk, influence on infant microbiome, 154, 294

breeding schedules for cows, seasonal versus year-round, 7, 17, 30, 42, 47, 50, 57, 122, 223

Brisbane, Arthur, 120, 124, 130

Brooklyn Daily Eagle, 81, 130

brucellosis, 297

bulk milk tanks, 256, 305, 324

butter, and cholesterol reduction campaign, 247; and creameries, 87, 250; displacement of manufacture from farm to factory, 84; Echo Farm, 86–88; and less well-paying milk manufacturing grades, 189, 317; in medieval England, 48–49; relative imperishability of, 49, 73; shifts in U.S. consumption of, 316

butterfat or milkfat, 18–19, 48, 86, 179, 243, 247

buttermilk, 45, 48, 52–176, 185, 276

Butz, Earl, 312

Cadogan, William, 66

Caird, James, 79–80

calcium, and alkaline phosphatase, 289; and bone formation, 179, 329; and casein, 18; and osteoporosis, 331–32; intake versus absorption, 330–332

Caldwell, Jacques R., 2, 3, 6, 327, 336

Campylobacter jejuni, 298, 305

Capra hircus, 35

Carnegie, Andrew, 116

Carqué, Otto, 274

casein, as allergen, 273; and β-casomorphin-7, 266–67; and curd formation through lowered milk pH or action of chymosin, 24, 29; and genomic attempt to create cows with reconfigured casein makeup, 272; and homogenized milk, 245; differing amounts in different mammals' milk, 98, 143, 273; structure of micelles described, 18; variant forms β-A1 and β-A2 in cow's milk, 266–68

cecum, 24

cellulase, 22

cellulose, 21–23, 25, 27, 215, 240

Centers for Disease Control and Prevention (CDC), 262, 305

centrifugal separation of milk, 250

certified raw milk, xii–xiii; and early differentiated price schedules, 188, 316; extra expense of, 133; and Henry Leber Coit, 109–10, 133–34; and standards of cleanliness in milk handling, 135, 192

Charles I of England, 54

cheese, simplest early versions, 24; broader regional and national marketing of cheeses in early modern times, 52; in Egypt and Sumer, 39; growth and decline of U.S. factory cheese manufacture, 86, 185; hard cheeses pioneered by Romans and adopted in northern Europe, 45; role of cheeses in Middle Ages, 47–49; twenty-first-century resurgence of U.S. cheese consumption and production, 324

Cheyne, George, as celebrity doctor, 59; on difficulties in digesting milk, 61–62; lacto-vegetarian diet of, 60–61; as specialist in nervous complaints 59–60

Chicago milk ordinance (1908), 114

child mortality, 72, 93, 95, 98, 105, 116, 121

child nutrition, xi, 64–65, 71, 95, 98, 181, 182, 329

childhood obesity, 281

China, milk in, 12, 270–72, 328

cholesterol, 247, 279, 280–81

chymosin, 24, 29

clabbered milk, 195

Clarke, Joseph, 68

clean-in-place systems, 261

clinical obesity, 281

coenzymes, 287

Coit, Henry Leber, certification system for raw milk, 109, 196; contribution to milk sanitation standards, 109, 135, 307; and Fairfield Dairy scandal, 133–35; opposition to milk pasteurization, 133

cold chain, 254, 256, 258, 262, 264

coliform bacteria, 307

Collier's Magazine, 169

Commodity Credit Corporation (CCC), 223, 323

Common Sense of the Milk Question, The (Spargo), 102, 137–38

concentrates, in animal feed, 27, 205, 216, 217, 222, 224

condensed milk, 76, 78–82, 183

confined animal feeding operations (CAFOs), 225–26, 229, 238–39

congenital lactase deficiency, 2

Conn, Herbert W., 152, 161

Copeland, Royal S., 187

Corday, Eliot, 249

Cornell University, 230–31

coronary artery disease, 247

cow-share agreements, 295, 300

cream, 48, 52–53, 86, 88–89, 114, 198, 250; and creamline in unhomogenized milk, 245; ultrapasteurized, 257

creameries, 88, 250

Crewe, Jennifer, ix

Crisco, 280

Croker, "Boss" Richard, 119

crossbreeding of dairy cows, 233–35

Cuatrecasas, Pedro, 2, 3, 6, 327, 336

cud, chewing of, 22–23

Dadirrian, Markar Gevork, 149–50, 157, 169

Dafoe, Allan Roy, 173

dairy cattle breeds and crossbreeds, Ayrshire, 212, 234; Brown Swiss, 212; Devon; 92; Guernsey, 212, 235, 245, 267; Holstein. See Holstein or Holstein-Friesian dairy cattle; Jersey. See Jersey dairy cattle; Montbéliarde, 234; Normande, 234; Shorthorn, 92, 212, 266; Swedish Red, 234; VikingHolstein, 237 VikingRed, 234

dairy cow population, U.S., 185, 191, 206, 313

dairy farm numbers, U.S., 206, 221, 313

Dairy Termination Program, 323

Dairymen's League,130

daughter-proven traits, 209

Davis, Adelle, 276

designer milk, 265

De Laval Company, 192–93

Dickens, Charles, 86

dietary enzymes, 287–88

Dietary Goals for the United States (1977 McGovern Committee Report), 248–49, 251

Dietary Goals for the United States— Supplemental Views, 249, 282

Dionne quintuplets, 173

"dirt farms," 108, 189–90

Dosch, Arno, 107

Douglass, William Campbell II, 288

drinking-milk, xii–xiv, 1, 3–10, 12–13, 30, 46; and associations with purity, 64; challenges of as target for pasteurization,105; and cold chain, 254–58; declining consumption of, 322–323; and developing nations, 227–29, 239, 264 ; and downward pressure on retail prices, 89, 182, 211, 224, 241; and farm price schedules, 188–89, 204–5, 313; and fat content gradations, 250–51; and gigantism, 177, 246, 264, 312; growing economic importance of, 69, 86,101, 184; hindrances to transportation of, 50, 66; medical endorsements of, 65, 179–81; as perpetual buyer's market, 201, 205, 211, 255, 313 ; production costs of, 176, 184, 197, 205, 211, 223–224, 313, 314 ; as substitute for mother's milk, 98; unique problems as cash crop, 211, 324 ; and urban-rural relationships, 37, 50, 53, 66, 73, 75, 113, 132, 189, 194

DSM (Royal DSM N.V.), 329

DuPuis, E. Melanie, 179

dystocia, 220, 233–34

Echo Farm, 85–89, 108, 192

Egypt, uses of milk in, 38–39

Elliott, Robert, 265–66

embryo transfer (ET), 209

Emerson, Haven, 180

emergent pathogens, 297–98, 303

Enig, Mary G., 279, 281–83

epidemic diseases, 111

epizootic diseases, 111

equids, digestive system of, 24

Escherich, Theodor, 153–54, 298

Escherichia coli (E. coli), 153–54, 298, 307

Escherichia coli O157:H7, xii, 298–300

Estes, William M., 152, 161

Eton, William, 148

eugenics movement, 10–11, 173

evaporated milk, 82

Fairfield Dairy Company, 133–34

Fallon, Sally. *See* Morell, Sally Fallon

Farm Echoes (Starr), 85–87

Farm to Consumer Legal Defense Fund (FTCLDF), 295–97

Farmer, Fannie, 146

fatty acids, *cis* and *trans* configurations, 279–80

Federal Milk Marketing Orders, 204–5, 277

Federal Trade Commission (FTC), 177–78, 200

fermented milk, varieties of, *amasi*, 335; *ergo*, 335; *gioddu*, 334; *ititu*, 335; *kivugoto*, 335; *kule naoto*, 335; *mursik*, 335; *nono*, 335; *nunu*, 335; *rob*, 335. *See also* kefir; koumiss; yogurt

Fertile Crescent, 32–34, 42, 240

Fesca, Albert, 105–6

fistulation, 28, 216

Fjord, Niels Johannes, 105–6

flash pasteurization, 106–7, 129, 132, 198, 246

flocculation, 29

flow cytometry, 307

Food and Drug Administration (FDA), 230–31, 278, 296, 300–301, 304

"Food Freedom," 285, 295, 302, 308–10

Food Safety News, 300, 320

forages, 215

Ford, Henry, 172

foregut, 22

foregut fermenters, 22

"foster mother of the human race," 98, 138, 176, 187

"foster mother of the world," 186

Frank, Leslie C., and 1924 Alabama draft milk ordinance, 194, 195–96; and United States Public Health Service Standard Ordinance and Code, 198

Frank Leslie's Illustrated Newspaper, 76, 81

"Frankenfoods," 268

Freeman, Rowland Godfrey, 110, 116, 118, 121, 123

freshening, 219

Friesian cattle. *See* Holstein or Holstein-Friesian dairy cattle

Fu, Jia-Chen, 174

full-lactose (i.e., unfermented) milk. *See* drinking-milk

Funk, Casimir, 179

galactopousia, 59

Garfield, James A., xii, 144–45

Gaulin, Auguste, 243–44

genomics and genomic sequencing, 3, 111, 161, 214, 237–38

germ theory of infectious disease, 104, 111, 275, 287–88

Gilroy, Thomas, 119

glass milk bottles, 88, 93, 246

Goldstein, Darra, x

Goodyear, Dana, 295

Grade A Pasteurized Milk Ordinance (1965), 198–99

"grade" cattle, 214

Grant, Hugh J., 116, 119

GrazeCross, 234

Great Depression, 177–78, 193, 199–204, 206

Great Steppe of Eurasia, 31–33, 39–42, 141–42, 228, 240

Greene, Robert, and Thomas Lodge, 51–52

Griffiths, J., 149

Grieve, John, 141–42

Grigorov, Stamen, 156, 159, 334

Guelph, University of, 269

Guiteau, Charles L., 144

Gumpert, David E., 302–3

Hamilton, Walton H., 200

hand milking 191–92

Hansen, Leslie B., 235–38

Hapgood, Cyrus Howard, 192

Harris, Walter, 66

Hart-Celler Act (1965), 333

Hartley, Robert Millham, exposé of New York "slop dairy" scandals, 73–74; on potential profits of clean country milk brought to city, 75

Hatch Act (1887), 91

Hauser, Gayelord, 276

hay, haymaking, 45, 49, 215–16, 222

Hearst, William Randolph, 121, 130–31

Hegsted, D.M., 331

Heins, Brad, 236

Heirloom Microbes Project, xiv, 338

heirloom yogurt starters,162

helplines for farmers, 314

Henderson, Mary F., 146

herd-share agreements, 295, 300

Herodotus, 40, 141

Hibben, Sheila,195

high-producing or high-performing dairy cows, 214, 217–18, 224, 231

hindgut, 22

hindgut fermenters, 22

Hoard, William Dempster, 98

Hoard's Dairyman, 98, 236

Holstein Association USA (formerly Holstein-Friesian Association of America), 237

Holstein or Holstein-Friesian dairy cattle, and β-A1-β-A2 milk debate, 266–67; and breeders' changing preferences in body conformation, 219–20; breeding programs based on genomic sequencing, 237–38; declining lifespans of, 229, 232; and developing-world dairying

Holstein (*continued*)
  programs, 227–28, 236; experimental
  outcrosses with other breeds, 233–34;
  and heat stress, 194, 226, 229; intensive
  breeding and management for higher
  milk yields, 213–17; as predominant
  U.S. dairy breed, 209, 220; recurrent
  disorders of, 217–20; Y chromosome
  bottleneck, 210, 236
Holt, L. Emmett, 181
homogenized milk, 242–47, 250, 253;
  disadvantages for cheesemaking, 245;
  reduced-fat gradations, 250–52
Hong Kong Medical Journal, 330–31
Hoover, Herbert, 98, 182–84, 187, 206–7
horses and horse-riding, 20, 25, 34, 39–40,
  337; and koumiss, 141–43; and pastoral
  nomadism, 41, 336
Howell, Edward, 287–88
Hyde Park, London, 54, 57
Hyde Park (play), 54
hydrochloric acid, 23, 67, 288, 293
Hylan, John F., 187

ice chilling of milk, 254–55
ice cream, 85, 114, 185–86
Iliad, the, 40
Illinois, University of, 212
Illinois state legislature, and tuberculin
  testing, 114
immune system, immunology, 290–92, 294
institutional economics, 200
intestinal microflora, xii, 154–55

Jack in the Box *E. coli* outbreak, 299
Jacobi, Abraham, 95, 99, 105, 109, 121, 131,
  133, 135, 165
Jagielski, Victor, 143–44
James I of England, 54
Japan, postwar, milk in school lunch
  programs, 270, 326
Jersey dairy cattle, 86, 194; experimental
  outcrosses with other breeds, 234; recent

inbreeding of, 234, 237; reputation
  for small yields and rich milk, 212–13;
  tolerance of hot climates, 194, 228;
  typical body conformation, 219
Johns Hopkins School of Medicine, 2
Jones, Judith, ix
Journal of the American Medical Association,
  132
Judd, Orange, 85
Julius Caesar, 44

kefir, 150, 164
Kellogg, Ella Eaton, 167–68, 174
Kellogg, John Harvey, xii, and
  autointoxication theory, 167–69, 170–71;
  and cereal flakes, 174–75; changing
  attitudes toward pasteurized and raw
  milk, 170–71; raw milk diet, 171–72; and
  Seventh Day Adventist Church, 166–70,
  172; and soy acidophilus milk, 172–73;
  and "water cure," 169–70
Kellogg, Will, 166–67, 174
Kennedy, Pete, 295
ketosis, 218, 234
Keys, Ancel, 247–49, 279–80, 316
Khövsgöl, Mongolia, 337–38
Kinkead, Alexander L., 117–18
kissélo mléko, 156, 159, 334
Knaus, Wilhelm F., 232
Koch, Robert, 72, 113
Koplik, Henry, 101–2, 109, 116
koumiss, 68, 141–46
Kummerow, Fred, 280–81
Kurlansky, Mark, 245

laban (yogurt), 148, 150–51
Lactaid, 327
lactase, 2–4; products and supplements
  containing, 327; secretion of 16, 17, 46;
  transgenic experiments with lactase-
  secreting cows, 271. *See also* adult lactase
  nonpersistence and persistence
lactase-phlorizin hydrolase, 343n1

lactase-treated drinking-milk, 327
lactation, 7, 15, 17; in high-producing dairy cows, 217–18
lactic acid bacteria (LAB), xii; ability to inhibit growth of some pathogens, xii, 6, 30, 42, 175, 195, 259; fermentation of lactose by, 4, 28, 139; mesophilic and thermophilic varieties, 147; and prehistoric dairying, 4, 27–30; reduction of milk pH by, 28; study of by microbiologists, 152–58. See also *Bifidobacteria*; individual *Lactobacilli*; and *Streptococcus thermophilus*
Lactobacillus acidophilus, 154, 158, 162–63; and acidophilus milk, 159
Lactobacillus bulgaricus, 156–63, 172
lactose, and adult lactase persistence/nonpersistence, 1–4; composed of glucose and galactose, 1–2; and lactic acid fermentation, 27–30; laxative effect of, 56, 143; manufactured lactose-reduced or lactose-free milk, 272, 327; and nursing infants' digestion, 16; varying amounts of in different mammals' milk, 20, 98–99, 143
lactose intolerance/tolerance. *See* adult lactase nonpersistence/persistence
Lakewood Preventorium, 123–24
laminitis, 218, 234
Lancet, The, 2, 79, 144
land-grant colleges, 84, 90–92. *See also* agriculture schools and experiment stations
Lederle, Ernst, 130, 132
Leprino Foods, 301
letdown reflex, 36, 38, 142
Linnaean classification system, 15, 25, 153
liquefying bacteria, 128
Lister, Joseph, 96, 144
Listeria monocytogenes, xiii, 261–65, 297, 303, 305
Lockwood, Dean H., 2, 3, 6, 327, 336
A Looking Glass for London and England, 51–52

"loose milk," 77, 113, 117, 127, 188
Lusk, Graham, 181
lysostaphin, 269

Macfadden, Bernarr, 275–77, 310
McAfee, Mark, lawsuit by Mary McGonigle-Martin and Tony Martin, 299–300, 306; and RAWMI educational program for raw milk farmers, 318–20
McCandlish, Andrew C., 216–17
McCann, Alfred W., 133
McCollum, Elmer V., 179, 181, 186
McGonigle-Martin, Mary, 299, 306
McGovern, George, 248
Macy's department store, 103, 115, 117, 126–27
Mammalia, 15
mare's milk, 40, 44, 141, 143
Markham, Gervase, 54, 86
Marler, William, 299–300
Marler Clark (law firm), 299–300, 319–20
Martin, Chris, 299–300, 306, 318
Martin, Tony, 299
Massie, Thomas 296
Massol, Léon, 156
matzoon (yogurt), 149–50
Max Planck Institute, 336
Mayor's Committee Report on Milk (New York City, 1917), 180–81, 185, 189, 211, 221
"medical milk commissions," 109, 133–34, 192, 196
mega-dairy farms, 12, 222, 227–29, 238–39, 271, 312
Mennes, Sir John, 55–56
mesophilic bacteria, 147, 259
methane emissions, 229, 239
Metchnikoff, Élie, xii, 155–60, 163, 166–68, 170
Michigan pasteurization law (1947), 198, 244
microbiome, concept of, 25; gut,154, 291–94; ruminal, 25–27, 216–18
microbiota, 291
microfibrils, 21
microvilli, 16

midgut, 22

midpoint herd size, 222

Milbank, Jeremiah, 80

milk. *See* certified raw milk, drinking-milk, homogenized milk, pasteurized milk, raw milk, skim milk, whole milk

milk allergies, 272–73

milk-borne pathogens, "emerging," xiii, 262, 264, 297–98; inhibited by lactic acid fermentation, 30, 140, 152–53; and milk pasteurization methods, 106–8, 110, 113; and refrigeration, 109, 261–63. *See also* milk testing, names of individual pathogens

milk cans, 77, 88, 113, 256

milk chemistry, 18–20

milk consumption, promotion of, 179, 180, 184–88, 201–2, 270, 322–23, 330

milk diet, of George Cheyne, 58–63; of John Harvey Kellogg, 171–72; of Bernarr Macfadden, 275–86

milk grades and classifications, 188, 317. *See also* Alabama Milk Ordinance

milk pasteurization, adjustment of recommended temperatures to eliminate brucellosis and Q fever, 297; and beliefs of Weston A. Price Foundation raw milk movement, 287–91; and bovine tuberculosis, 112–13; early criticisms of, 107–8; early debates over, 104; early methods, 105–6; and enzyme denaturing, 289; high-temperature-short-time method (HTST), 246, 257, 260; and Louis Pasteur,104–5; mandatory, 114, 132–33, 198, 244, 285, 306; and *New York Herald*, 124–29; surreptitious use of, 109; ultrapasteurization (UHT), 257–58; wins out over certification, 188

milk price supports, 178, 204, 223–24, 322

milk prices, and agricultural depression of 1920s, 184–85; chronic downward pressure on, xii, 9, 211, 224; Commodity Credit Corporation (CCC) as attempt to stabilize, 224, 323; consumer resistance to increases in, 182; effect of mega-dairies on, 239; and Great Depression, 202–5; imbalance between retail and farm prices, 241; and independent small farmers, 224, 323; milk dealers force down in 1870s; and New York Mayor's Committee on Milk investigation of World War I increases in, 180–81

milk production, overall U.S., 206, 220, 298, 322

"milk question," 98

Milk Question, The (Rosenau), 181

Milk Reporter, The, 127

milk sanitation, and Alabama draft ordinance, 193–97; and antiseptic principles of Lister and Pasteur, 96; and example of Nathan Straus's operations, 121; and F. Ratchford Starr, 86–88; and Gail Borden, 83; and Henry Leber Coit, 109–10, 135; and J. Cheston Morris, 89; and Mark McAfee's RAWMI program, 319–20; and Milton J. Rosenau, 191; at Straus's first milk depot, 117–18

milk surpluses, xiii, 12, 89, 202, 322–24

milk testing for bacteria, by coliform count, 307; by culturing and standard plate count of sample, 106–9, 127–28, 196, 306–7; by flow cytometry, 307; by gene sequencing, 307

"Milk Week" (New York City), 187

milk yield per cow, U.S., 203, 206, 213

milkfat. *See* butterfat

milking machines, 192–93, 206

milkshed, 179

Mills, William Wirt, 120, 130

Minnesota, University of, 233–34, 235–37

Mitchel, John Purroy, 180

Mitchill, Samuel Latham, 67

Mongolia, Inner, 271

Mongolia, People's Republic of, 337

Monsanto Company, 230

Moore, Edward Duke, 79–80

Morell, Geoffrey, 283

Morell, Sally Fallon, xiii; and Campaign for
Real Milk, 284; and dietary enzymes,
287–88; and "Food Freedom," 295;
influence of Weston A. Price, 282; and
online media, 284; opposition to germ
theory, 288–90; publishes *Nourishing
Traditions*, 283; stresses value of meats
and animal fats, 283; and Weston A.
Price Foundation, 283–84

Moro, Ernst, 154, 158, 291

Morrill Act (1862), 84, 90

Morris, J. Cheston, 89–90, 92–93

Mycobacterium bovis, 111–13

Mycobacterium tuberculosis, 111–13

N-Zime capsules, 287

Nason, Annie, 129

Nathan Straus Pasteurization Laboratories,
120

National Dairy Council (NDC), 185, 187–88,
197, 202, 315

Nature Genetics, 3

naturopathy, xiii, 274–77, 282–83, 287–90

negative energy balance (NEB), 217–18

Newton, Isaac (USDA Commissioner), 84

New Trends Publishing, 283

New York City Board of Health, 94, 113, 117,
121, 127–28, 130, 165

New York City Park Commission, 116–17,
119

New York American, 129

New York Herald, 124–132. *See also* Bennett,
James Gordon

New York Journal, 120

New York Medical Journal, 107

New York Times, 129, 165, 168, 187, 236, 260,
283

New York World, 118

New Zealand, 265, 271

nonfat milk. *See* skim milk

North, Charles E., 107, 206–7

Nutrition and Physical Degeneration (Price),
282

"nutrition ideology," 179, 185, 187

oligosaccharides, 294

Organic Pastures, 299, 306, 318

Orland, Barbara, 214

osteoporosis, 331–32

Ovis aries, 35

oxen, 38, 40, 44, 50

oxytocin, 36

Panic of 1893, 116

parity (agricultural price yardstick), 184, 205

parity (dairy cow's reproductive status), 232

partial hydrogenation, 280

Pasteur, Louis, xii, 72, 96, 289

pastoral nomadism, 40–42

Paul, Rand, 296

Paul, Ron, 296, 310

Pearson's Magazine, 107

pediatricians, attitudes toward
pasteurization; 105, 109, 121; and
developments in baby feeding, 97–99,
101–2

pediatrics, growth of discipline, 95, 97;
precursors of, 64

Penn State University, 236–37

pepsin, 23

Pepys, Samuel, drinks fresh milk in Hyde
Park, 54–55; frequents Whey-House, 55;
and unpleasant digestive effects of milk
or whey, 55

per capita milk consumption, U.S., 322

Percival, Bronwen and Francis, 28

Perdue, Sonny, 313–14

Phelps, William Lyon, 136

Piffard, Henry G., 164–66, 176

Pingree, Chellie, 296

placental blood supply, 17

plant-based milk substitutes, 172–74, 322,
332–33

plastic milk jugs, 260

Platter, Thomas, 53
Plimmer, R.H. Aders, 176
Pliny the Elder, 44
Plumb, J.H., 63
podkvassa, 159, 162
polymorphism, 36, 46, 336
polysaccharides, 21, 294
Pool, David de Sola, 136
population demographics, xiv, 323, 333
Posilac, 230–31
Postnikov, N.V., 142
powdered dried milk, 189, 203, 270, 317,
    325–26
prebiotics, 293–94
Price, Weston A., 282–85, 289–90
Printer's Ink, 127
probiotics, 154, 292
ProCROSS, 234
psychrophilic/psychrotrophic bacteria, 259,
    261, 263
Public Citizen (advocacy group), 278
public health, emergence of as issue, 70, 83,
    94–95
public health authorities, positions on milk,
    113, 174, 178, 181, 193, 277, 301–4; and food
    rights movement, 308–9. *See also* United
    States Public Health Service
Purchas, Samuel, 147

Q fever, 297

railroad transportation of milk, 75–77, 255–56
RAW FARM, 318
raw milk, x–xiv; and Bernarr Macfadden,
    275–77; and bovine tuberculosis,
    110–13, 123; and Chris Martin legal case,
    299–300, 306, 319; emergence of as
    political cause, 276–78, 295–96, 308–10 ;
    evolving medical disapproval of, 132–33;
    and Henry Leber Coit, 109, 133–35; and
    John F. Sheehan, 301–3, 306–8; and John
    Harvey Kellogg, 170–71; and Nathan
    Straus, 117, 119–20, 123, 133, 135; and

naturopathy, 274–76, 287–88, 290; and
    RAWMI program, 318–19; and Sally
    Fallon Morell, 283–84. *See also* certified
    raw milk; *Escherichia coli* O157:H7;
    "Food Freedom,"; "medical milk
    commissions,"; milk testing; Weston A.
    Price Foundation
Raw Milk Institute (RAWMI), 319–21
rBST or rBGH, 230–31, 236
Recommended Dietary Allowances (RDAs),
    329
refrigerated milk trucks, 256
refrigeration, 109, 135, 253; of bulk milk
    tanks, 256; limitations of for ensuring
    food safety, 263–65; and recommended
    temperatures for milk storage, 255; and
    psychrophilic/psychrotrophic bacteria,
    259–6. *See also* ice chilling
rennet, 24
rennin, 24
Rettger, Leo F., 159–60, 172
Rice, Andrew, 236
Richardson, Samuel, 62
Rodale, Jerome, 276
Roosevelt, Franklin Delano, 189, 204, 223
Rosenau, Milton J., on consumer resistance
    to increases in milk prices, 182; on
    difficulties of dairy farmers, 181–82;
    on possible germicidal action of raw
    milk, 126–27; on sanitary protocols
    for milking, 191; on situation of small
    farmers, 190–91
Rotolactor, 193
Rousseau, Jean-Jacques, 63
ruminal acidosis, 27, 218–19, 224, 234
ruminant digestive system, 22–24, 74;
    abomasum, 23–24, 215; omasum, 23;
    reticulum, 22–23; rumen, 22–23, 215
ruminants, 22
Rusk, Jeremiah M., 91

Salmonella enterica, 298, 305
Saudi Arabia, 226–28

Scientific American, The, 145
SCOBY (symbiotic community of bacteria and yeasts), 150
Scott, Walter, 67
"scrub" cows, 186, 190–91, 194, 214, 228
Scythia, 39–40, 141
sedentism, 36–39, 41
Select Sires, 238
Seventh Day Adventist Church, 166–69, 171–73
Sheehan, John F., xiii; enforcement of prohibition on transporting raw milk against state lines for retail sale, 301; at FDA Center for Food Safety and Applied Nutrition, 301; at Leprino Foods, 301; opposition to legal sales of raw milk, 301–4, 306–9; "Russian-roulette" comparison, 301, 307–8
Sherman, Henry C., 179, 181
Shiga, Kiyoshi, 298
Shiga toxin-producing *E. coli* (STEC), 298
Shirley, James, 54
Shurtleff, William, 173
Sifton, Elisabeth, ix
silage, 122, 190, 216
Sinclair, Sir John, 68, 139
Singer, Peter, 231
single nucleotide polymorphism, 3, 6
skim milk or nonfat milk, 48, 235, 242–43, 248–51, 257
"slop milk," 75
smoked milks, African, 335
solids-nonfat or solids-not-fat (SNF), 235, 246, 250–51
sour milk, medical distrust of, 67, 68, 163; rehabilitation of, 140, 152, 164; ubiquity of in early dairying regions, 4; use of in medieval England, 49
Soxhlet, Franz, method of sterilizing milk for infants,100; and Soxhlet extractor, 99
soybeans, 172
soy acidophilus milk, 172–73

soy milk, 172, 174, 273, 322
Spargo, John, *Common Sense of the Milk Question*, 102, 137; on competing claims of milk pasteurization proponents and opponents, 137–38
Staphylococcus aureus, 269
Starr, F. Ratchford, 85–90, 192
Steagall Amendment, 204
Strabo, 40–41, 45
Straus, Isidor,115
Straus, Lina, 117, 124
Straus, Nathan, xi; and Abraham Jacobi, 121, 131, 133, 135; and Alexander L. Kinkead, 117–18; article "Helping People to Help Themselves," 118; and James Gordon Bennett, Jr., 124–32; and first New York City pasteurized milk depot, 117–18; and Henry Leber Coit, 121, 133–35, 178, 316; and Lakewood (NJ) Preventorium, 123–24; and Macy's department store, 103, 115, 117, 126–27; manifestos on pasteurized milk, 120; and Nathan Straus Pasteurization Laboratories, 120, 123; and New York City Board of Health, 121, 127–28, 130; and New York City mayoral race, 119; and New York City Park Commission, 116, 117, 119; and *New York Herald*, 126–29, 132; and Panic of 1893, 116; polarizing legacy of, 115, 135; and Tammany Hall, 116, 119, 121; and tubercular family cow, 102–3, 111; and Washington, DC, 140
Straus, Oscar, 115
Streptococcus thermophilus, 160, 162
Strong, William, 120
substrate, 22, 27, 262
suicide prevention hotline, 313
Sumer, uses of milk in, 38–38
"summer complaint," 77, 116, 149
sustainable agriculture movement, 232
"swill milk," ix, 76
Sydenham, Thomas, 59

Tacitus, 45

Taft, William Howard, 131, 136

Tagesspiegel, Der, 227

Tammany Democrats, 116, 119, 121

Tatars (Tartars), 141–43

Taylor, Dr., of Croydon, 58–60

thermophilic bacteria,147, 259

Till, Irene, 200–202

Tissier, Henry, 154–55, 163, 172, 291

Total Mixed Rations (TMR), 224–27

transgenic experiments with cows, 268–73

triglycerides, 18, 279

tubercles, 112–13

tuberculin testing of cows, 113, 125–26

tuberculosis, as bovine-human
      zoonosis,111–12; and koumiss, 142; and
      Robert Koch, 113; and Straus family
      cow, 103, 111; unique status in milk-
      pasteurization debate, 112–14, 123

"turbo-cows," 214, 233, 240

Twain, Mark, 145–46

Twichell, Joseph Hopkins, 145–46

Type 2 diabetes, 281

ultra-high-temperature (UHT)
      pasteurization, of cream, 257; of milk,
      258

United States Census, 132

United States Department of Agriculture
      (USDA), founded, 84; promoted
      to cabinet status, 91; publication of
      informational bulletins, 92; recognizes
      growing importance of drinking-milk,
      101

United States Public Health Service
      (USPHS), 177, 194; draft of Alabama milk
      ordinance, 194–98; Grade A Pasteurized
      Milk Ordinance, 198; Standard Milk
      Control Ordinance and Code, 198

United States Sanitary Commission, 94

vaccines, 274–75, 277, 309

Valenze, Deborah, x, 63

VikingGenetics, 237

vitamin D fortification of milk, 242, 244

Walker-Gordon Company, 192–93

Wallace, Henry Agard, 199–201, 203–4, 270

Warinner, Christina, 337

Washington, DC, 140, 153

weaning, 15–16, 64, 73, 97, 98, 294

Weingarten, Debbie, 313

Wen Jibao, 270

Wesley, John, 63

Weston A. Price Foundation (WAPF), xiii,
      283–84, 288–90, 295, 297, 300, 302–4, 319

whey, 29, 49, 52, 55–57, 325

Whey-House, 55, 57

White, Ellen G., 166–67, 173

White, James Springer, 166–67

whole milk, 247, 249–52, 276, 285

Wickard, Claude, 203–4

Wilckens, Martin, 89

Wiley, Andrea S., x

Wiley, Harvey W., 130

Willard, Xerxes A., 82

Willich, A.M., 67

Wilson, Woodrow, 180

Winters, Joseph E., 126

Withers, Robert, 147

World War I, 177, 180–82, 186, 204–6, 221,
      224

World War II, xii, 112, 177, 198–99, 205–6,
      213, 220, 221, 232, 254, 270, 276, 329

World-Wide Sires, 236, 238

Wright, Robert A., 260

yaourt, 147–48, 157

yogurt (*also spelled* yaghurt, yoghurt), ix,
      xii, 5, 29, 147–51, 156–63, 168–70, 176, 185,
      334. See also yaourt

zebus, 228, 334

Zoolak, 149, 157, 164

zoonoses, 111–12, 297

zymotic disease, 93